*Gentle Birth Choices*

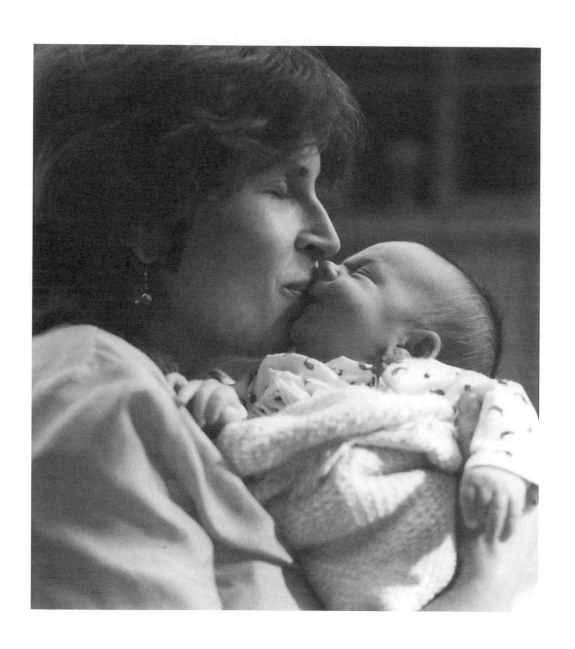

# Gentle Birth Choices

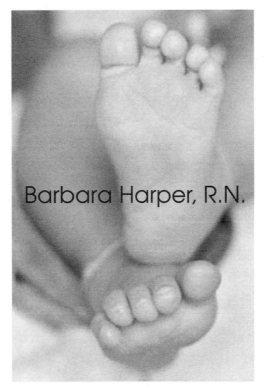

Barbara Harper, R.N.

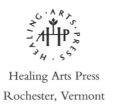

Healing Arts Press

Rochester, Vermont

Healing Arts Press
One Park Street
Rochester, Vermont 05767
www.InnerTraditions.com

Healing Arts Press is a division of Inner Traditions International

*Note to the reader: This book is intended as an informational guide. The remedies, approaches, and techniques described herein are meant to supplement, and not to be a substitute for, professional medical care or treatment. They should not be used to treat a serious ailment without prior consultation with a qualified health care professional.*

**Library of Congress Cataloging-in-Publication Data**
Harper, Barbara, 1952–
      Gentle birth choices / Barbara Harper.
            p. cm.
      Includes bibliographical references and index.
      ISBN 1-59477-067-0
   1. Natural childbirth—Popular works. I. Title.
      RG661.H369 2005
      618.4'5—dc22

                                                              2005005713

Printed and bound in Canada by Webcom

10 9 8 7 6 5 4 3 2 1

Text design and layout by Jonathan Desautels
This book was typeset in Sabon with CaflischScript as a display font

*This book is dedicated to my
daughter, Beth Elaine Braunstein, who has
become the most loving, caring, sensible mother that
any child could ask for. Even though my grandson, Alex
Nathan, was born very prematurely by emergency cesarean, Beth
applied all the skills and knowledge of gentle birth and newborn consciousness that she had learned and instinctively knew. I have watched
her blossom into a strong advocate for all birthing mothers. The love and
care that she provides for her postpartum doula clients and their babies
in Portland is incomparable. I would wish that all mothers have such
fulfilling and close relationships with their daughters. Let us initiate
our daughters into the beauty and mystery of being strong and
confident women who claim their right to give birth and
raise their children with dignity, power, love, and joy.*

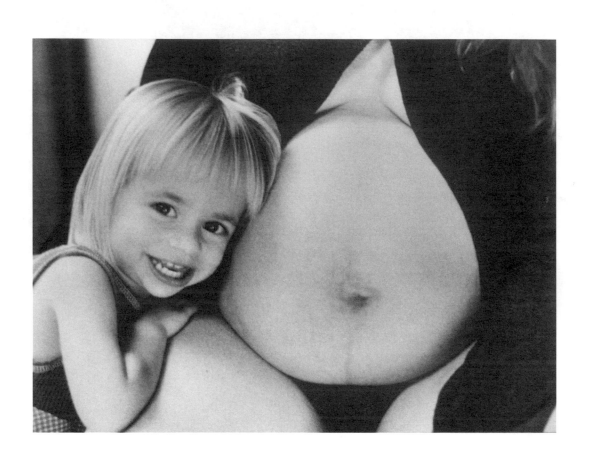

# Contents

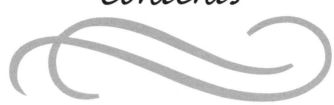

CHAPTER 4

## A Gentle Revolution 106

CHAPTER 5

## Midwifery In America: A Growing Tradition 129

CHAPTER 6

## Waterbirth 149

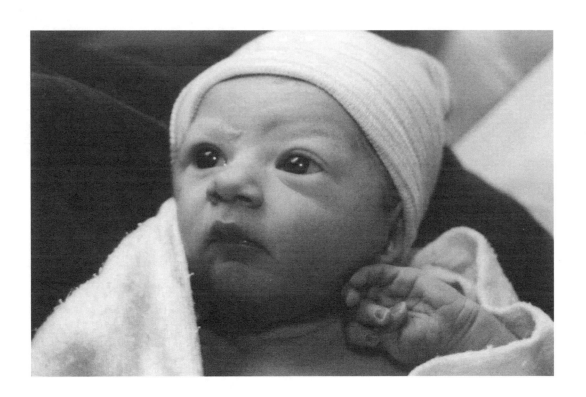

# *Foreword*

This gentle book beautifully conveys the magic, wonder, and excitement of birth as it can be—when women approach it as a natural process they can trust, and when practitioners remember to honor its sacredness. One of the book's strengths is its comprehensiveness. Barbara Harper lays out the spectrum of alternatives and possibilities available to today's women so that they will be empowered to make real choices. Here she performs an invaluable service in a culture that tries hard to channel birthing women into the "straight and narrow" way of technocratic birth.

We in the United States live today in a *technocracy*—a society organized around an ideology of technological progress. We value technology for all that it enables us to do and for the sense of safety and control over nature that it provides. Thus it is easiest for us to believe that "managing" birth with technology is far safer than allowing birth to flow. But just as damming rivers profoundly alters natural ecosystems, intervening in birth profoundly alters this natural process and can cause problems that require more technology to fix them—one of the major reasons for the inexorably rising cesarean section rates in the United States and around the world.

To have the safest and most rewarding birth experiences, women must have enough information to evaluate medical recommendations for intervention. Medical practitioners believe deeply in the power of technology to improve birth outcomes because that is what they are trained to believe. They rarely if ever see births that are not technologically managed, so they have no way to develop a sense of trust in the effectiveness of the birth process. They do not usually enable women to make truly informed choices by providing full information about the risks of interventions or about the potential benefits for women giving birth on their own with the support of low-tech aids like doulas, massage, eating and drinking during labor, walking, and immersion in water. Why use all of those when you can simply have an epidural and read a magazine until your baby comes? You will hear very little from physicians about the problems epidurals can cause women and nothing at all about their negative effects on the baby and on breast-feeding. Likewise, you will hear little from medical practitioners about the magic, joy, and overwhelming sense of accomplishment and connection with their bodies and their babies that women who give birth on their own experience.

But you will read about all of that in this book. Whatever choices you do make for childbirth, reading this book will enable you to make them with your eyes wide open. You will discover that hospital birth is far riskier than you thought and that midwife-attended birth at home and in freestanding birth centers is far safer than you may have imagined, and so your range of options will increase. If you choose hospital birth, you will learn from this book how you can work to make your hospital experience the best it can be. When you are truly and fully informed, you will find yourself empowered to evaluate medical suggestions and to know what is right for you.

This is not a book designed to perpetuate the simplistic technocratic notion that high technology makes birth safer. Rather, it is designed to inform women about all the things that really do make birth safer, as well as better all around for mother and child. Barbara writes of the possibilities for women to take charge of their birthing experiences by finding the setting and the practitioner(s) who will truly nurture them as they labor. Ideally, these should and can be people to whom it does not occur to take the baby away from the mother, who would never dream of asking her to give birth lying flat on her back, who will hold her, dance with her, laugh and cry with her, and facilitate her choices and desires. So pervasive is the technocratic model of birth, so intensive the training of most medical people in that model and those techniques, that it takes a book like this one to let American women know that such options do exist—such choices can be theirs.

Hospital-based childbirth classes usually do not teach women about the wonder and mystery and sweaty, intense power of birth, but rather prepare them for each and every hospital procedure by educating their intellects instead of honoring their bodies. By contrast, in this book Barbara Harper speaks of the deep mind-body connection that comes when women let go of fear and plunge deep into the flow of birth, allowing their bodies to be their teachers, their guides. Birth wisdom, as Harper shows, comes most completely not from the outside but from deep within the woman's physiology.

Harper takes on the medical myths that support the technocracy's efforts to make us believe that babies are best produced by science and technology, not by women. She challenges long-held assumptions: *the hospital is the safest place to give birth; maternity care should be managed only by a physician; babies should be born on or before their due date; vaginal births after cesareans are very dangerous; pain-relieving drugs won't hurt the baby; women should not eat or drink during labor; birth is more difficult the older you get,* and more. Some readers may be shocked at the challenges this chapter presents to their long-held assumptions, but I urge them to continue. Barbara is unafraid to expose these myths and the real harm they do to mothers and babies.

This book is exactly the sort of guide that pregnant women need to help them sort through the myriad number of choices and options confronting them in the new millennium. Women themselves have been instrumental in creating these options and alternatives, and Barbara Harper is one of those women. Her own quest for alternatives to the technocratic norm led her to be one of the first women in the country to give birth in the water—an enlightening embodied experience that inspired her to want all women to know the true range of their choices. This led her to create the Global Maternal/Child Health Association and write the first (1994) edition of this book. Women's reactions to the book and the acompanying video have been nothing less than life-changing when they realize just how much power they have in making their own decisions and choices about where, how, and with whom they can give birth. It is my hope that mothers, fathers, and birth practitioners will choose to be guided by the information, the loving and accepting attitude toward women's bodies in all their untrammeled fluidity, and the profound wisdom that Barbara Harper offers them in these pages.

ROBBIE DAVIS-FLOYD, PH.D.
AUTHOR OF *BIRTH AS AN AMERICAN RITE OF PASSAGE*

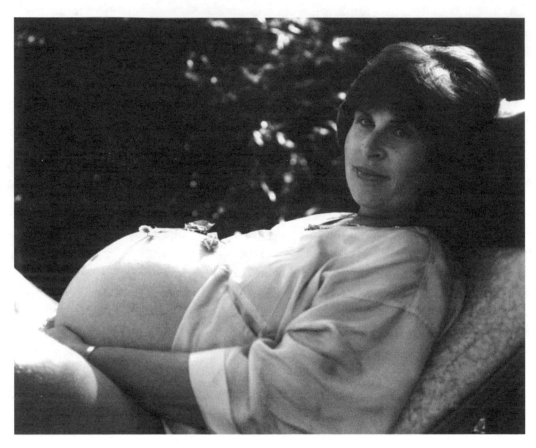

*Author Barbara Harper relaxes in the sun between contractions, just a few hours before her son Abraham is born at home in the hot tub.*

# Acknowledgments

I am indebted to and grateful for so many wonderful people in my life. As I get older, the list gets longer and longer. First, and foremost, are the women who have sought my personal care and guidance over the past ten years. I must thank them for sharing their most intimate moments, thoughts, and fears with me and in doing so giving me the opportunity to witness the divine nature of birth and the power of the Holy Spirit. Each birth teaches me more about myself, and each child brings a renewed hope for a kinder, gentler way of being with one another in this life.

I must also thank all of the mothers, fathers, and providers who have been inspired by the first edition of *Gentle Birth Choices*. For ten years I have been blessed with letters, phone calls, and e-mails praising this work. These compliments and, more importantly, the triumphant stories of how women have been changed and empowered by both the book and the video have inspired me to continue my work, even through the rough spots.

My own children, whose births inspired this work, have given me unparalleled support, understanding, encouragement, joy, only a tiny bit of angst, and a whole lot of love. My daughter, Beth, has grown into a loving and attentive mother of her son, Alex, and a postpartum doula. She has cared for me in ways that I will never be able to repay. Sam has wisdom beyond his years and a heart to match. His gentle spirit has been a testament to what gentle birth and parenting can mean in a person's life. Abe is a quiet, generous, thoughtful young man, whose talent has no limits. All of them have accepted that parts of me belong to the families who call upon me for support. I love listening to their stories about the people who have come through our lives because of the work of birth. I can't wait to read their autobiographies some day!

Writing this edition would not have been possible without my support staff in the offices of Waterbirth International. Melissa Boyd came to my rescue in 2003, first as a volunteer, and then accepted the job of keeping me organized and helping me run the organization. I am grateful for her enthusiasm, intelligence, commitment, and daring. I respect her choice to obtain the best possible midwifery education and know she will be a dynamic midwife. Michele Adams, our first office manager, inspired by the thousands of women we have served, decided to make it personal, becoming a childbirth educator. Her daughter, Claire, will always be a gentle birth advocate, having taken her first steps in our offices. And Claire's grandmother, Jan Lauer, went from being the doula for our 2000 Waterbirth Congress to providing doula services to the families of Portland. Jackie Tanguy, although new to our organization, provides an invaluable service by watching our bottom line. Lisa Durrell artfully assisted us through the 2004 Waterbirth Congress and provided a sense of stability so I could concentrate on the manuscript for this book. Jackie Wheatley taught me that even passions need to have a business plan. Gertrude Welsh gets a special commendation for making me look good in front of an audience. She midwifed me into the multimedia age and taught me how to go through transitions—the PowerPoint kind, that is.

Jake Summers, Daniel Fellin, Findlay McLaughlin, Jonathan Digby, and Brian Edwards all graduated from Wilsonville High School in 2002, and decided to bless us with their talents and energy while they attend community college. These young men clean, pack, and ship all of our birth pools and spas. They also help considerably with our Web site. Without them I could not devote my time to research, writing, and consulting. I so enjoy watching them become dynamic young men and strong advocates for gentle birth and waterbirth. I will be curious to see what kind of influences they will have on their partners when they prepare for being fathers in the future.

Reading, editing, and computer skills were provided by my book doulas for this edition: Kerstin Cathcart, Debra Catlin, Ray and Marie Rainbolt, Lisa Bourlon (and baby Marin), Ronica Briggs, and my close friend and spiritual sister, Sandra Bardsley. Their input and patience with my writing process is to be commended. Thank you for the support, inspiration, and friendship, and the reminders of why I needed to do this. I must also thank Carol Gautschi for keeping my mind focused on the blessings of Christ by sending me scripture daily and Shelley Weid for her constant support and her unique talent for wordplay. Fiscal support always comes when I most need it and I have been blessed by the generosity of many, especially Karen Beesley, Barbara Brittingham Powers, Sigrid Morton, and Bill and Win Sweet. Their belief in the power of my message and their hope for all parents to have lives filled with joy is an inspiration to me.

The community of birth advocates, who have supported my work and with whom I share a professional passion to create undisturbed natural birth spaces and to protect babies, includes so many people that it would be impossible to list them all. I do, however want to thank those whom I know I can ask for prayer support, comfort, and advice whenever I need it: Mark and Shelley Albini, Suzanne Arms, Zina Bakhareva, Janette Breen, Rae Davies, Robbie Davis-Floyd, Laura Erickson, Kitty Ernst, Anne Fry, Jennifer Gallardo, Judith Halek, Breck Hawk, Tracey Johnstone, Kathleen Kett, Kip Kozlowski, Rita Ledbetter, Lisa Lederer, Gloria Lemay, Roxann Mitchell, Sister Angela Murdaugh, Joni Nichols, Debra O'Conner, Michel Odent, Diana Paul, Debra Pascali-Bonaro, Brenda Ramler, Angela Ripley, Roberta Scaer, Rachel Schallman, Holly Scholles, Carol Schumacher, Karen Strange, Yon-Erik Strole, Jack Travis, Jan Tritten, Nancy Wainer, and Laurel Walter.

My editors at Inner Traditions, Jeanie Levitan and Vickie Trihy, woke me up one morning and reminded me it was time to birth the next edition of *Gentle Birth Choices.* I am glad they allowed the process to unfold, just like all births should. They have been great midwives.

None of the work would have progressed this far had it not been for the constant support of my dear friend and business consultant, Penelope Salinger. Her skilled guidance and intuitive counseling stretched me beyond my perceived limits and enabled me to harness my passion and creativity. She helped to gently birth my pool manufacturing company, Waterbirth Technologies, kept our nonprofit organization, Waterbirth International, focused, and helped me considerably with creating

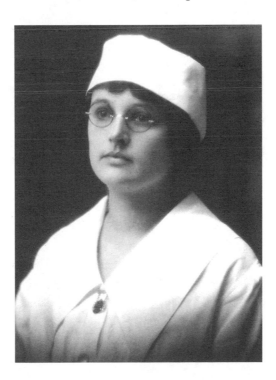

*The author's grandmother, Estella Harper Lemunyon. Graduation photo from Lima Memorial School of Nursing, 1921.*

this book. I am so gratified to see her wonderful talents extend to many more people through her professional consulting business.

Endurance and persistence are always rewarded. I have to thank my mother, Ruth Lemunyon Protsman, and grandmother, Estella Harper Lemunyon, for those great Midwestern values. My grandmother watches over me daily along with a group of eleven other nurses. Their framed photo, from the 1921 graduating class of the Lima Memorial School of Nursing, hangs in my office. Those twelve women are my Angel Team watching over birth and letting me know that what I do is important. My grandmother, midwife and nurse for forty-five years, explained to me before she died that the "little ones" need protecting. I now completely understand what she meant and for this I am eternally grateful.

BARBARA HARPER
MAY, 2005

# Introduction

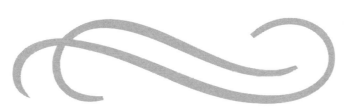

Women the world over are seeking true choices in childbirth: not which hospital to go to or what the decor of the birthing room will be, but a variety of options for laboring and giving birth without interference. Women want to be in control of their bodies during birth and in charge of their babies after birth. The pendulum, we hope, has swung as far as it can in the direction of the medicalization of birth and is now swinging back to a more sensible, humanistic, mother- and baby-friendly approach.

So often, women and their families live with humiliation and a sense of powerlessness forced upon us by modern technology. Our births have been taken away. Birth is the continuation of a healthy female sexual cycle, yet many women and most young girls think of birth as a process that is bloody, sickening, and painful. This sad state of affairs seems to me utterly unnecessary and unacceptable.

I have seen the deep, deep scars that women were left with after giving birth in the conventional hospital setting, not just in the United States but all over the world, and I have scars of my own. Even though I was a thoroughly informed pregnant woman in 1978, and had completed nurse's training in 1974, my involvement in decisions during the birth of my first child was shockingly limited, and the experience left me frustrated and angry. When I became pregnant with my second child, I vowed I would be as informed as possible about gentle options for childbirth, and totally in charge.

During my second pregnancy I became fascinated by one such option: waterbirth. The thought of laboring in water suddenly made the experience of labor seem tolerable for thousands of women. When my son Samuel was born this way I experienced the kind of birth I had wanted for so long.

But waterbirth did more than liberate me and other individual women to experience powerful births; it also sowed the seeds for change on a broader scale.

It began to shock people out of their complacency about birth. If a woman thought she wanted a waterbirth she had to educate herself on the best possible way to obtain the birth she desired. Couples began to work to create options for themselves that previously did not exist. More and more couples sought the services of midwives or doctors who were willing to listen and who agreed that women should be allowed to be in charge of their birth experiences. Sometimes couples would take on the task of educating their practitioners about what they wanted. Women were taking responsibility for their own health and well-being, not just handing their birth decisions over to someone else and saying "Okay, Doctor, whatever you say." Women and men began to "just say no" to controlled and managed childbirth.

This was the scenario ten years ago when I first wrote *Gentle Birth Choices*. I looked at the task from two perspectives—the mother's and the baby's. I wanted mothers to know that there were many options for creating an ecstatic birth experience and that support was available for achieving that goal. I also wanted to put an end to the acts of violence that were part and parcel of the treatment of laboring mothers and newborn babies.

My involvement with birth has been continuous since the first edition of *Gentle Birth Choices* came out in 1994. In response to this book—which has been translated into French, German, Russian, Korean, and Spanish—providers, both midwives and doctors, have written to me and asked for assistance in teaching others about gentle birth, especially waterbirth. Invitations to share the hope of gentle birth came from many distant parts of the world. I have had the privilege of attending births in homes, hospitals, and birth centers around the globe.

The life of this book has had many convolutions and turns, but it has continued to lead me on a path of discovery and awareness. There is an urgency underlying my desire to communicate the message of *Gentle Birth Choices*. It is an urgency that I share with millions of women and those active in the childbirth reform and pre- and perinatal psychology movement. I have realized through my work that I have more than a job or a dream—I have a calling. The more I surrender to it, the more I accomplish. It is the same in birth.

When I established the nonprofit organization Global Maternal/Child Health Association (GMCHA) in 1989 and created the first portable pool rental service in North America through Waterbirth International Research, Resource and Referral Service in 1990, it was the realization of a dream for me. My dream was to help women empower themselves with information and awareness about their own abilities and all their options. GMCHA and Waterbirth International provide families with information and resources. We strongly support the belief that women have the ability to have a natural gentle birth experience and that midwives should be the primary care providers for maternity care. Our office now processes thousands of requests for information and assistance each month through our Web site. Over three thousand women have sent us birth stories that resoundingly testify to the fact that when labor is left alone and not medically managed, the majority of women will birth instinctively with power and dignity.

My personal vision statement is an ambitious one, but one that I know will eventually happen. Waterbirth will someday be an option for all women in all birth settings and children will be treated as the most precious resource on our planet. My hope is that women's and children's health care reform becomes the top priority of our government. My prayer is that we all work together to restore authenticity to birth, to respect pregnant and birthing women by giving them choices, and to revere all children for the enlightened, joyful souls that they came here to be.

# CHAPTER ONE

# Gentle Beginnings

Human birth is the most miraculous, transformational, and mysterious event of our lives. It is also an experience that is shared by every single member of the human race. The birth experience indelibly imprints itself in the lives of both the mother who is giving birth and the baby who is being born. In today's high-tech, industrialized, computer-run world, our cultural perspective of birth depends greatly on who controls the birth experience.

For centuries medicine has been trying to investigate, calculate, and predict within a certain degree of probability the outcomes of birth. In the twenty-first century, doctors poise themselves, ready to intervene at any given moment, needing to know what is happening at all times during the birth process. It has never been a priority of obstetrics to consider birth from the mother's perspective or to ask what could be done to make her birth more fulfilling.

A gentle birth begins by focusing on the mother's experience and by bringing together a woman's emotional dimensions and her physical and spiritual needs. A gentle birth respects the mother's pivotal role, acknowledging that she knows how to birth her child in her own time and in her own way, trusting her instincts and intuition. In turn, when a mother gives birth gently, she and everyone present acknowledge that the baby is a conscious participant in his or her own birth. The experience empowers the birthing woman, welcomes the newborn child into a peaceful and loving environment, and bonds the family. The goal of a gentle birth is to reclaim the wonder and joy that are inherent in the beginning of a new life.

Gentle births occur throughout the world: in homes, where births have traditionally been natural and without intervention; in birth centers, which are becoming more popular as women demand greater freedom in giving birth; and in hospitals that are responding to the needs and desires of today's families. Women

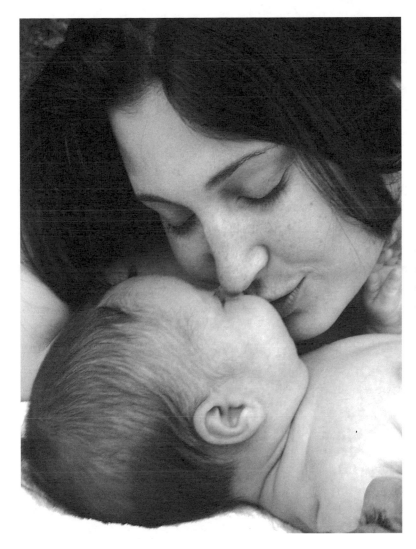

*In a gentle birth, the newborn experiences a peaceful and loving welcome.*

worldwide are seeking more natural, family-centered ways to birth their children and experience this passage into motherhood as life-affirming, without the suffering and trauma that have been traditionally associated with labor and delivery. Women are realizing that their births do not have to incorporate the biblical "curse of Eve," that is, birth as a painful burden that women must endure in order to have children. Instead, more and more women and their families are viewing labor and birth as one of the most extraordinary experiences of their lives, a time when they can witness the strength and sensuality of the female body. Women also know that birthing a baby can be hard work, the type of exertion that will test their endurance both physically and emotionally. Because of this they want optimal education and support.

Today, with advances in medical technology, drugs for pain relief during labor and birth, and an increase in the number of neonatal intensive care units, people might think that women have more birthing options than ever before. They may also believe that birthing is safer than at any other time in history. This is not necessarily true.

The United States offers the most technically advanced obstetrical care in the world. Ninety-eight percent of all births in the United States take place in hospitals, and the majority of them are attended by physicians. Yet when this country is compared with others worldwide, it ranks only thirty-first in maternal and infant mortality and morbidity rates, with 6.63 newborn deaths for every 1,000 live births.[1] (Mortality reflects the number of deaths and morbidity reflects the number of illnesses associated with birth.) Every single European nation has better maternal and infant outcomes than the United States. As of 2004 one of the safest countries in the world in which to have a baby was Sweden, with only 2.7 deaths per 1,000 births. The majority of the industrialized nations that have good statistics have one thing in common that the United States lacks—midwives, and lots of them, who see birth as normal and natural and are the gatekeepers for all pregnant women.

While there are additional factors to consider when comparing birth outcomes in different countries, such as socialized medicine and access to care, it cannot be denied that there is a strong case for reconsidering the consequences of the "medicalization" of childbirth. Two basic questions many parents and health care professionals ask as they reassess the medical model for modern birth are (1) What have we sacrificed for technology's promise of safer births? and (2) Can we trust birth to be a normal and safe process that flows naturally, or must we "control" the process with technology? The truth is that birth, like death, is an innate part of life and in most cases does not require the medical intervention and control we have been told is necessary.

Armed with understanding, knowledge, and choices, women are making their own decisions about how their births should be. Consider Kathy's quest for a gentle birth for her daughter, Amber.

During the seventh month of Kathy's pregnancy, she and her husband, Stephen, realized that the kind of birth they envisioned for their second baby was not likely to happen. This time Kathy wanted to labor and give birth without any drugs. She had given birth to her son, Stephen Jr., at a local hospital where, upon the recommendation of her doctor, labor had been induced around her due date. The contractions had been so painful that she had received an epidural to assist her in coping with her pain. However, she experienced great discomfort with the insertion of the needle and the medication only numbed one side of her body. To correct this, the anesthesiologist gave her more medication, only making matters worse. She felt that her recovery from the epidural took many months, as she experienced headaches and nausea while trying to care for her newborn son.

This time she wanted to do things differently. When she expressed her concerns to her obstetrician during her prenatal visits, they were brushed aside. The couple felt that their needs were being neglected, so they decided to confront the physician about their desire for a "natural" birth, which might include laboring and birthing the baby in water. Kathy's doctor informed her that it would be necessary for her to have continuous electronic fetal monitoring and an intravenous (IV) line in her arm; she would be allowed no food or drink; and he preferred to use stirrups during his deliveries, although she could sit almost upright in the new hospital bed designed to help women "push" their babies out. Kathy was also told she might be able to use the shower during labor but that she would need constant monitoring, especially since her blood pressure had been so low during her last birth (an effect of the epidural).

The response from Kathy's obstetrician crushed her expectations but strengthened her resolve to have a normal, natural, gentle birth. Home birth was not a viable option for Kathy due to her husband's concern over possible complications. Her next step in the search for a gentle birth was to seek support and information from Global Maternal/Child Health Association (GMCHA). She asked for a referral to a provider who would listen to how she wanted to birth her baby. She was given several names of midwives and encouraged to call them to discuss which doctors in her area were more open to alternatives. She was also advised to consider attending an alternative childbirth class other than the one that was being taught in the hospital.

Kathy and Stephen made an appointment with a new doctor after receiving a referral from a local midwife who also offered labor support in the hospital. The doctor had actually read some things about natural childbirth and the use of water to help manage pain and anxiety in labor.

On Kathy's first visit no one talked about IVs or fetal monitors. Kathy was treated like a healthy pregnant woman without a history of a "medical condition." Kathy's options had expanded, and she felt she was in charge again. She made an appointment to tour the hospital and meet the nurse manager to ask if she could bring a portable pool into the hospital with her when she was in labor. That is when difficulties began to arise. Even though her doctor was in favor of her use of water, the nurse manager was reluctant to consent, stating that she would have to make a policy change and didn't know if there was enough time to do so in the two months that Kathy had left before the baby was born. But she would at least try to get it pushed through.

During this time Kathy met several times with the midwife, whom she had now hired to be her doula (trained labor assistant) for the hospital birth. Upon her doula's recommendation, Kathy and Stephen took a "Birthing From Within" childbirth preparation class. The class reinforced the naturalness of labor and birth and helped them sort out what had happened in their first birth that had caused Kathy to feel powerless and angry. Her "homework" included creating an art project, with Stephen assisting, to express her desire for a completely natural birth with this baby.

The couple watched birth videos together and openly discussed their fears, both of home and hospital birth. As much as Kathy wanted to please her husband, she began to feel that the hospital experience was something that she wanted to avoid instead of embrace. Stephen revealed through process work with the doula that his mother had almost died during his own birth from a terrible hemorrhage and that, if anything like that were to happen to his wife and baby, he could never live with himself. Just knowing the origins of his anxiety and fear and discussing the safety issues with their doula helped the couple look more objectively at the choices before them.

By the beginning of Kathy's last month, the nurse manager still had not gained the approval from all the hospital departments to allow her to bring in a portable pool. After carefully evaluating all her options, Kathy made the decision to have a home birth just ten days before her due date. Her doula, with whom she now felt quite comfortable, became her midwife. She announced her plans to her doctor who actually encouraged her to stay home so that she could be completely in charge of her experience. He even went so far as to volunteer to make a house call after the baby was born.

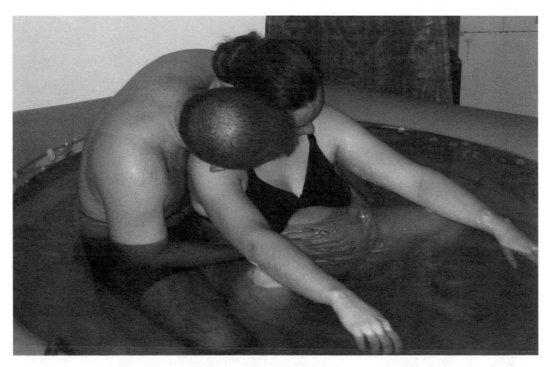

*Laboring in water helps women get comfortable and relaxed, and to tune in to their instincts.*

The baby was due on Christmas Day, and when she waited a day before deciding to make her entrance, everyone was grateful. Once Kathy's active labor began, it progressed quickly, as she moved about freely and sipped water or ate as she needed to. Stephen, a restaurant owner and gourmet chef, had stocked the kitchen with all kinds of Christmas delights for the midwives, as well as his wife. The midwife and two assistants came and helped set up the birth pool, which had arrived a few weeks before in hopes that the hospital would approve its use. They offered encouragement and reassurance.

Kathy walked around and sometimes sat in a rocking chair; she found that her most comfortable position for labor was sitting on the toilet. She was surprised that sitting upright and relaxed on the toilet could be so comfortable. Kathy handled the intense work of labor well, but felt instantaneous relief the minute she sank into the deep water of the birth pool. After only four hours of active labor, Kathy realized that the baby was ready to be born. She leaned back in the water and the baby slid out into Stephen's waiting hands. Kathy and Stephen both had tears of joy in their eyes as he lifted their new daughter into Kathy's waiting arms. Their three-year-old son shared in the awe of those first moments with this delightful new little being.

Kathy called GMCHA a few days after her birth to thank the staff for all the support she had received. As she relates her birth story, it's clear how pleased she was with her choice:

> After my first birth experience I doubted that I could trust my body. Yet, this time I instinctively knew what to do to birth my baby. No one told me how to breathe or how to sit or what to do. I felt the energy of the birth moving through me, and I just let it happen. It was so incredible. I'm so happy that we made the decision to stay home. It was great climbing into my own bed right after the birth. The midwives cleaned everything up and came back to visit us for several days after the birth. Now I know that I can do anything!

Kathy took the empowering experience of her birth and applied it to mothering her baby. She knows she will be able to do whatever it takes to be a mother. Every day thousands of women, like Kathy, seek a birth experience that they intuitively know will be best for them and their babies. They know that there is far more to birth than just getting the baby out of their bodies. That is one of the reasons women are asking for gentle births.

The idea of women having choices when birthing their babies has slowly developed as a woman's right over the past twenty-five years. Until recently it did not occur to most women to question or challenge a physician's procedures during labor and delivery or a hospital's policy in the maternity ward. To do so implied that you were not a caring mother and that you were willing to risk your baby's safety for your own selfish needs. However, in recent years many parents, childbirth educators, midwives, and physicians have asserted the need to again treat birth as a natural process, saving technological intervention for births that are truly high risk. Many doctors throughout the world feel that if birth is allowed to proceed normally, at least 75 percent of the time it will take place without any complications that require intervention. But in hospitals in the United States, interventions are routinely used in more than 90 percent of all births.[2]

A growing number of medical studies strongly indicate that the excessive use of technology in childbirth has contributed to a rising cesarean rate and other unnecessary complications. Ironically, the countries with the highest number of obstetricians and the lowest number of midwives have the highest cesarean rates. In 1970 the cesarean rate in the United States was 5 percent; in 1990 it was 25 percent, and in 2003 it reached a record high of 27.3 percent. That means that almost one out of every three women give birth by undergoing major surgery. And if you lived in one of five southern states you were guaranteed a 1 out of 3 ticket in the cesarean lottery. If you were an African-American woman in one of 16 states, your chances increased another 1–7 percent. A 1994 report citing individual hospital cesarean rates named over one hundred hospitals in the United States that had rates from 35 to 53 percent.[3] The World Health Organization (WHO) has called for a reduction in the cesarean rate because of the increased risk of maternal and neonatal mortalities. They recommend that no hospital should have a cesarean rate over 15 percent each year and maintain that those who do are intervening too often in the birth process.[4] The U.S. National Health Service has a stated goal of reducing the primary cesarean rate (for first-time mothers) to no more than 15 percent by the year 2010.[5]

Dr. Edward Hon, inventor of the electronic fetal monitor (EFM), has said, "When you mess around with a process that works well 98 percent of the time, there is potential for much harm."[6] In response to a survey conducted by the GMCHA, Dr. Josie Muscat, an obstetrician and the director of the St. James Natural Childbirth Center on the island of Malta, stated that he has found that 98 percent of all births at his clinic are natural and without complications when women are not disturbed with medical procedures during labor but instead encouraged with love and support.[7]

The elements that make up a gentle birth are certainly nothing new or revolutionary. Many have been a part of childbirth for thousands of years. However, many of the traditions of gentle birth wisdom have been lost or devalued, particularly during the twentieth century, as medical technology and procedures have transformed birth into a medical event.

## WONDERFULLY MADE

A gentle birth relies on the understanding that labor is part of a mysterious continuum of physiological events, beginning with conception and continuing well into the first year of life. Mother and baby, inseparable and interdependent, work together as a unit from the fertilization of the egg until weaning from breastfeeding takes place. Mothers the world over know that the physical and psychological connections that bind our children to us last a lifetime.

How babies are created is nothing short of miraculous and women's bodies are perfectly designed to bring forth this new life. The hormonal changes that a woman's body experiences assist her in letting her baby be born gently. Early in pregnancy her body doubles its blood volume to be able to pump nutrient-rich blood to her growing baby.

Once the baby is implanted in the wall of the uterus, a hormone called human chorionic gonadotrophin hormone, or hCG, is released into the blood stream. The hCG level starts off very low but rapidly increases, producing physical pregnancy signs in the woman. Within two weeks of conception the breasts begin to grow larger, due to the increase in blood volume and also to the hormonal signal to start mammary gland production of milk.

A gentle birth is dependent on growing a healthy and vibrant placenta. The placenta, a pancake-shaped organ, attaches to the inside wall of the uterus and is connected to the fetus by the umbilical cord. The placenta produces many pregnancy-related hormones, including estrogen, hCG, and progesterone. Nourishing the placenta with the right foods and supplements will help to ensure a normal pregnancy and a gentle birth. Folic acid has been identified in the past few years as being a vital link to preventing early birth defects in the neurological growth of the baby.

Every placenta is a life-support system that supplies the baby with the essential nutrients for critical brain and body growth. Small blood vessels carrying the fetal blood run through the placenta, which is full of maternal blood. Here a wondrous exchange takes place: Nutrients and oxygen from the mother's blood are transferred to the fetal blood, while waste products are transferred from the fetal blood to the maternal blood, without the two blood supplies ever mixing.

The umbilical cord is the tether that connects the baby to the life-supporting placenta. The thick, beautifully crafted ribbonlike rope has three internal strands of blood vessels—two small arteries from the baby to the placenta and a larger returning vein from the placenta to the baby. The umbilical cord can grow up to a length of about twenty-four inches. Most cords are shorter. But even short cords give the baby plenty of room to be active—rolling, turning, twisting, and somersaulting within its protected home, the amniotic sac.

The fluid-filled bubble that protects and nurtures the baby for the duration of its stay begins with about six teaspoons of fluid at ten weeks and by the thirty-sixth week there can be as much as 200 teaspoons. Where does all this fluid come from? The baby makes all of its fluid and recycles it, too. Fetal urine and lung secretions make up most of the fluid in later pregnancy. The baby swallows almost as much as it pees and toward the very end of pregnancy, it swallows even more, decreasing the amount of fluid.[8] Today there are tests which assess the volume of fluid present around the baby, but this varies on a day-by-day basis.

Progesterone, produced by the placenta, keeps the uterus relaxed, as well as the bladder, bowels, and veins, so they can adjust to more volume. This hormone is no longer needed in high doses at the end of pregnancy, so its production drops off just when the baby is signaling that it is time to be born. Oxytocin, like the CEO of a major corporation, then steps in and orchestrates the progress of labor, birth, and breastfeeding. Oxytocin is produced in the hindbrain, or "back office," where the pituitary and hypothalamus work overtime secreting all the necessary chemicals to make labor normal. The "front office," the neocortex, is the thinking part of the brain, which must take a break—a vacation—for the duration of labor. This process starts during late pregnancy and causes women to become less intellectually focused, sometimes forgetful, but more focused within. This condition of late pregnancy is affectionately termed "placenta brain."

The mother's ligaments stretch more in pregnancy because of another hormone, relaxin. The softened ligaments open up the bones of the pelvis to allow the baby to pass through.[9]

This incredible interplay of hormones, changing body, and growing baby all culminate with the labor and birth. Let's take a closer look at how these forces come together and influence where and how you can create the perfect environment in which to give birth gently and naturally.

## INGREDIENTS FOR A GENTLE BIRTH

Before describing the important elements of gentle birth, I want to point out that these are merely suggestions. Gentle birth is not a method or a set of rules that must be followed. Rather, it is an approach to birth that incorporates a woman's own values and beliefs. Every birth is a powerful experience—sometimes painful, always transformational. Each birth is as unique as the woman giving birth and the baby being born. There is no illustrated owner's manual.

For many women, early social conditioning creates the belief that they are unable to give birth normally. This misconception must be replaced with an understanding of the philosophy of gentle birth and the science behind it. When women realize that their bodies really know how to give birth and that their babies know how to be born, they gain confidence. Only then is gentle birth a possibility.

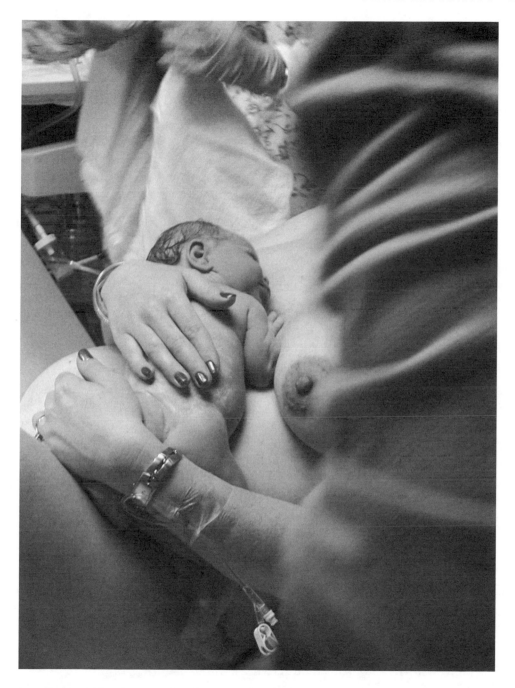

*A gentle birth can take place even in the hurried routines of the hospital.*

A gentle birth takes place when a woman is supported by the people she chooses to be with during this most intimate time. She needs to be loved and nurtured by those around her so she can feel comfortable and secure enough to follow her natural instincts. A birthing woman must be trusted so she in turn can trust herself, her body, her partner, her baby, and this process of giving birth. Her intuition must be respected. During a natural gentle birth, a woman feels and senses the power of the birth and uses this energy to transform every part of her own being. A gentle birth is not rushed. The baby emerges at its own pace and in its own time, and is received into the hands of those who love and recognize it for the divine gift that it is.

Some of the most important ingredients for a natural gentle birth are described on the following pages. Each woman has individual needs and preferences, so again, use these elements only as guidelines.

## Preparation

The education that best prepares a woman for a gentle birth is one that empowers her by providing information and a belief in her ability to give birth naturally. The original childbirth educators were mothers who labored in front of their children and included them in the folk medicine of the day. Pregnant women asked their mothers about a pain or an ache, and the mothers responded by saying, "Oh, I had that with all three of you." For a daughter to experience her mother giving birth is worth a whole course in childbirth education. In sharing her mother's labor and giving birth, she learns about the essence of this miracle firsthand.

Today childbirth educators have taken over the job of mothers whose memories of birth were obliterated by drugs, unconsciousness, and the medical treatments of the day. There are many styles of education and preparation for birth. One of the most important components for all methods of childbirth preparation is a healthy attitude. Women pay attention to their bodies throughout their pregnancy by eating healthful foods, avoiding stress, sticking to a physical exercise program, being cautious about exposing themselves to harmful chemicals or toxins, and maintaining a positive emotional outlook. While preparing for a gentle birth, it's important to keep an open mind as to how the birth may actually proceed. Flexibility is essential, because in some cases medical intervention may be necessary.

I recommend that a woman look into her attitudes, ideas, and beliefs about birth. This may include exploring her feelings about her sexuality, her relationship with the baby's father, and her relationships with her parents. A woman who is comfortable with her sexuality will feel less inhibited during the birth. A woman who has examined her own birth and its impact in her own life will not be likely to repeat the pattern of that birth in the one she is preparing for. A woman who has a good sense of herself will not be easily swayed from what she knows to be right for herself and her baby. A woman who is at peace with her partner and her family members will find comfort in and draw strength from those bonds and will want to include those people in the birthing experience.

## A Reassuring Environment

When a woman is in a comfortable, distraction-free, reassuring environment, she is more likely to shift into a more instinctive level of concentration or consciousness that will enable her to labor spontaneously. Making this shift helps tremendously in reducing the sensation of pain. The levels of certain brain chemicals, called endorphins, increase throughout pregnancy, reaching a peak during labor.[10] These endorphins are part of what Michel Odent describes as a "love cocktail" of hormones that are released with oxytocin, which have a major effect on the perception of pain and feelings of well-being. They are the body's natural painkillers and tranquilizers, which aid and enhance the birth experience. As the body responds to the natural oxytocin that causes the uterus to contract, more endorphins are released into the system, reducing the pain and creating a sense of well-being. Runners describe a similar response in long-distance running, which they refer to as a "runner's high." Lovers experience an overwhelming feeling of well-being with orgasm, as the same chemical cocktail is released in the body.

The uterus by the end of pregnancy is a very large muscle with a difficult job, but endorphins work in cooperation with the uterus. As the contractions of the uterus become longer and stronger, more endorphins are released. However, if a laboring woman is treated impersonally in a hospital's cold surroundings, bombarded by IV hook-ups, medical paraphernalia, bright lights, loud noises, and separation from her loved ones, her response will be one of fear and inhibition. The body responds to fear by tightening, thus blocking the release of endorphins and releasing the chemical adrenalin, which influences the body's "fight or flight" response. Adrenalin can actually slow or stop labor altogether. It sends mixed signals to the laboring body, sometimes causing a racing heart and an intensification of pain. In *Birth Reborn* Dr. Michel Odent writes:

> For the body's natural powers to come into play, they must be left alone. . . . Giving women painkilling drugs and synthetic hormones [artificial oxytocin] during birth, as is common practice in most modern hospitals, destroys the hormonal balance on which spontaneous labor depends. Certainly pain itself can slow labor down, but when drugs are not used, the body can defend itself effectively and naturally against it.[11]

Equally disruptive to a laboring woman is the imposition of time constraints for birthing the baby. When a woman in labor shifts into a deeper level of concentration, she removes herself from concepts of time. Unfortunately, laboring women are often threatened with various kinds of interventions if they are "taking too long": the artificial rupture of the amniotic sac, the administration of synthetic oxytocin (Pitocin), or a cesarean section. Generally the intention is to help quicken the birth process and to ensure the mother's and child's safety, but often the greatest assistance comes from simply letting the mother continue with her labor, unhurried and undisturbed. Midwives traditionally allow labor to unfold in whatever time is necessary, especially if the mother is active, rested, and eating and drinking, and if the baby shows no signs of stress.

On one occasion a certified nurse-midwife (CNM) in California had been attending a woman during her first birth, at home, for over thirty hours. She suggested to the woman and her husband that perhaps a change of scene was in order and drove the couple to the beach for an early-morning walk. The woman's contractions actually slowed down and she was able to sleep for several hours. When she woke up, she ate, showered, and went for one more walk. By that time it had been almost thirty-six hours. Her contractions increased, and after forty hours she birthed her baby in warm water. The mother's level of energy and her confidence and trust that everything was normal never swayed. The midwife had faith in the woman's ability to birth her baby without intervention.

In hospitals the length of time a woman can labor without having interventions used has decreased over the last two decades. Doctors used to let women labor for up to forty-eight hours and not think it was abnormal. It is now not unusual for interventions to be used to speed the labor after only six or twelve hours.

## Freedom to Move

If a woman is physically active during labor, her baby is constantly repositioning in the womb, readjusting and descending, preparing for the birth. Movement helps the pelvis to open wider and changes its shape, making it easier for the baby to move through.[12] Requiring a woman to be in bed during any part of her labor and decreasing her ability to move increases the need for interventions.

There is great benefit to be derived from being upright and active during labor. A growing body of evidence supports the observation that unrestricted movement in labor assists the woman in managing her pain and making her labor more efficient.[13] Educators and providers alike share the conviction that the worst possible position for giving birth is the traditional "lithotomy," or lying-down position, a posture still insisted upon by most Western doctors. Women are commonly 'attached' to the bed with many devices that keep them from assuming positions that are comfortable.[14] Past president of the International Association of Obstetricians and Gynecologists Dr. Roberto Caldeyro-Barcia has stated, "Except for being hanged by the feet, the supine position is the worst conceivable position for labor and delivery."[15]

When lying on her back, the woman's enlarged uterus compresses the major blood vessels and diminishes the amount of oxygenated blood available to the placenta, possibly placing the fetus under distress. Additionally, the lithotomy position forces the woman to push against gravity during the actual birth. Rarely does a woman choose to lie down during labor or delivery because it is so painful. Most of womankind will give birth in the vertical position if there is no obstetrician or labor nurse around to make them lie down.

The two most widely chosen birthing postures throughout the world are kneeling and squatting. In cultures where women still control childbirth, women naturally squat, kneel, or lean against a support person in a semisitting position. These same women who squat or kneel during the birth are also active and moving throughout their labors.[16] Taking a woman off her back and putting her upright does more than merely change her position. It gives her control of her body. It removes her from being a patient upon whom the birth is performed and empowers her to become a woman giving birth.

It appears that the lithotomy position remains in favor today in Western medical practices only because it is convenient for the attending physician. By sitting on a stool at the end of a bed or table, he or she can easily observe the development of the delivery, intervening as needed—and besides, "that's the way it's always been done." Dr. Lisa Stolper, chief of obstetrics at the Cheshire Medical Center in Keene, New Hampshire, observes, "We learned that if you want the birth to be normal, the woman must be encouraged to be active. It pains me to see women lying down on a bed while in active labor."

A 1998 study by a group of researchers looked at the effects of walking in labor. Even though the labors were no shorter than for women who did not walk, 99 percent of the women who were active stated that they would like to walk again during future labors.[17]

After Mark Albini and his wife experienced their own natural birth in water, he sought to change the birth practices at St. Mary's Hospital in Waterbury, Connecticut, where he was chief of the Obstetrics Department. He helped create the BirthPlace at St. Mary's, a freestanding birth center within the hospital where women with uncomplicated pregnancies may labor and give birth without all the medical routines. He grew more and more confident and learned to trust what he was witnessing—that women instinctively know how to give birth and, when not impeded by medical interventions, do so in their own way and in their own time.

Albini, and the midwives who work with him, took birth out of the labor ward with its narrow obstetrical bed, and created a private, homelike atmosphere for birthing women. A laboring woman at the BirthPlace is encouraged to remain active and to take any position she wishes, whether standing, sitting, or squatting, on the floor, on the bed, or in the bath—whatever feels right for her. Albini believes that a woman in labor needs a place where she can do exactly as she likes, where she can feel free physically and emotionally. Laboring women are not forced into positions or told to be quiet or to control themselves. They are supported with calm reassurance, understanding, and tenderness. The birth is not hurried. When allowed to take its own course in this way, the birth usually progresses easily and spontaneously for mother and child.

## Quiet

An important element for a gentle birth is quiet, not only for the laboring mother but for the baby. It may seem a difficult requirement at first, but in a quiet, hushed atmosphere the mother remains undistracted, able to stay centered within herself. In a calm environment a laboring woman can concentrate during the contractions, and in the time between the contractions, she may rest and sometimes even sleep. A sense of intimacy can be extremely important to the woman, knowing that when she comes out of a contraction, there will be a pair of loving arms to hold her and the privacy to hug, kiss, share a joke, or mend a hurt with her partner. While in labor a woman can shift back and forth from deep concentration during contractions to a lighter, playful state between contractions. Intimacy and the ability to concentrate enhance a woman's endurance and ability to focus on the work of birthing her child. Unnecessary chatter by the doctor, midwife, nurses, or others present can be distracting to a woman in labor.

A baby born into a quiet environment is not startled by the intensity of sounds and voices. If you stop and listen for just a moment and pretend you have never heard any sounds before, you get an idea of how terribly frightening the raw, unfiltered sounds of a conventional delivery room might be to the newborn. Imagine hearing for the first time the crackling sounds of a hospital intercom, the exuberant cry of observers, and the clanging of stainless-steel basins and instruments.

Ideally, the baby is best welcomed into a quiet place, a safe place, an environment that is free from bright lights and jarring loud noises. By maintaining a quiet atmosphere the mother can better move into her deep recesses and draw upon her inner strength and wisdom. Today's birth rooms are generally private and can be as quiet as the staff will make them.

A nurse on a busy labor unit was heard commenting about a birth in which the mother had used hypnosis. She was initially disturbed by the lack of sounds from the mother because she had no way of judging what the mother's experience of pain was. The parents had explained to the nurse that they wanted as few disturbances and as little talking as possible. The mother was completely and utterly silent, focusing on her breath and meditating between the rushes of the uterine contractions. As the birth neared the mother began a low moaning sound, which her husband matched in tone and intensity. The nurse described the chorus that was created in the silence of the birth room as almost angelic in nature. She had never experienced anything like it. Her routine had always been to chat with the mother about things in her life or her experience as a labor and delivery nurse, which she thought reassured her patients. She now had a new perspective.

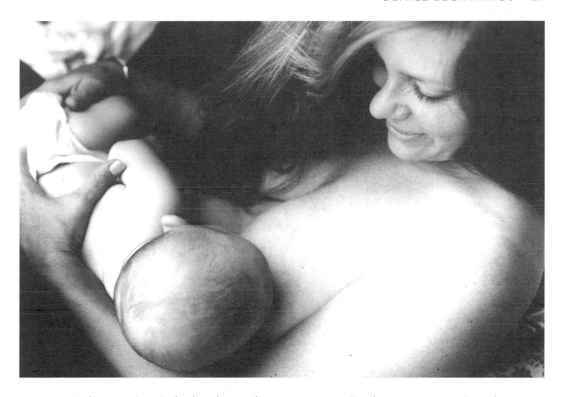

*Birthing in low light heightens the senses, especially the perception of touch.*

## Low Light

Low light is soothing. We seek it as a refuge from the bright light of the workplace and from the fluorescent lights of institutions. We return to low light to rest, reflect, relax. We meditate or pray in the dim light of holy places. We make love in candlelight, in the moonlight, or in darkness. When ill, we recover our strength in the dim light of our sick room.

During the birth process, low light provides the most comfortable environment for mother and child. Low light creates a relaxing and private atmosphere in which a special, intimate event can occur. A room lit with natural light, candles, or very low wattage electric light provides an ideal ambience for a laboring woman. After the birth, the child's eyes are spared from bright lights. The most amazing thing has been witnessed in darkened birthing rooms: Newborn babies almost immediately open their eyes and gaze at their mothers. Gazing into the eyes of your newly emerged child, who seems peaceful and present, is an unforgettable moment.

This approach to birth was introduced to the world by Frederick Leboyer, as we will see in chapter 4. Dr. John Grover, one of the first physicians in the United States to undertake a Leboyer-style delivery in a hospital, observed:

I noticed immediately that babies born in this peaceful, twilight atmosphere seemed calmer and more alert than those I had delivered in the past. After a while the nursery nurses began to comment, "Ah, you've brought us another gentle birth baby!" without my having to point out the fact. When I asked them how they could tell, the reply was, "Oh, most babies are either asleep or crying most of the time; yours look about more, they seem to follow us with their eyes."[18]

Many physicians experience no trouble attending births with reduced lighting. Not only does the human eye adapt to dark, but other senses become keener. Midwives report that perceptions, especially the sense of touch, are actually heightened in low light. A midwife from Ohio related that her attention was much more focused on the mother when the room was dark and quiet. It was actually easier for her to sense changes in breathing, which can be the very first signs of distress or tension. The midwife could then talk to the mother and help her relax.

Births that take place at home by firelight or candlelight may seem to some like a return to the Dark Ages, but the participants, including the care providers, view these births as sacred events. Dr. Bruce Sutherland, an obstetrician in Australia, describes feeling privileged to be able to witness the tenderness of a two-second-old baby gazing into his mother's eyes. Sutherland openly wept when he said, "They [the other physicians] don't know what they are missing."[19]

## Continuous Labor Support

Gentle births are easier when the mother chooses and trusts the people around her during her labor. Very few women desire to go through labor alone. There is comfort and ease in sharing the experience and having a loving touch, a cool drink, a smile or embrace when it is most needed. Fathers can provide this type of care and relish being there when the baby is born, but women sometimes desire the presence of another woman, someone who is experienced in labor and birth to provide support and assistance. Experienced mothers, sisters, and friends can easily step into that role if the mother chooses them and feels safe with them. Some mothers seek the services of a doula, a trained labor assistant.

The professional doula is a relatively new addition in hospital birth rooms. Women have been caring for each other during childbirth since the beginning of time. Even when a woman is armed with education, the intensity of labor often takes her by surprise. A doula can bring reassurance to both the mother and father that everything is progressing normally. She can suggest position changes, provide massage, or employ other techniques to assist a woman in avoiding drugs in labor.

Nurses on busy maternity units often cannot stay in a labor room due to the fact that they have many duties and care for more than one woman in labor at the same time. Having a midwife in the hospital can sometimes provide a mother continuous support, but more often the reality is that she is responsible for many other tasks. A midwife or physician is making decisions and evaluating the medical aspects of the labor, whereas a doula is there solely to provide physical and emotional comfort and support.

A doula will help a mother achieve the birth outcome that she desires. Often meeting with a family a few times before labor begins, the doula becomes familiar with what a mother and father want out of their birth experience. She will work very diligently to establish an environment that is conducive to an undisturbed birth. A doula does not make decisions for parents about their care, but helps them understand the implications of certain procedures so that they can make an informed choice. Her presence gives couples confidence in their choices. She will support women in all their choices for pain management and see that every effort is made to keep the mother and baby together immediately after the birth. A birth doula will stay with the family from the time that her presence is requested in labor until a few hours after the birth, assisting with the initiation of breast-feeding, if needed.

A doula's purpose is to help a family create a positive and loving birth memory, fostering a great start for this precious little new being. I received a letter in the mail from a very young teenage mother for whom I had served as a doula a few months before. Handwritten on school paper, she wrote:

I am back in school and taking my baby with me to class. I thought it was about time to send you an update on us. My birth was an incredible experience, hard . . . but I got through it. I would tell you that your being with me made it easier, but in reality, the baby was going to come out no matter what. You kept telling me that and I finally believed you. After that it got easier. I think every mom should have a doula.

Sometimes all that is needed to keep a birth normal is simply to be present—not just physically, but in the moment with the mother. Holding the energy of the birth space is an important job that is more easily accomplished by someone outside of the emotional or the medical aspects of the birth.

## Labor Starts On Its Own

In a gentle birth labor begins naturally, without the use of drugs or interventions to make it start. During the last few weeks of pregnancy, the mother's body prepares for labor and birth. The baby "drops down" into the pelvis, the cervix softens and moves forward, and the uterus begins to tighten more regularly. The occasional contractions help thin the cervix and even begin to dilate it slightly.

The rise in hormone levels which causes all these changes is also good for the baby, who reacts to the changes by slowing his movements. By slowing his movements, he reserves more oxygen for the birth.[20]

The last few weeks of pregnancy allow the baby to add a bit more protective fat and to mature her lungs. Many researchers believe that labor in the mother is actually initiated by the release of a small amount of hormone from the baby's pituitary gland. In the majority of cases, it is only when both the mother's body and the baby's body are ready that the powerful hormones release and the process of labor begins.

Allowing labor to begin naturally is the best way to assure that the baby is ready to be born. One of the biggest problems with inducing labor is that due dates are never accurate. Babies who are born even two weeks prematurely have a much higher chance of dying within the first year of life.[21] A gentle labor that starts on its own and continues without medical intervention increases the possibility of a positive birth memory and immediate bonding with the baby. Experiencing natural contractions produced by the body's hormones increases the opportunities for movement, being in charge, and making your own decisions about your labor and birth.

When a doctor suggests induction for medical reasons it is usually not to ensure a safe birth for the baby. More often the reason for induction is convenience or simply fitting it into the doctor's schedule. A nurse manager on a busy labor unit in Columbus, Ohio, remarked that doctors used to schedule inductions only one day of the week and now they schedule inductions Monday through Friday mornings. This change reflects an attitude that suggests more reliance on technology than on women's bodies.

According to a national study on birth trends in the United States, the induction rate in 2002 was 36 percent.[22] Mothers may become impatient toward the end of pregnancy, but doctors and midwives need to reassure women that it is normal and desirable to wait, not tell them how easy it is to get things going with drugs or technology.

## The First Breath

Once the child is born and comes into contact with the air, his breathing begins naturally. There is rarely a need to artificially stimulate a healthy, normal newborn's breathing, especially by suctioning and vigorous rubbing. If stimulation is necessary, a gentle rub on the back or on the feet is usually enough. With the first expansion of the chest, air enters the baby's nose and throat. As the lungs expand to accommodate the air, the fluid that earlier filled the tiny air sacs is absorbed into the blood and lymphatic circulation.

Some practitioners feel that the first breath can be gradual or abruptly painful, depending on when the umbilical cord is cut. When a baby takes his first breath,

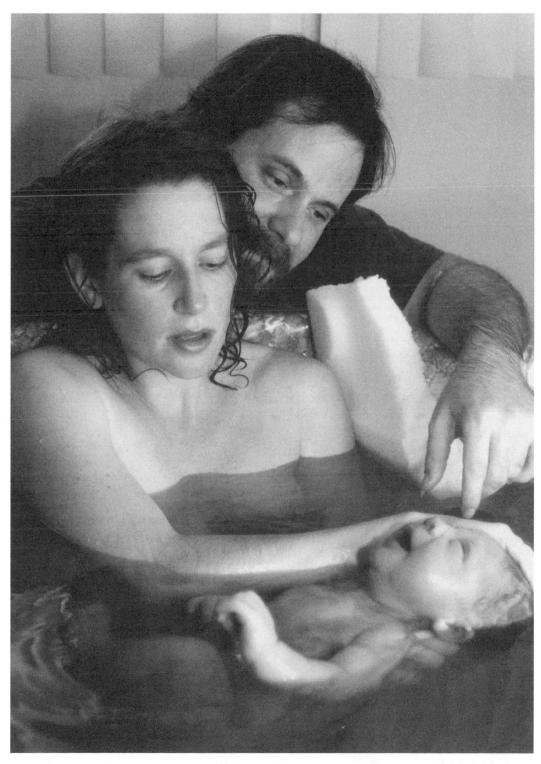

*A baby starts breathing as soon as she is exposed to air.*

he crosses a threshold to a new world. Until this moment, the mother is supplying the baby with oxygenated blood through the placenta and umbilical cord. Now the baby's heart closes off the connection between the placenta and the baby's own circulation and begins pumping blood directly into the lungs for oxygenation. By keeping the newborn attached to the umbilical cord while it is still pulsating, the transition to breathing with the lungs is gradual and gentle. The newborn begins to breathe through newly operating lungs while simultaneously receiving oxygen from the placenta via the umbilical cord. The baby can fill her lungs gradually, coming to terms with the new substance, air. The extra blood from the placenta is an essential element, enhancing the baby's health and vitality. It usually takes ten to fifteen minutes before the blood flow through the cord decreases substantially and stops. Physicians are traditionally in a hurry to cut the cord in order to speed the process of the delivery of the placenta. In a gentle birth the cord is often not cut at all until the placenta has been expelled by itself.

During the time between the birth of the baby and the cutting of the cord, the newborn is placed on the mother's abdomen, face down, arms and legs folded under. If the mother is upright, the baby can be held in the mother's arms, where essential body contact between the two is maximized. This period of tranquility marks important transitions for both: The baby moves from being breathed for to breathing alone, and the mother experiences the infant who was once inside her as an individual beside her, separate but still deeply dependent.

## The First Caresses

The newly emerged baby who is placed in his mother's waiting arms receives the immediate benefit of skin-to-skin connection. The baby is slowly massaged, caressed, or held with loving hands. The mother is simply there with her child, communicating with her touch that this child is welcomed, loved, and long-awaited. This simple act has the power to calm and soothe a newborn like nothing else. An unhurried and undisturbed interaction immediately after birth is one of the most critical times in the life of a new baby.

Touching and massaging the newborn is beneficial for both mother and baby. The mother's instinctual reaction is to smell and lightly touch the baby with her fingertips. In a gentle birth the mother is asked to determine the sex of her baby either by looking or feeling under the warm blankets. Finding this part of the baby's body can be part of a whole-body massage. The natural hormones that have flooded the mother's body during birth are shared by her baby. The oxytocin gives them both a sense of bliss, of oneness. The presence of her baby on the mother's chest evokes another chemical response that is more powerful than any synthetic drug. Within the first few moments of birth the mother's body will experience the high of a lifetime. This blissful feeling, which comes from a gentle birth, is nature's

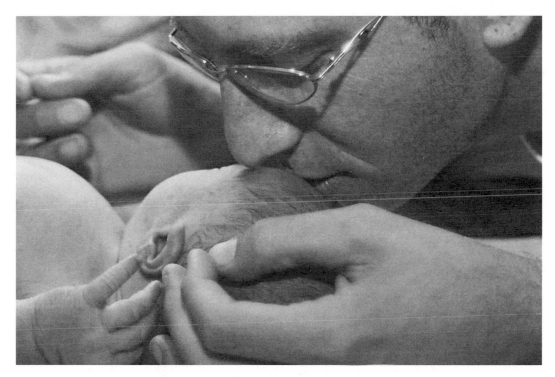

*A father drinks in the smell of his newborn son.*

way of making her fall completely and desperately in love with her tiny infant. No matter what her fear, or what level of pain she experienced, as soon as her baby is on her chest, warm and wet and helpless, she has the overpowering urge to protect it. This is the beginning of attachment.

How a baby is received and experiences these first few moments is utterly important and completely remembered. Babies have what is known as implicit memory. They record everything and store those images, sounds, and sensations and their emotional response to them in their mind and body. The baby comes out with a genetic encoding, a preprogrammed expectation, which activates certain areas of his brain and nervous system when placed on or near his mother's left breast. Mothers throughout all cultures and geographic locations instinctively cradle their babies in this position where the baby is in contact with her heart rhythm.[23] Joseph Chilton Pearce, a well-known researcher and philosopher, states that "this awakening of maternal capabilities is well known among animal researchers, who link it to the action of pregnancy and birth hormones on the brain of newly delivered mothers." He continues describing what the baby experiences: "[W]hen in contact with the mother's heart rhythm a cascade of supportive confirmative information activates every sense, instinct and intelligence needed for the radical change of environment . . . thus intelligent learning begins at birth."[24]

Touching and holding the baby in the moments after he has been born is extremely important for fathers, siblings, and other family members as well. Hospitals no longer require family members to wear a gown and mask while in the birth room, but do require covering up for a cesarean birth. There is an artificial modesty that prevails in the birth room, though. Women are often draped and covered and no one usually suggests that fathers remove their shirts. This creates an artificial barrier for skin-to-skin contact between parents and their new babies, as well as between the partners.

Fathers can often feel overwhelmed by the intensity of the birth experience. Some feel excluded; some remain distant, not wanting to "get in the way." Fathers can be encouraged to remove their shirts so they, too, can pick up their babies and hold them against their skin. For many fathers, the child is not real until they hold the baby in their arms or touch the baby in the moments after birth.

One father related his experience while returning his birth pool a few days after the birth of his child. Aaron described feeling the baby emerge into his hands under the water and seeing the baby's eyes open while still submerged. "The whole experience was so incredibly awesome and overwhelming. But it wasn't until I was in the shower a few minutes later [that] it hit me. I just started weeping and sank down on my knees realizing, I'm not Aaron anymore . . . I'm River's DAD! It was just all so amazing." For parents touching and gazing at their new child, this is when birth becomes real; emotions surface and unbreakable bonds are formed.

## The Baby at the Breast

The ideal time to begin breast-feeding your baby is within the first moments after birth. When the mother is awake and aware and has given birth to an alert baby, it is easy to watch for the early cues that the baby is seeking the breast. The baby's head will turn, his mouth will twitch and form an oval shape, and his tongue will move in and out. This is called rooting. If the baby is in his mother's arms these signs can't be missed, and the baby is gently guided to the nipple. Researchers have documented that newborns left on the mother's belly will actually crawl to and attach themselves to the breast within the first twenty minutes following birth.[25]

If the baby is not put to the breast within the first hour after birth, she may lapse into a drowsy state that can continue for up to twenty-four hours, making nursing more difficult. For early nursing to develop easily, the baby's senses must be stimulated to function fully. In a gentle birth, mother and child are free to communicate with each other without inhibition. The cuddling, talking, stroking, and loving that take place immediately after the birth provide the mother and baby with the opportunity to continue the symbiosis that began nine months before, in the womb.

Babies enjoy nursing immensely. When you see a baby at the breast, it is clear that he is engrossed in a most wonderful, sensuous activity. Breast-feeding contributes to a baby's emotional life. All the smells, tactile sensations, sights, and sounds of nursing enrich the experience. While breast-feeding, a mother communicates her feelings and emotions to her infant in many different ways. The way she looks into the baby's eyes, the way she touches and holds him, her movements, her voice, her breath—and even the taste, smell, and feel of the breast from which the warm, nurturing milk flows—all communicate love and acceptance to the baby.

By issuing statements about the benefits of nursing, the World Health Organization is working to reverse the trend to bottle-feed, which started in the mid-1950s. Statistics show that infant mortality rose proportionally, especially in developing countries, when bottle-feeding replaced breast-feeding. In a poor country a bottle-fed baby is twenty-five times more likely to die than a breast-fed one. In an effort to reduce infant mortality, one of the goals of WHO is to see infants worldwide breast-fed exclusively for the first six months by the year 2010.[26]

The routine hospital practice of separating infants and mothers and giving infants glucose water or formula has actually been shown to cause harm to the infant. The infant may suffer from an irritable bowel, or may inhale the glucose into the lungs, which can be very dangerous.[27] In addition, offering the baby something other than the breast interrupts the natural rhythm that needs to take place for breast-feeding to work. Breast-milk supply is dependent on the amount of stimulation the nipple receives from sucking. The rhythm and flow of breast-feeding is a delicate balance that can be easily disturbed by supplements or glucose bottles or even pacifiers.

The first breast milk, colostrum, is a very nutritious, balanced substance ideal for sustaining new life. Colostrum is higher in protein and lower in fat and carbohydrates than mature milk, so the baby needs very little to get off to a good nutritional start. Colostrum is also high in natural antibodies that protect the baby from infection. The baby needs to be exposed to the mother's, and ONLY the mother's, bacteria. The germs that the mother possesses are friendly to the baby because mother and baby share the same antibodies. A lifetime of protection comes in the first hour of life and cannot be replaced. There is absolutely no rationale for denying the baby this invaluable resource.

Colostrum, besides supplying the baby with normal flora for the gut, acts as a laxative, which helps to ensure that the baby's bowel is cleared of meconium, the sticky, tarry first stool. If the first bowel movement is delayed more than twenty-four hours, a baby is more likely to develop jaundice, probably because the meconium is reabsorbed through the intestines.

The process of encouraging the baby to nurse shortly after birth is extremely beneficial for the mother. The baby's sucking at the breast stimulates the immediate release of two hormones in the mother that are important for postnatal recovery and health. The hormones, oxytocin and prolactin, work together to stimulate milk production. Oxytocin also causes the mother's uterus to contract, which is important in preventing hemorrhaging, and stimulates the uterus to return to its normal size. Prolactin helps prepare the breasts for milk production and is secreted as a direct result of the baby's sucking so that milk can flow.

Prolactin has been called "the mothering hormone"; some scientists think that during breast-feeding it produces an aggressively protective behavior.[28] This hormone is thought to create a passion in the mother for her newborn, making her hypervigilant and impelling her to put the baby's needs first. Prolactin also inhibits ovulation—breast-feeding has been used worldwide as a natural form of birth control, although it is not considered a reliable contraceptive. Breast-feeding can also increase a mother's feelings of well-being and give her an immediate sense of her ability to mother. It is a special and satisfying feeling for nursing mothers to know that they can feed and nurture their babies with their own milk.

There is a direct correlation between difficulty in establishing breast-feeding and interventions in birth, especially the use of an epidural.[29] Anything that makes the birth more difficult for the mother results in more difficulty in getting the baby to the breast.

## Bonding and Attachment

Perhaps no aspect of conventional birthing has caused as much distress for new mothers, fathers, and babies as hospital policies that require enforced separation at a time when the parents most want and need to be with their babies. There is no good medical reason to separate a healthy newborn baby from his mother. The separation of mother and child immediately after birth harkens back to the days when mothers were routinely drugged for labor and delivery and were virtually unconscious. It was felt that they needed time to "sober up" before they could relate to or care for their babies.

Dr. Robert Bradley, an American obstetrician and author, wrote, "I'm sure the humane society would and should arrest me if I did to animal mothers what we do to human mothers—take their babies away from them at birth and put the babies in a big box with a glass window where the mothers could see their babies but couldn't hold them or touch them."[30]

Sheila Kitzinger, well-respected British childbirth educator and author, noted, "A screaming baby alone in its cot or lined up with rows of other screaming newborns is a neglected baby. He cannot know that help is near, that milk is coming in half an hour, or twenty minutes, or even five minutes. He cannot know that loving arms are waiting to hold him. He is to all intents and purposes completely isolated and abandoned."[31]

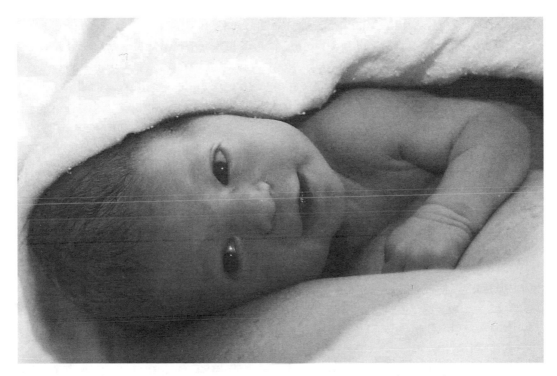

*A newborn is fully conscious and needs to relate to her mother.*

When Santha was seeking an alternative approach to her previous hospital birth, she recalled her three-year-old son telling her, "I remember [when I was born] they put me in this box and they made me go to sleep and I wanted my mommy." Santha responds, "That was really sad to hear. I remember wanting to be with my son, but he couldn't be with me because he had to go through all these hospital procedures."

In a gentle birth the child is not suddenly taken away from her parents to be weighed, measured, and cleaned far from her mother, who is the only person in the world safe and familiar to her. There is no reason or justification for such a practice. In a gentle birth the mother is awake and aware, highly conscious, energized by having given birth, and extremely eager to spend time with her child—touching, looking, feeding, resting, or sleeping together. The newborn needs and wants the comforting presence of her mother, her warmth, touch, sound, and smell. After a gentle birth most mothers experience an incredible high that helps them overcome their exhaustion. They come alive immediately upon seeing the baby. If a mother really is too tired or too uncomfortable, she can rest and the father or other family members can hold and love the baby.

Amber managed to have an unmedicated, rather quick birth in the hospital—so quick the doctor didn't even make it to the room until the baby was already halfway out. But after a completely natural birth the doctor kept the baby just out of Amber's reach. She explains:

I think the main thing that bothered me about Cora's birth was it seemed like an eternity before I was allowed to hold her. He was cleaning her off and I had my arms outstretched and he just would not hand her to me until she was "clean". . . then he had to wait for a nurse to bring a towel (like I cared that I might "get dirty"!). I only had her on my chest for about three minutes, then the nurse came and took her to do all the newborn stuff. I was devastated and I won't let that happen again.

A baby controls himself by attuning to his mother. The mother must be physically present and emotionally available for the baby to be able to interpret where he is in the world. The mother tunes in to the baby and responds to his cues. It is only through this interaction that the baby will be able to shape his response to his new physical body, and his relationship to self, other people, and the environment around him. The baby who receives quiet responses, attaches to the breast, is touched with care, and is in attunement with his mother is secure in his knowing. He thinks and feels that his birth has happened for a good reason with the roots of his spiritual being intact.

The first hours and days after birth are extremely important ones; they can deeply affect the future relationship between the child and the parents. Time spent together during those first few hours and days after the birth lays the groundwork for a profound relationship with one another. Becoming securely attached is vital for the family and can be wonderfully satisfying to all.

One might ask, why should it be any other way?

# CHAPTER TWO

# The Medicalization of Childbirth

Parents who seek a more gentle, family-centered birth experience ask many questions before deciding how they would like their birth to be. They want to identify the medical procedures and technological advances that make sense and the ones they feel are unnecessary. In order to evaluate the efficacy of modern obstetrical practices, it is important to first understand how some of these technical interventions originated and what attitudes they reflect. How did childbirth evolve from a woman-centered, integral part of home life to a hospital-centered, physician-controlled medical event? How did a natural process come to be seen as a pathological state that required the intervention of doctors, drugs, and medical technology? How and why did the reproductive processes of women become the realm of male physicians?

## OUR LEGACY OF BIRTH

Until the twentieth century, birth, like death, generally took place at home. Some of our grandmothers and most of our great-grandmothers were born at home, naturally and without interventions. Giving birth was unique to women, binding them together. This bond crucially influenced how their emotional and physical strengths were defined. Women eagerly supported one another through the birth process, often traveling long distances and staying for days or weeks to aid their birthing relatives or friends. Older daughters assisted at their mothers' births and mothers, in turn, were commonly called upon to attend their daughters' births.

31

Women who were experienced with the birth process and who often had birthed children themselves came to be known as midwives, respected and sought after for their knowledge and services. It was not uncommon for a woman to be pregnant or nursing for half her lifetime, particularly when the average life expectancy was so low.

Women of these times struggled with conditions that complicated pregnancy, birth, and recovery. Diets were less than adequate, sanitation poor, and housing often substandard. The lack of birth control and frequent pregnancies yielded a high infant and maternal mortality rate. Deaths from maternity-related causes at the turn of the century were approximately sixty-five times greater than they are today. The largest single cause of death in 1900 was systemic infection after birth, commonly known as childbed fever or puerperal fever. These infections, especially in women in early charity hospitals, most frequently resulted from physicians' ignorance of the effects of bacteria.[1] The fever was spread from patient to patient by medical personnel, and the use of unclean instruments and linens greatly contributed to the problem. Surgery during pregnancy had an equally high rate of infection and death. As a result, a woman's greatest fear in birth was death; during each pregnancy she coped with the thought that she may only have a few more months to live.

Women eventually traded their comfort and shared experience of childbirth attended by midwives for the promise of safer, faster, and less painful labors and births. This process evolved gradually over centuries, but it can be seen most dramatically beginning in the 1860s with the movement of the physician into the birthplace and the evolution of routine hospitalization for childbirth. The rapid development of the field of obstetrics in the late 1800s and early 1900s, coupled with the growth of related medical technology and hospital procedures, began to make women feel inadequate about their ability to give birth. They no longer trusted their bodies, their instincts, or the wisdom of their grandmothers. Doctors increasingly discredited women birth attendants and eventually controlled the education and licensing of midwives. While 95 percent of American births took place at home in 1900, only 50 percent did so in 1939.[2] By the end of World War II only a third of babies were still born at home, mostly in the rural South.[3]

Today 98 percent of American babies are born in hospitals, with a perinatal mortality rate that still remains higher than in thirty other countries.[4] Hospitals have made remarkable changes, especially in décor, and adopted policies which make integrating natural birth options easier, but most institutions continue to treat birth as a potentially dangerous, life-threatening medical problem rather than a naturally occurring life process. The medicalization of childbirth can be traced to the gradual shift not only from home to hospital but from attending midwife to attending physician.

## FROM MIDWIFE TO PHYSICIAN

Physicians were gradually introduced into the birthplace, due in part to early restrictions against midwives' use of any kind of instruments and to the eventual professionalization of the field of medicine. As early as the thirteenth century, midwives called on male "barber-surgeons" to remove a fetus in a long or difficult labor. These early surgeons were really no more than barbers with sharpened blades and instruments—instruments that women were banned from using by the Catholic Church.[5] In cases where the baby died in the womb, barber-surgeons used an instrument to perforate the infant's skull. The cranial contents were removed and the dead baby was delivered, sometimes after being surgically dismembered. Occasionally this action spared the life of the mother; in other cases it only prolonged her death. Cesarean sections were sanctioned by the Church in order to attempt to save the baby when it appeared that a mother was dying any time during her pregnancy or labor. Instruments were also created to infuse water into the uterus to baptize an unborn baby being buried with a dead mother.

The Church was extremely influential in the lives of all people in Europe during this time but especially in the lives of women. Women healers and midwives were often targets for Church-sanctioned public condemnations or witch hunts. The use of metal instruments would have made midwives more powerful than men, and the Church was determined to prevent their use at any cost.

Forceps were invented in 1588 by Peter Chamberlen. Their original purpose was to remove dead babies and speed the process of labor by pulling babies out through the birth canal. The Chamberlen family kept the design, manufacture, and use of forceps a well-guarded secret for almost a century. Doctors themselves, the Chamberlens did not want the tool to be used by other birth attendants, especially midwives. It became known in London that if a woman was experiencing a prolonged labor, the birth could be effected with quick dispatch if one of the Chamberlen doctors were called in. Arriving with a bundle beneath his coat, the doctor would use the instruments under blankets or sheets, never exposing the clanking metal to wary eyes. After handing the baby to someone, he would wrap up the instruments and collect his fee. The device became known as the "hands of iron" due to all the clanking metal.

By the seventeenth century, forceps were being used by surgeons to try to save babies from dismemberment and death. Lives were saved, but mothers and infants suffered from a host of forceps-delivery complications, including unspeakable pain, infections, and permanent injury. Physicians classified forceps as "surgical instruments," and the same restrictions on their use by women continued. Cost was perhaps as limiting as the actual restrictions—most midwives, who were usually paid in the form of a bartering arrangement, could not afford to have a set of forceps forged for themselves. Thus, midwives and the families they attended were forced to rely on "specialists" for difficult births.

By the early 1800s urban middle-class women in England and the United States began inviting these "technically" superior men with their surgical instruments to attend their births, along with the traditional midwife. The inclusion of these barber-surgeon midmen (as some women called them) quickly turned childbirth into a successful business, whereas previously it had been women serving other women.

Medical education was standardized in America in the nineteenth century, and men entered medical schools in great numbers. Women, particularly midwives, were excluded from this formal training as a result of the prevailing attitude that women were "inherently incompetent."[6] The Victorian ethics and mores of the day restricted male students to mere book knowledge as far as female anatomy was concerned; thus many physicians graduated without even examining a pregnant woman or seeing an actual birth.

As advances were made in all areas of science and technology, it became easy to convince the public that medicine offered a superior way of both explaining and controlling the human body. In their new role as technically superior advisers, physicians were summoned more frequently to the bedsides of upper-class birthing women. In Philadelphia from 1815 to 1825, a span of just ten years, the call for midwives vastly decreased while the number of physicians increased greatly.[7] The only voices to protest this takeover were a few supportive physicians and midwives who believed that men and their technology had no place around birthing women. In the 1820s midwives in England organized, and they charged the new male doctors with "commercialism and dangerous misuse of the forceps." Physicians responded by demeaning midwives as ignorant "old wives" who were unscientific and superstitious.[8] Thus began the battle between physicians and midwives—a struggle that unfortunately continues to this day.

Nineteenth-century doctors felt obliged to offer women the technology of the day. Rather than let nature take its course while attending a birthing woman, they needed to prove themselves as physicians by doing something. They often used bloodletting to relax a woman in labor, sometimes draining her blood to the point where she fainted or lost control. The use of opium or opiate derivatives to minimize the pain of childbirth also gave physicians an advantage over midwives. (Playwright Eugene O'Neill often referred to his opium-addicted mother as a tragedy of his own birth; her doctor had given her opium during and after the birth, thus setting the stage for addiction.)[9] Doctors commonly used forceps, bloodletting, and opium for perfectly normal labors.

Ether and chloroform, developed in England in 1847, were introduced in the birthplace. Sir James Simpson of Edinburgh, together with two friends, discovered the anesthetic value of chloroform by experimenting on themselves. No sooner had Simpson announced that the pains of childbirth could be relieved by this new drug than a storm of condemnation swirled around him. It came primarily from the

British clergy and members of the medical profession, as well as from the public. Everyone argued that pain relief was unnatural and would bring great harm to mothers and babies. He, however, painted a picture of a woman going peacefully to sleep from the first twinge and waking with a baby in her arms; the doctor who would deny her this right was shamefully neglecting his duties and more than cruel.[10]

In the 1850s Queen Victoria of England went against public opinion and the teachings of most Christian churches by accepting the use of chloroform during the births of her seventh and eighth children, setting the trend for her countrywomen. Even though medical opinion worried about unpredictable complications, by the end of 1848 these drugs were used in more than half of all births attended by physicians in Britain.[11] It was difficult for doctors to stand by and witness what they saw as immense suffering when one whiff of a chemical could alleviate all memory and pain. Women readily complied with this new practice.

## THE PROMISE OF SCIENCE

Motivated by fear of death and permanent injury, women in the late nineteenth century embraced the promise of improved birth outcomes through the use of "science." Families who could afford specialists with the latest technology readily sought them out. Women saw the use of drugs in childbearing as a gift that released them from the pain and suffering biblical tradition had taught them was their lot. Rather than giving up control, they saw themselves as retaining control over a frightening and potentially harmful experience.

Hospital births, which also began in America in the mid-nineteenth century, extended the promise of science to women of low social classes. Unmarried, poor, or immigrant women who had neither family support nor the financial means to afford a specialist turned to charity hospitals for their time of "confinement." These institutions welcomed even destitute women as birthing patients to supply the new, more clinically oriented medical programs with "teaching material." In these first charity hospitals, birthing women encountered the male physician, usually in training, who could not do much to aid them. In many cases the only reason the physician took charge of charity cases was to gain knowledge and experience. It was unusual for student doctors to actually participate in the birth process due to Victorian codes of modesty.

As medical technology developed during the 1920s and 1930s, there emerged yet another group of women who chose to birth in hospitals. Upper-middle-class and wealthy women hired specialists, soon to be called obstetricians, from urban medical schools. Their ability to pay gave them access to the latest technology in private, newly built maternity hospitals or in private suites in general hospitals. The place of birth moved rapidly from home to hospital, with hospitals becoming the setting for half of all U.S. births by 1938.[12]

The experience of my grandmother, Estella Harper Lemunyon, exemplifies this trend. She graduated from a relatively new nursing program in Lima, Ohio, in 1921, then worked in a rural area of northwestern Ohio, attending home births alongside a country doctor. Throughout the Depression she drove her horse and buggy from house to house to take care of the medical needs of families, from birth and childhood diseases to more serious conditions. However, by the end of the 1930s it was unusual for her to call on a family outside of the Otis Hospital, where she worked until she retired in 1966.

American physicians and midwives were increasingly in direct competition for patients. Midwives were shut out of an ever more exclusive medical establishment in the United States. The Flexner Report, a privately funded national survey of American medicine in 1910, criticized the lack of uniform licensing procedures for physicians and the inadequacy of their training. This led to even stricter admission standards, higher tuition, and longer periods of training at U.S. medical schools.[13] There was deliberate discrimination against African Americans, Jews, women, and working-class poor students; the role of the physician was thus reserved for primarily white upper-class men who had the money and the social status to meet medical school requirements.

Meanwhile, the American Medical Association (AMA) launched an "educational" campaign in the 1920s and 1930s to improve the quality of health care as well as the status of doctors. Midwives, still banned from attending medical schools because of their sex, were labeled "uneducated, low-class and non-medical."[14] Physicians throughout the United States actively pursued the elimination of the midwife. Articles against the practice of midwifery were written in professional journals, and lobbyists were hired to urge legislatures to enact strict laws governing the licensing of midwives. The public was warned with exaggerated stories of the dangers of birth outside the control of doctors and hospitals. From 1910 to 1920 the majority of midwives practicing in places like New York City were European immigrants who had been well trained in their native countries. However, the AMA saw them as a threat to the new field of obstetrics and denounced foreign-born midwives as "uneducatable [sic] and a threat to American values."[15]

As a result of this campaign and other factors already mentioned, attendance at childbirth not only shifted from midwives to doctors but from the jurisdiction of women to that of men. The Sheppard-Towner Maternity and Infancy Protection Act of 1921 addressed the problem of rising infant and maternal mortality rates and the lack of proper care for the underprivileged and poor. Fourteen states used federal funding to establish midwifery education programs and care for all pregnant

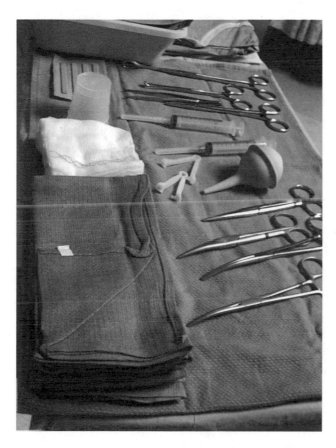

*An instrument table is set up at the foot of every bed, even for an anticipated normal vaginal birth.*

women and children. But in 1929 the AMA was effective in lobbying against the use of midwives, and the bill failed to be renewed.[16] By 1930 midwifery was virtually eliminated in the United States, except among the poor of the rural South. In 1935 midwives attended only 11 percent of all American births, but only 5 percent of those births were of white babies.[17]

As the midwife disappeared, the obstetrician/gynecologist, a specialist dealing only with female patients and their reproductive processes, brought forth a new era of childbirth. In 1930 the new American Board of Obstetrics and Gynecology refused to certify any doctor who did not exclusively treat female patients. This eliminated an enormous number of doctors whose practices dealt with gynecological problems and birth as part of the treatment of entire families. The object in establishing this specialty branch of medicine was purely economic. The specialty decreased the competition, thus increasing the chance for a monopoly. With the midwife gone and the family practitioner barred from entrance into this specialty, the field of obstetrics began to expand into the branch of medicine it is today. Ironically, the word obstetrics is derived directly from the Latin *obstetricius,* which means midwife.[18] The French derivation means "to stand before," thus our words "obstacle" and "obstetrics."

The idea that childbirth was inherently dangerous and needed constant technical intervention grew with the development of obstetrics and the medical profession. A 1920 article by Dr. Joseph B. DeLee in the new *American Journal of Obstetrics
and Gynecology* outlined the horrors of birth for both mother and baby. According
to DeLee, labor was a crushing force that threatened the baby and was responsible
for "epilepsy, idiocy, imbecility and cerebral palsy" as well as death. For the mother,
DeLee compared giving birth to "falling on a pitchfork, driving the handle through
her perineum." He believed that "only a small minority of women escape damage
during labor." DeLee concluded that labor itself was abnormal: "[T]he cause of the
damage, the fall on the pitchfork and the crushing of the door is pathogenic, that
is, disease-producing, and anything pathogenic is pathologic or abnormal."[19] DeLee
recommended the routine use of episiotomy and forceps to spare women from
these potential afflictions.

The episiotomy is an incision made into the thinned-out perineal tissue in
order to enlarge the vaginal opening. Its purpose is to avoid overstretching, undue
damage to the pelvic floor, or trauma to the baby's head. DeLee claimed that the
stretching and tearing of the perineum resulted in such gynecological conditions
as a prolapsed uterus, tears in the vaginal wall, and a sagging perineum. Though
first tried in Ireland in 1782 by Dr. Fielding Ould, the episiotomy was not used
in the United States until a century later and only became popular with DeLee's
endorsement.[20] American physicians, who found tearing of the perineum to be a
problem in hospital births, began to insist that the clean, surgical cut of the episiotomy was easier to repair than a natural jagged tear. What they failed to realize
is that tearing was largely due to the doctor-enforced lithotomy position in which
women lay on their backs with their knees elevated, causing undue stress on the
perineum. In addition, as soon as the baby's head was visible the doctor would
often grab it with forceps and pull, causing the baby's big, blunt shoulders to rip
the woman's perineum. Doctors also believed DeLee's claims that the episiotomy
would restore "virginal conditions" and make the mother "better than new,"
implying that women were irreparably damaged in normal childbirth and thus less
sexually desirable.

What person could resist such arguments, given the state of knowledge about
childbirth and women's health at the time? Even the media sold women on the
advantages of medical science and technology in childbirth. As early as 1920 articles in *Ladies' Home Journal* and *Good Housekeeping* urged women to "see an obstetrician early. . . . Choose a doctor you have faith in. . . . You can trust him to guide
you through." Women remained haunted by their underlying fear of permanent
injury or death. At the same time, midwives were hampered by laws limiting the
extent of their involvement or even their right to practice at all. They occasionally
had to stand by while birthing mothers hemorrhaged or died of childbed fever,

knowing that if they could practice as they wished, they could save them. It was precisely these situations that led women to be swayed by the promise of safer and less painful childbirths. They surrendered some of their most valued traditions in childbirth, traditions that included the support and comfort of their families, a basic trust in their bodies, and the right to be attended in birth by other women. All of these traditions were traded for what they thought would be the protection of life and health during birth.

## PAIN RELIEF: THE ERA OF "TWILIGHT SLEEP"

The promise of complete pain relief probably brought more women into the hospital than any other reason. "Twilight sleep," introduced in Germany in 1914, appeared to solve many problems connected with birth, from both the doctor's and the patient's points of view. Twilight sleep consisted of a combination of morphine for pain relief in early labor and scopolamine, an amnesiac that often caused hallucinations. Under twilight sleep a woman could still feel and respond to her contractions but supposedly would not remember what happened. The amnesiac component of twilight sleep separated a woman from her body, which could writhe, toss, and even feel pain but all outside her cognizance. The birth itself was not part of the mother's conscious experience because the increased use of scopolamine as labor progressed usually resulted in a heavily sedated mother who was totally unconscious for the delivery. In addition, women had to be carefully guarded from hurting themselves, which sometimes required them to be strapped or tied to the bed for hours as a result of the hallucinogenic side effects of the drug. If that wasn't bad enough, the effects on the baby were even worse. Most of the babies needed assistance in breathing and smaller babies just didn't survive.

Many of the early supporters of pain relief in childbirth were suffragists with strong beliefs in women's rights. Suffragists, many of whom were women physicians, organized the National Twilight Sleep Association in 1915 in the United States. They sponsored rallies in department stores so that ordinary women would be able to hear about the drugs that could ease them through their trial. They published articles and led women's groups, dealing with such topics as pain relief and the "new science" of obstetrics. Women's magazines of the day extolled the benefits, imploring women to "ask for it. Demand it. Tolerate no other way . . . than Twilight Sleep."[21]

Just as ill-informed feature articles can seize public attention today, the "fashion" of painless childbirth captured people's imaginations, not their common sense. Through these efforts the public learned of the possibility of a shorter and less painful labor. The suffragist twilight sleep supporters claimed it was the dawning of a new age in childbirth.[22] Little did they know that by insisting on physician-attended births and the use of twilight sleep as a painkiller, they were actually giving up the control over their births that they were fighting so hard to obtain. More and more women began requesting twilight sleep. Physicians readily agreed to the public demands and institutionalized the use of anesthesia in obstetrics. By the 1930s public and medical opinion were in agreement that some form of narcotization should be used for every labor. Scopolamine continued to be used until the 1960s when the drugs were gradually replaced by analgesics, such as Demerol, and anesthetics administered through spinals, caudals, and epidurals.

The era of twilight sleep is described in nursing school today as the age of "knock 'em out, drag 'em out obstetrics." A mother of five and grandmother of six who recently attended her daughter's home birth commented that although she had given birth five times, she had never seen a birth or a newborn baby. "All my labors went really fast," she recalled. "With my first one, I got to the hospital and knew that the baby would be born soon. I could feel it; I wasn't scared. But just as I was about to have what felt like the biggest orgasm of my life, they put a mask over my face and I missed the whole thing. I can't believe that I let them do that to me!" Shortly after her new granddaughter's gentle arrival, this woman, while rocking the baby with tears rolling down her face, exclaimed, "I had no idea birth could be so beautiful!"

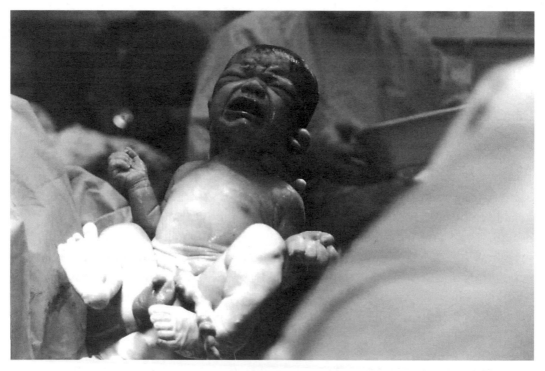

*The first moments of birth can be terrifying for a baby who is not immediately placed on its mother.*

## HOSPITAL BIRTHS FOR EVERYONE

The promise of painless childbirth, seen as a right by some women in the early part of the twentieth century, became the standard of obstetric care. The uniform approach to childbirth in the hospital provided an appearance of safety but robbed women of their freedom. Every woman was treated the same way, even though every labor and birth was unique. The standard of care required that women be the passive recipients of all that medical science offered, for her own good and the baby's well-being.

Obstetrics placed great emphasis on the ability to predict complications in labor and birth. Every case was seen as a potential disaster, with every physician playing the role of a potential hero. This view of birth stripped women of the chance to experience the emotional and social aspects of childbirth. Women became baby machines, treated like repositories for little uteruses that contained little fetuses, all of which were subject to the control of the physician.

During the 1940s, 1950s, and 1960s, the birth process was turned into an assembly line managed by skilled technicians and machines. Time limits were established for the first and second stages of labor, with some hospitals actually instituting the policy that a woman could only be in the delivery room for a specific length of time.[23] With the development of oxytocic drugs to induce or speed up labor, doctors could manage birth even more effectively. Drugs were given to slow a labor until the doctor or the delivery room was ready; then Pitocin could be used to get the labor going again. Cesarean sections replaced the use of high forceps, and fetal monitors helped detect fetal distress that resulted from the use of drugs and anesthesia. One intervention inevitably led directly to the next, until every birth was a medically managed, staged, and produced event.

By 1950, 88 percent of all births in the United States occurred in hospitals; five years later 95 percent of all births took place in the hospital setting. In 1960 it was almost unheard of for a woman to give birth anywhere but in a "modern" obstetrical unit in a hospital.[24] With hospital births for everyone, women had given the responsibility for decisions concerning their births to physicians who promised less pain, fewer deaths, fewer fetal injuries, and no birth defects from difficult and long labors. Women voiced their primary concern like this: "Doctor, give me a healthy baby. I don't care how you do it." They rationalized, "I may lose control over certain aspects of my birth, even my independence, but the promise of a perfect baby is worth the trade-off."

## UNMASKING PRENATAL TESTING

Prenatal testing has become routine for all pregnant women, even mandated in some states, despite the fact that the majority of the tests were created to screen for conditions that are common only in high-risk pregnancies. Prenatal tests involve obtaining a sample of amniotic fluid, chorion, fetal blood, or mother's blood. We have all been reassured by the medical profession that most tests are without risk, but many of them have never been thoroughly studied and may actually bring harm to either mother or baby. Waiting for test results and basing decisions on them can produce unnecessary anxiety for many women. Results can sometimes be vague or downright misleading.

The tests are done to provide information on the health of the fetus. When testing actually reveals a fetal disability, the mother is confronted with an array of complex decisions, such as whether to continue the pregnancy and prepare for the birth, fetal surgery, or organ donation, or to end the pregnancy with an abortion. With the rise of in vitro fertilization there have been discussions about testing parents who participate in these programs and may have genetic risk factors. Testing of preimplanted embryos might ensure that only embryos free of genetic diseases or problems are placed into the uterus.

Women need to inform themselves about the latest technological advances that are applied during pregnancy and childbirth. Well-informed women who know the risks and benefits of tests and procedures can decide which ones make sense to use in their particular situations. Many diagnostic procedures are performed merely to provide documentation in the event that an alleged physician error leads to a malpractice case. Understandably, the doctor or midwife desires as much information as possible about the chemical and physiological aspects of a woman's pregnancy. Unfortunately, when tests are performed without regard for each individual's situation, a subtle message is transmitted to the woman that tells her she cannot possibly be considered normal until her health has been verified by tests. This message now has a name—"the nocebo effect." The word comes from the Latin *nocere,* to harm, and so has a literal meaning of "I shall cause harm or be harmful." The word explains the negative effect that some treatments or tests can have upon a normal situation (i.e., pregnancy). Routine testing assumes that abnormalities will be found and that a physician will be needed to manage them.

## *Ultrasound*

Ultrasound is the most commonly used prenatal diagnostic procedure. High-frequency sound waves are beamed into a pregnant woman's uterus through a transducer. The sound waves rebound and are converted into a "picture" of the baby.

The ultrasound test, which usually takes only a few minutes, displays information on a television monitor, usually in full view of the parents. The technology has progressed to the point where 3-D detailed photos can now be instantly printed or emailed to eager family members around the world.

In the case of complications or questions during a pregnancy, ultrasound provides valuable information that can assist a physician in making a diagnosis. Undeniably the most cost effective, least invasive of all prenatal tests, ultrasonic diagnosis has some valid uses. These include judging the age of the fetus when there is a difference between the actual and expected size; determining a fetal presentation and assisting in turning the baby if it is in a breech position; viewing the placenta and fetus when there has been vaginal bleeding; looking for spina bifida, heart defect, or cleft palate; determining a multiple pregnancy; monitoring fetal growth when it is suspected that the fetus has not been growing normally (fetal growth retardation); and determining if an inactive fetus is still alive.

If a woman has none of these concerns during pregnancy, ultrasonic diagnosis should not be routinely performed. Although initial studies show no side effects from the use of ultrasound, there have been no conclusive long-term studies on its effects on the fetus. There have been studies, however, which have shown definitively that there are no better outcomes for women who have had one or more routine ultrasound examinations during their pregnancies as compared to those who have had none.[25]

More and more physicians routinely use ultrasound on every prenatal visit, which is not a judicious use of this device. The test has a very high rate of false positives when used so frequently. Aside from the early ultrasound picture for the baby's memory book, repeated use of the technology is simply not warranted. This is evident in a joint UK study on all health technologies released in 2000. After over a year of evaluation it reported that routine ultrasound "has not been shown to confer any benefit to either mother or baby."[26]

## AFP and Triple Screen

The AFP test, sometimes called the MSAFP or maternal serum AFP, requires a blood sample which is drawn from the mother between fifteen and twenty weeks of pregnancy (preferably at sixteen to eighteen weeks). The test is used to determine levels of alpha-fetoprotein, which is a naturally produced chemical excreted in the mother's blood where it can be easily tested. When an abnormality occurs in the fetus's neural tube, an excess of AFP is released into the amniotic fluid. Neural tube defects result from a lapse in the prenatal development of the brain (anencephaly) and spinal cord (spina bifida). The incidence of these defects in the United States is approximately 1 per 1,000 live births. High AFP levels can also indicate a multiple pregnancy, fetal death, and low birth weight. A few other prenatal diagnoses include placental complications, digestive system problems, and urinary tract defects. A low level of AFP is a signal that Down's syndrome may be present.

Another test called the Triple Screen requires a sample of blood which is drawn from the mother to measure three things: the levels of hCG (human chorionic gonadotropin) and estriol, which are produced by the placenta, and the level of AFP, which is produced by the fetus. The levels of these three substances in the blood can help doctors identify a fetus at risk for certain birth defects such as spina bifida and chromosomal abnormalities like Down's syndrome. This test, which is beginning to replace the standard AFP test, poses no risk to either mother or baby. The major drawback of Triple Screen testing is its high rate of false highs or lows, as great as 98 percent, which can often lead to more invasive testing or extreme worry for the mother. Because this test does not identify the existence of any specific abnormality, but only the presence of chemicals that may indicate risk, its results are inconclusive and open to interpretation.

Physician-researchers at Boston's Brigham and Women's Hospital, after studying 87,584 pregnancies, reported that an elevated AFP level in conjunction with a normal ultrasound scan implies a less than 0.1 percent chance that the baby will have one of the four most common birth defects, including Down's syndrome and spina bifida.

Whether or not to have the AFP or Triple Screen test is a very hard decision and a very personal one. Some women feel that no matter what is wrong they would not terminate the pregnancy, and therefore do not want the test, while others are very eager to receive the "normal" results, even knowing that there are no guarantees. If you decide not to utilize the AFP or Triple Screen test, you may be asked to sign a waiver refusing the test. Your provider is obligated by most states to offer you the test and information about it.

## Amniocentesis

Amniocentesis is a fairly invasive procedure that tests for genetic defects in the fetus. Until recently amniocentesis has been regarded as a routine procedure for women over thirty-five years of age because genetic defects tend to increase with maternal age. The American College of Obstetricians and Gynecologists now recommends the Triple Screen for all pregnant women and only suggests an amniocentesis if there is an indication of risk.

Amniocentesis involves inserting a hollow needle into the mother's abdomen and removing a sample of the amniotic fluid that surrounds the baby. The amniotic fluid contains cells excreted by the fetus that reflect its genetic makeup. These cells are analyzed to detect genetic defects. The most common disorder screened for through amniocentesis is Down's syndrome; other genetic disorders targeted by the test include hemophilia, sickle-cell anemia, and Tay-Sachs disease.

There are accompanying risks to performing amniocentesis. Ultrasound is used along with the procedure to ensure proper placement of the needle, but fetal movement can sometimes result in injury to the baby. The risk of miscarriage is 1 in 200.[27] Fetal death sometimes occurs and has been reported up to four to eight weeks after the amniocentesis. And, needless to say, the procedure is extremely painful and anxiety-producing for the mother. The testing will not guarantee a normal child. It cannot detect most nonchromosomal genetic defects, nor can it detect defects of body structure, such as harelip, cleft palate, congenital heart disease, clubfoot, or congenital hip dislocation. Defects caused by exposure to toxic substances will also not be detected by amniocentesis.

In light of the finding that amniocentesis itself carries a 0.5 to 1.5 percent chance of spontaneous abortion,[28] researchers have concluded that "many women may choose not to have an amniocentesis when informed that the risk of pregnancy loss is substantially greater than the likelihood of finding an anomaly."[29]

The use of amniocentesis has also been associated with early sex determination and the controversial practice of selective abortion if the fetus is not the preferred sex. According to the latest reports, parents throughout the world still desire male babies twice as often as female babies. India banned the use of diagnostic ultrasound in 2004, in an effort to reduce the number of abortions caused by sex selection only. In addition, women will sometimes accept a diagnosis that indicates severe handicaps and choose to abort what turns out to be a perfectly normal fetus. Even when abortion is chosen for the "not medically perfect" baby, couples may experience an enormous amount of guilt, influencing subsequent pregnancies and births. Consenting to amniocentesis is a decision that warrants careful and thoughtful consideration.

## Chorionic Villi Sampling (CVS)

Chorionic villi sampling (CVS) is used for very early detection of possible chromosomal (genetic) abnormalities. It can be performed as early as the ninth week of pregnancy. It requires a small sample of the chorion (the outer sac that surrounds the embryo during the first two months of pregnancy) along with the villi (hairlike tissues that protrude from the chorion) to be gathered for analysis, which may be obtained either through the abdominal wall or through the vagina and cervix.

Most recent studies indicate a greater risk of miscarriage in women who undergo the CVS procedure than in women who do not, and a much greater risk of damage to the baby than that associated with amniocentesis. There have been no conclusive tests proving its safety and accuracy. Recent studies have suggested that it may actually *cause* a birth defect, missing limbs or digits.[30]

## The Glucose Tolerance Test (GTT)

The glucose tolerance test (GTT) is used to rule out gestational diabetes, which is sometimes referred to as gestational glucose intolerance. This "condition" of pregnancy is being called into question. The explanation of gestational diabetes is that the hormones of pregnancy suppress insulin release, allowing a mother's blood sugar to be higher during pregnancy and thus providing more glucose to nourish her fetus. This is a normal consequence of pregnancy and one that is established to provide for the baby. Occasionally, the pancreas, where insulin is made, cannot handle the stress of pregnancy and the insulin/glucose levels become severely unbalanced, causing the blood sugar to remain too high during part of the pregnancy, primarily in the last trimester. Prolonged exposure to this high blood sugar level may cause the fetus to grow excessively large, resulting in such complications as premature birth or respiratory distress.

A GTT is usually recommended at twenty-four to twenty-eight weeks and repeated around thirty-two to thirty-four weeks in women who are considered high-risk. The woman drinks a sweet liquid called glucola, and her blood sugar is checked one hour later. If the one-hour test is positive, a more accurate three-hour test is done. The reliability of a test that has a woman drink a concentrated sugar substance on an empty stomach, however, is questionable. The GTT is done under abnormal conditions and, therefore, often shows unnatural results. An alternative is to measure the blood sugar levels two hours after a heavy meal and to encourage the woman to do normal activities to help her body process the glucose.

Some physiologists and researchers believe that normal pregnant women should not be tested using the same standards as nonpregnant women, since the pregnant metabolic condition is not being taken into account.[31] The fact is, no studies have proven that high blood sugar leads to problems in pregnancy or larger babies. It has been estimated that only 30 percent of women with an abnormal glucose tolerance test will have larger-than-average babies. One clinical trial, which studied the outcomes of women who had elective cesarean sections because of gestational diabetes, showed no better outcomes than the control group and a significantly higher incidence of mortality for the babies.[32] The label of gestational diabetes subjects mothers to many more tests and interventions including cesarean sections.

Gestational diabetes should not be confused with a preexisting diabetic condition. Gestational glucose intolerance is more common in obese women, older mothers, or those with a family history of diabetes. These women may require close monitoring throughout their pregnancies to prevent stillbirth and congenital defects. If detected early enough, a mother's diet may be adjusted to keep her blood sugar from getting too high. Occasionally extra insulin is needed.

## Group B Streptococcus (GBS)

In the past few years midwives and doctors have been very concerned with the detrimental effects of the bacterial infection Group B Streptococcus (GBS) on newborn babies. Identified in the 1970s, GBS is not the same infection that causes strep throat. In pregnant women, GBS can cause bladder and womb infections and stillbirth. Before prevention methods began to be used, about 8,000 babies in the United States contracted GBS infections every year, and about 5 percent would die. Some estimates of newborn death are even higher, taking into consideration babies up to three months old.

Between 5 and 35 percent of pregnant women will carry GBS in their bodies without developing any symptoms. The most common places for the infection are in the vagina or rectum. When the baby moves down the birth canal, it can become infected by the bacteria, which can lead within a few hours to pneumonia, sepsis (infections of the blood or tissues), or meningitis. Some think that a considerable number of cases of Sudden Infant Death Syndrome (SIDS) could be attributed to GBS, especially before it was widely known that babies could be at risk.

It is now routine practice to test pregnant women for the presence of GBS in late pregnancy, between thirty-five and thirty-seven weeks. This is done by swabbing the rectum and vagina. A culture is grown in the lab and the results come back in three to five days. A positive result does not necessarily mean that you will pass the bacteria on to your baby during the birth. The degree of risk has been studied and researchers found that fewer than 3 out of 100 babies will become ill. If the positive test is combined with other risk factors, such as a fever during labor, prolonged rupture of membranes, or premature labor, your provider will give you the opportunity to receive IV antibiotics during labor. Most women in hospitals who have tested positive will receive the antibiotics even if they have no other risk factors. The Centers for Disease Control (CDC) recommends treating all women who tested positive with a dosage of Penicillin or ampicillin every four hours in labor.

A few hospitals have stopped testing mothers and begun offering routine antibiotics to all newborns.[33] Since the use of antibiotics was introduced in the early 1990's, GBS in newborns has declined 70%. However, we are now seeing that there is a connection between increased antibiotic use and more severe or antibiotic resistant strains of infection in newborns.[34]

The test has some record of false positives and some women request a retesting after following a strict diet protocol. There are some naturopathic physicians and midwives who have more natural treatments for ridding the mother of the GBS infection before birth.[35]

## Informed Consent

Any test or procedure used in maternity care must be explained, clearly outlining the risks and benefits of participating in or not doing the procedure. The Informed Consent Doctrine requires that medical practitioners provide a mother with all relevant information about a proposed procedure or treatment prior to obtaining her consent to carry out the procedure or treatment. These four items of information must be provided:

- the nature of the procedure
- the risks
- the benefits
- the availability of alternative treatments (including no treatment) and the risks and benefits of those

Not only do you have the right to refuse any test or procedure for you or your baby, in some cases you may even have the legal ability to charge your provider with assault if a procedure is done against your will.

Today's parents have a difficult task in sorting out all the evidence that supports or refutes the arguments for common medical interventions in childbirth. It is no easy job, especially under the stress of labor. Attending an independent childbirth education class, researching interventions online, talking to your provider, and reading books on normal birth will help protect you from the overuse of medical interventions.

## MEDICAL LEGAL DILEMMAS

Within the medical model of maternity care there is an underlying promise of perfection. Decisions are made by evaluating risk factors, but who is at risk and who is ultimately responsible when the outcome is not what everyone wanted? There can never be any guarantees with human reproduction. Babies die. It is a sad fact of life. Babies sometimes have genetic defects that are not predicted or expected. However, the technocracy has developed to the point where protection of fetuses now takes precedence, sometimes under court order, over the well being of the mother and wishes of parents. Well-intentioned parents who refuse treatment or testing in some instances are now at odds with their providers who order treatments for the protection of the unborn baby.

Imagine a law declaring that a pregnant woman gives up her rights to bodily integrity, life, and liberty. Such a law would certainly bring many objections, but in fact state and federal laws have been passed that put fetal rights above those of the mother. This has resulted in some bizarre court cases. For instance, a mother in Utah was jailed after the death of one of her twins because she refused to undergo a cesarean, resulting, the doctors alleged, in the death of the smaller baby.[36] A woman dying of a serious illness was forced, after the hospital obtained a court order, to undergo a cesarean to save the life of her baby. Her doctors implored the hospital not to proceed, stating that it would surely kill the mother. The baby and the mother both died as a result of the operation.[37]

Consider the work of personal injury attorneys who bring cases of cerebral palsy to courts and collect big awards for parents, when the most significant research shows that cerebral palsy is a condition of the first trimester of development and not related to birth trauma or asphyxia. In a cerebral palsy case in Texas the parents were awarded over $11 million in damages. The lawyer for that case proclaims on his Web site that vaginal birth after a cesarean, or VBAC, is inherently more dangerous than a repeat cesarean and that ominous things happen when busy nurses don't monitor every single contraction a woman has. The fear of lawsuit propels the medical model even further down the slippery slope of guaranteeing good outcomes by applying more technology.

The wrongful birth cases that our court system has allowed to develop present an interesting dilemma. In 1996, a law firm in New Jersey obtained a $1.5 million settlement in a wrongful birth case when the mother's HMO failed to disclose the abnormal results of an alpha-fetoprotein test until pregnancy termination was not an option. The infant, now 10 years old, was born with a brain injury, and is partially blind and suffers from seizures.[38] In a similar case in Ohio, the Supreme Court dismissed the legal action stating that the court could not define the quality of a life or determine who should be alive and who should not.

With a great deal of discussion and argument about stem cell research and many more parents opting for in vitro fertilization, we are now faced with more complex moral, legal, and ethical choices about the essence of life. We are starting to hear terms like selective reduction (performed when too many embryos have been implanted) and the aforementioned wrongful birth, and there will likely be many more to follow.

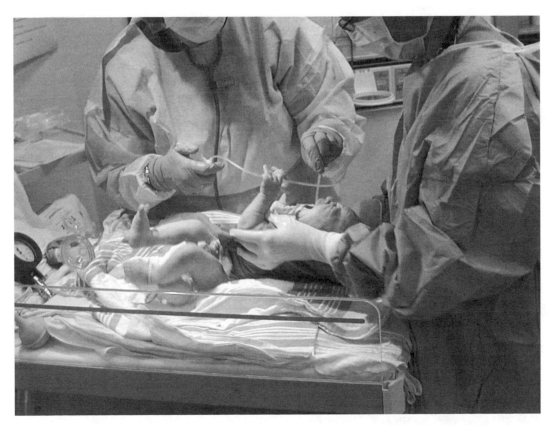

*The baby is seen as the product, upon whom routine procedures are performed.*

# THE RESULTS OF MEDICAL INTERVENTION

What are the results of medical manipulation of a normal physiological process? Have technology and medical intervention lived up to their promises? During the period in which childbirth became a medical event, there was a great decrease in the number of infant and maternal deaths. There are many possible explanations relating to the advent of technical intervention that could explain this decrease. New antibiotic drugs spared women from septicemia. Hospital blood banks were established, along with blood typing and transfusion techniques, in the late 1930s.[39] Housing and sanitation conditions improved. Most pregnant women's diets were healthier than their mothers' and grandmothers' had been. Neonatal resuscitation was developed and neonatal intensive care units were built. Birth control and abortion helped control the timing and number of pregnancies. Yet even though the obstetricians claimed medical superiority, the infection and complication rates were much higher in hospital births than in home births. Women who have needed technology can attribute the safety of their lives and their children's lives to the advancement of medical science and obstetrics. But the labor and birth experiences of the majority of women with normal pregnancies, as well as the birth experiences of their babies, have been affected in many unforeseen and permanent ways.

What price have we and our children paid for this supposedly advanced technology? Women who sought to liberate themselves from the more uncomfortable and sometimes lethal aspects of childbirth lost much in the process. Women and families must cope with children who have obvious birth-related injuries as a result of the use of forceps or drugs, or through mishandling of the labor. How do families rationalize the child whose abilities to love, trust, and learn may have been impaired by the drugs given to the mother during birth? How has the use of drugs altered women's perceptions of childbirth? What are the personal costs for women who experience intimidation, loss of freedom, humiliation, and even abuse while giving birth?

Interventions in childbirth are usually administered by kind, well-intentioned hospital personnel for what they consider appropriate medical reasons. Unfortunately, those reasons do not alleviate the humiliation a woman feels when she is rendered helpless and attached to monitors and IVs, preventing her from moving. It doesn't lessen her embarrassment when she is asked to remove her clothes and put on a hospital gown, or her helplessness when her loved ones are excluded and she labors alone. A woman's trust in her own body and her ability to birth normally is shattered by repeated vaginal examinations in order to assess her "progress" during labor. A mother's self-confidence wavers when her newborn is taken away to the nursery to be cared for by "medically superior" professionals.

The American system of maternity care sends women the message that they are not capable of giving birth without the help of physicians and hospitals. From rules that prohibit eating and drinking during labor, to constant electronic fetal monitoring and subsequent interventions for fear of malpractice suits, the medicalization of childbirth has become the norm.

In a plea for the de-medicalization of normal birth, Dr. Richard Johanson, just prior to his death, published a paper in the *British Medical Journal (BMJ)* in April 2002. He asked his colleagues, "Has the medicalization of childbirth gone too far?" He stressed that routine interventions in normal birth have increased without evidence of their effectiveness.

With our concern for comfort and our sincere interest in protecting our children's lives, we have helped create the modern medical myths concerning childbirth.[40] Dr. Johanson's suggestions to his colleagues for turning this tide are: educate women on their choices, practice only on the basis of the available evidence, work as a team, and embrace midwifery. In response to this opinion, he received the highest number of letters to the editor that the *BMJ* had ever received.

The emotional richness, the transformational power, and the amazing energy of birth have been ignored in favor of advancing technology. Centuries of feminine wisdom about the birth process have been lost in the creation of a new medical mythology. Medical myths and the technocracy they have spawned have drastically altered women's self-perception and have given society a distorted view both of womanhood and of the birth process itself.

# CHAPTER THREE

# Dispelling the Medical Myths

A wealth of information and research shows that the medicalization of childbirth has been detrimental on many levels to mother, baby, and family. Yet the dichotomy between practice and the ideal remains. The medical management of birth continues; women yield to physician and hospital control; there have been only minor adjustments aimed at achieving the changes that research and instinct tell us are necessary. Is it possible to view birth as a normal physiological process with the birthing woman in control, or is it necessary to approach every birth as a potential emergency "just in case"? How can we overcome the attitude that birth is dangerous and begin to protect the woman's right to birth in privacy and peace? How can we honor the sacredness of the mother/child continuum and acknowledge the impact that disruption of this continuum has on the health and well-being of the individual?

Childbirth and women's advocates as well as parents who are looking for alternatives to today's medical model for birth are asking many questions similar to these the world over. There is a growing understanding and appreciation of childbirth as a normal and natural process, one that offers a unique opportunity for emotional, spiritual, and personal growth for the mother, baby, and family. Proponents of gentle birth are reevaluating the standard obstetrical practices of hospital births. Each one of the practices has been studied and researched. The stacks of data accumulate, and when they are all read and evaluated, they all say the same things. These findings, coupled with a greater understanding of the normal progression of labor and birth and the latest research on the developing infant brain, indicate that the prevailing practices and beliefs about childbirth are based on false, outmoded, or unverified assumptions.

In order to be able to give an informed consent, a woman requires necessary and individually appropriate information to be given to her in a way that enables her to grasp the implications of her decision. The information needs to be based on unbiased evidence, not the typical "that's the way it is done here" explanation. All of the options in maternity care need to reflect "best practice" or "evidence based" principles. If evidence drawn from across the disciplines shows a particular form of care has proven to be beneficial, it needs to be incorporated into practice. Those practices which have been proven to be either of no benefit or harmful should be discarded.

Several decades ago, Iain Chalmers and his colleagues began to organize a register of controlled clinical trials, assembling an extremely important body of work known as the Cochrane Pregnancy and Childbirth Database. An exhaustive search of all relevant literature was begun and over 40,000 obstetricians in eighteen countries were asked to submit unpublished research that might be used as protocols for various aspects of maternity care, culminating in the publication of the massive two-volume set of books *Effective Care in Pregnancy and Childbirth* in 1989.[1]

A second *Effective Care* book was published which summarized the analysis of the clinical trials and research data in a user-friendly guide for creating policy in all aspects of maternity care.[2] With the advance of the Internet, an electronic database was begun in 1993 and launched in 1995 and is continually updated. The Cochrane Library[3] is available online to anyone for a subscription fee. They encourage consumer involvement, providing an e-mail list and newsletter and sponsoring meetings both in Europe and the United States. This database has helped many childbirth advocates by giving them access to the most up-to-date reliable evidence on the benefits and risks of health care and obstetrical interventions. It is in this evidence that we see the downside to many hospital procedures that are still considered standard practice today.

The unnecessary procedures and outdated attitudes concerning women and childbirth rob a woman, her baby, and her family of the emotional and spiritual opportunities inherent in life's most creative and powerful experience. The general public's perceptions about childbirth practices are unfortunately based on myths that support the belief that the more physicians can monitor and control the birth process with up-to-the-minute technology, the better the chances for a "successful" birth. Only in recent years has anyone acknowledged women as the center of the birth process and babies as conscious participants.

For many years most women have accepted the myth that their bodies are inadequate to birth their babies without a physician's directions and interventions. Women are encouraged to doubt their bodies' wisdom, their physical strength, and their intuition. In labor and birth a woman waits for the doctor to tell her when to "push" and accepts that an episiotomy may be best or that childbirth is unbearable without pain medication.

The language of childbirth reveals whom we see as the person in control of the birth process. It is common to say the doctor or nurse delivered the baby, when in reality it was the woman who birthed her baby. When women accept their primary role in the birth process and acknowledge the ability of their bodies to birth their babies into the world, they will reject this ideology. Our language will then reflect this fundamental shift in the perception of childbirth, and our children will have a different understanding of birth.

In this chapter we will look at what could be considered the "medical myths" of our time. These myths concerning childbirth include justifications for commonly used obstetrical practices that are unnecessary and that actually interfere with the normal physiology of the birth process. You must become an informed consumer and decide for yourself what makes sense in childbirth.

## MYTH: THE HOSPITAL IS THE SAFEST PLACE TO HAVE A BABY

In 2004, 98 percent of all births in the United States took place in hospitals. Everyone is familiar with the modern image of birth as seen on many TV shows as that of a woman lying in a bed in a hospital, draped for modesty, hooked up to various monitors and equipment, with a physician or nurse "directing" or "coaching" her through the process as though it were an athletic event.

When a woman today asks a physician about the possibility of birthing her baby at home or in a birth center, it is very likely that she will be discouraged by her doctor, who will state that the hospital is the only place that will guarantee a safe birth. This attitude has not wavered over the past twenty-five years. It is important to clarify that safety is usually measured by death (mortality) or illness (morbidity) during the labor and birth process and shortly thereafter. The United States has consistently high maternal and perinatal mortality and morbidity rates compared to other industrialized countries. In 2003, the United States was ranked thirty-second by the National Center for Health Statistics, which publishes the mortality and morbidity statistics.[4] This means that there are thirty-one countries where it is safer for women to give birth than in the United States.[5]

The countries with the lowest mortality and morbidity rates are those where midwifery is an integral part of obstetric care and where births more commonly take place outside of large hospitals (see chart on page 55). Japan has had a consistently high ranking among all countries since the 1970s. In 1996 perinatal mortality in Japan reached an historic all-time low: 3.8 deaths per 1,000 live births. The United States experienced 7.3 deaths per 1,000 live births that year, reflecting a 48

## INFANT MORTALITY FOR 2003

### (Infant deaths per 1,000 live births)

| | | | |
|---|---|---|---|
| Singapore | 2.28 | Belgium | 4.76 |
| Sweden | 2.77 | Liechtenstein | 4.77 |
| Japan | 3.28 | Canada | 4.82 |
| Iceland | 3.31 | Luxembourg | 4.88 |
| Finland | 3.59 | Netherlands | 5.11 |
| Norway | 3.73 | Portugal | 5.13 |
| Malta | 3.94 | Gibraltar | 5.22 |
| Czech Republic | 3.97 | UK | 5.22 |
| Germany | 4.2 | Ireland | 5.5 |
| France | 4.31 | Greece | 5.63 |
| Switzerland | 4.43 | San Marino | 5.85 |
| Spain | 4.48 | New Zealand | 5.96 |
| Slovenia | 4.5 | Italy | 6.07 |
| Denmark | 4.63 | **United States** | **6.3** |
| Austria | 4.68 | Cuba | 6.45 |
| Australia | 4.76 | Taiwan | 6.52 |

from the CIA World Fact Book

percent difference. The United States has reduced infant mortality since 1965, but we still consistently have much higher rates compared to almost all other industrialized nations.*

In most of the industrialized countries of the world midwives attend more than 70 percent of all births, with many of them taking place in homes or birth centers. Japan has seen a resurgence of the midwife-run small community birth center in the past decade, and as we have seen their infant mortality rate is relatively low. For U.S. midwife-attended births the mortality rate drops to 2.1 deaths per 1,000 live births as compared to the overall U.S. figure of 6.3 deaths per 1,000 live births.[6] While there are additional factors to consider, such as socialized medicine and prenatal care, when comparing birth outcomes between Japan (or other countries with low infant mortality rates) and the United States, the data makes a strong case for home births attended by midwives. Dr. Michel Odent authored a 1991 report for the World

---

*There are several different ways to define mortality. Infant mortality includes deaths from birth through the first year of life. Neonatal mortality includes infant deaths from birth to less than twenty-nine days. Perinatal mortality refers to fetal deaths from twenty-eight weeks' gestation up through infant deaths of less than seven days. In the United States perinatal mortality is defined as deaths of the fetus from twenty weeks' gestation up through infant deaths of less than twenty-eight days.

Health Organization in which he stated, "The priority must be to challenge the universal propaganda that home birth is dangerous. . . . The best means by which to challenge the current beliefs are the statistics from the Netherlands (where midwifery and home birth are prevalent)."[7]

One of the most common rationalizations for the choice of couples wanting to give birth in the hospital is the number of emergency cesareans they hear about from all their friends who have recently had babies. Women will often say, "I'd like to stay at home or go to a birth center, but this is my first baby, and I just want to be in a hospital in case something goes wrong." Eighty-five percent of birthing women in the United States are considered low-risk as they enter the hospital, but 100 percent of women receive at least one intervention in labor.[8] The sad fact is that the majority of cesareans are the *result* of being in the hospital. Routine interventions used in hospital births produce a "cascade effect" which causes cesarean rates to climb. In out-of-hospital birth settings, the focus is on the mother, not the technology. Undisturbed birth leads to healthier babies and happier mothers.

One of the largest studies comparing outcomes of hospital births and out-of-hospital births, which includes home and birth-center births, was conducted by the U.S. Centers for Disease Control between 1974 and 1976. Although now thirty years old, the newer data is comparable. North Carolina was the site of the study, which included over 242,000 hospital births and 2,200 out-of-hospital births. In this study it was necessary to differentiate between out-of-hospital births that were planned by women who received prenatal care, and births that happened accidentally (for example, while en route to the hospital) or where there was no preparation or qualified person in attendance. The results of this two-year study showed that the infant death rate in hospitals was 12 per 1,000 live births, whereas the death rate for planned, attended home births was 4 per 1,000 live births. The infant death rate in unplanned or unattended home births soared to 120 per 1,000.[9] This study demonstrates that if the birth is planned for and attended by doctors or midwives who are experienced with the birth process, birth is safer at home.

In 1991 the British government formed a committee with members of parliament to investigate maternity care that was in place through the National Health Service (NHS). Their report, submitted in 1992, offered sensible suggestions for improvement, which included the statement that "the policy of encouraging all women to give birth in hospitals cannot be justified on grounds of safety." It went on to conclude that maternity care in Britain should no longer be based on a "medical model of care."[10] This historic report, along with consumer demands, established the groundwork for a committee that included mothers, practitioners, and administrators, all working for the common goal of providing women with choices, including the option of home birth.

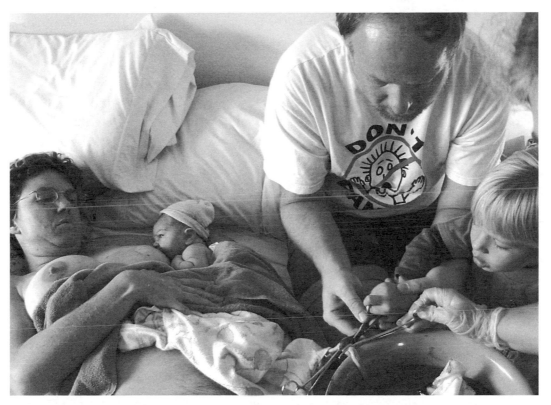

*In a home birth everyone participates, including young children.*

In 1976 Dr. Lewis Mehl-Madrona and a group of researchers at Stanford University conducted a comprehensive study that focused on the differences between planned home births and planned hospital births. They studied 2,092 births, half of which were planned home births and half of which were planned hospital births.[11] The women in the study were also matched in terms of age, socioeconomic level, and risk factors. Researchers analyzed each birth for length of labor, complications, and infant health after birth, as well as all procedures that were used during the course of labor and delivery. In the entire study there was only one infant death, and that death occurred in the hospital. The results of this particular study show that the mortality statistics for hospital birth and home birth were identical.

Aside from similar mortality rates between hospital and home births, this study also dramatically revealed that complications and interventions during birth were far greater in births that took place in the hospital than in births that took place at home. Five percent of home-birth mothers received some form of medication, whereas 75 percent of hospitalized mothers received medication. There were three times as many cesarean sections in hospital births as there were in the planned home births with subsequent transfer to hospital. Hospital-born babies suffered more fetal distress, newborn infections, and birth injuries than home-birth babies. The episiotomy rate was ten times higher for mothers in the hospital, and they suffered twice as many severe perineal lacerations. The increased episiotomy rate and severity of perineal lacerations for hospital births was most likely the result of the use of forceps and the lithotomy position for birth. Another interesting aspect of the study was that physicians attended 66 percent of the home births, implying that when childbirth can be removed from a hospital setting where a birthing woman is considered a "patient" and placed in an environment where birth is treated as a natural event, there is less likelihood of intervention. Mehl updated this study in 1997 by comparing births attended by direct-entry midwives (non-nurse midwives with formal training) and family physicians with outcomes for matched control groups of similar women who had either home or hospital births attended by physicians, with similar results.[12]

A more recent 1992 review of the outcomes of the midwife-attended planned home births from The Farm, an intentional community in rural Tennessee, revealed extremely good midwifery statistics including a cesarean birth rate of less than 2 percent. Dr. Mark Durand, the author of the study, admitted after comparing 1,707 home births from The Farm with over 14,000 physician-attended hospital births that there is "some evidence that elective interventions, which are used more frequently in hospitals, may increase the risk of various adverse outcomes in low risk women." In addition, the report concluded, "it is possible that the unfamiliar setting and the presence of unfamiliar personnel, the limited presence and role of family members, and the restricted freedom of movement of the laboring woman may all create an atmosphere at a hospital birth that undermines self confidence and encourages passivity on the part of the laboring woman, diminishing her ability to deliver spontaneously."[13]

One of the safest alternatives to hospital birth is to give birth in a freestanding birth center. The National Birth Center Study (NBCS), conducted between 1985 and 1987, studied 11,814 women who gave birth in freestanding birth centers in the United States. The results demonstrated that for basically healthy women with no prenatal complications, birth centers are a safe and economical alternative for childbirth. Certified nurse-midwife (CNM) Kitty Ernst, founder of the National Association of Childbearing Centers, helped design and participated in the study with the Center for Population and Family Health and the School of Public Health at Columbia University. The study was undertaken in reaction to statements from the American College of Obstetrics and Gynecology (ACOG) that discouraged the use of birth centers because of the lack of data proving their safety. The overall infant mortality rate for the eighty-four birth centers in the study (which constituted 52 percent of all birth centers in the country) was 1.3 deaths per 1,000 live births. There were no maternal deaths. The rate of cesarean births that took place in the backup hospitals was 4.4 percent, compared to a 1999 national average of 22.8 percent.

The birth centers studied in the National Birth Center Study used few invasive, uncomfortable, or restrictive procedures. Many offered measures to provide comfort and support for the women during labor. The midwives who attended the women during labor and birth had also provided prenatal care to the women throughout their pregnancies. The women who used birth centers expressed great satisfaction, and the general consensus was that they would use a birth center again.[14]

A few doctors objected to the validity of the National Birth Center Study because the general population giving birth in birth centers is low risk and cannot be compared to the overall hospital population. Women who use a birth center are low risk at the time of birth because they had consistent prenatal care; women who needed the attention of specialists were screened for hospital births. Ernst suggests that this study demonstrates the effectiveness of birth centers in their continuity of care rather than their questionable safety.

Birth centers are now an integral, yet still small, part of the medical care system. Each center in the United States has a relationship to an acute care hospital, which ensures that if the mother or the baby develops a problem they can receive the level of care that they need. Home-birth midwives also must, in most states, provide a backup doctor and have a plan for transport to a medical center in case of complications.

A 1996 Netherlands study concluded that childbirth can be safe outside a hospital environment, provided a woman has consistent prenatal care and is supported by a midwife or a physician during labor and birth.[15] In order to prepare for a gentle birth environment outside a hospital, it is important to first reexamine the generally held belief that hospitals are the safest place to birth. In a lengthy review of all the literature on out-of-hospital births I could not find one single study that proved that hospital birth was safer. On the contrary, the safety of home and birth center births is unquestionable for women who are low risk, prescreened, and give birth with trained professionals in attendance. More women would choose to birth out of the hospital if they understood that there is just as much harm from unnecessary medical interventions as the lack of them. In addition, the rate of home and birth center births would go up if insurance companies provided adequate coverage for births taking place out of hospitals.

## MYTH: MATERNITY CARE SHOULD BE MANAGED ONLY BY A PHYSICIAN

Because most births in the United States take place in a hospital, it is assumed that physicians provide the only competent maternity care available to women. However, studies have shown that Certified Nurse-Midwives (CNMs) offer equal if not better maternity care for pregnant women. As of 2005 there were fifty accredited freestanding birth centers in the United States, and another 170 known birth centers that were not accredited.[16] Almost all of them employed CNMs and nurses for maternity care. There are over 6,000 certified nurse-midwives employed in hospitals or birth centers as well as 850 certified professional midwives who offer home or birth center services in the United States.[17] Some nurse-midwives also offer home birth services. Statistical records show that nurse-midwives attended fewer than 20,000 births in 1975 and over 300,000 in 2002.[18]

Although midwifery is practiced throughout the world, in the United States only 10 to 12 percent of all births are attended by midwives.[19] Countries with the highest rate of midwife-attended births (the Netherlands, Scandinavian countries, and Japan) also have the best maternal and perinatal mortality statistics. For every 250 midwives in Japan there is just one obstetrician. Maternity care in these countries is based on a midwives model that emphasizes competent prenatal care and education and empowerment for the woman giving birth (see chapter 4). The midwives model of maternity care assesses all the circumstances—physical, emotional, and spiritual—that may influence the outcome of a pregnancy. Midwives refer clients to physicians only when there is a medical problem.

A common argument against the use of midwives is that they have less formal education than doctors. While it is true that doctors' formal medical education is more extensive in the area of obstetrics, they are not necessarily more experienced than midwives when dealing with normal labor and birth. Dr. Michael Rosenthal, a retired obstetrician in Upland, California, admits, "I didn't learn about women in childbirth by going to medical school but rather by watching women giving birth normally." He adds, "Doctors are trained to intervene. Midwives aren't trained to do cesareans—it's not in their realm. Subsequently they utilize other methods to guide a woman through a vaginal birth."

Nurse-midwives may spend up to seven years or more obtaining the education necessary to become licensed in some states. In most European countries where midwifery is the norm for pregnancy care, those wishing to become midwives enter directly into specialized midwife training programs. Here in the United States, nurse-midwives must first graduate from an accredited school of nursing before specializing in midwifery. There are currently forty-three accredited programs of nurse-midwifery in the United States, all of which provide excellent graduate education for midwives.

In addition to their medical competency, it's important to consider the psychological support that midwives provide. The majority of midwives are women, and many have given birth themselves. Their firsthand knowledge of giving birth and their sharing of that experience, woman to woman, is invaluable. Pregnant women are also less likely to be overly dependent on a midwife, who generally assists women in becoming educated about the birth process and encourages them to trust their instincts. In comparison, it is common for pregnant women to see their doctors as authority figures and for doctors to readily assume that role. Even the language that most midwives use differentiates their views of childbirth from those of physicians. Physicians have patients but midwives have clients. A physician "delivers the baby," which implies control, while a midwife helps the woman "birth her baby." A midwife is continually with a woman in labor, a doctor is not. When women are supported and comforted in labor, they request less pain medication or anesthesia and their rates of breast-feeding are higher.

A physician's experience of labor is typically very different from that of a midwife's. A physician in New York called my office toward the end of her own pregnancy wanting to know some of the things that she herself should do to cope with labor. She admitted that in her years of attending births she was normally only there for the last thirty minutes to an hour, usually while the mother was pushing her baby out. She had no idea what to do in an unmedicated labor and she knew her personal physician would not be of any help either. Compassionate care and continuous labor support are not skills usually associated with doctors, but are often experienced by recipients of midwifery care.

The development and implementation of midwifery training programs in Canada only began in the 1990s. In Ontario, an original group of sixty-five midwives registered in 1994 has grown to 220 in the year 2000, and is increasing at approximately 30 per year. The demand for midwifery services continues in most settings to be greater than the supply.[20] The midwifery movement in Canada was born out of consumer frustration with lack of choices in maternity care. Grassroots consumer groups petitioned and put pressure on the government to provide midwifery services.

The statistical data in Ontario comparing midwifery practice to that of obstetricians tell a very important story. Midwives spend an average of forty-five minutes with clients for each prenatal appointment compared to five minutes that doctors typically spend for prenatal visits. Midwives visit women postpartum, whether they have had a home or hospital birth, three times the first week, and three or more times in the first month, while physicians only see a woman at two weeks and six weeks postpartum. Ninety percent of midwife clients were breast-feeding at six months compared to 50 percent of physician clients. The lower breast-feeding rates can be directly linked to interventions during birth, which interfere with attachment and bonding and successful breast-feeding. During labor, midwife clients use epidurals about 25 percent of the time; physician clients use them 80 percent of the time.[21] This one comparison alone speaks volumes. Even though the profession of midwifery is in the very beginning stages in Canada, we can learn a great deal from their successes and the challenges that have ensued from implementing such widespread public health care policy change.

The World Health Organization (WHO) and the International Confederation of Midwives (ICM) support the use of midwives for pregnancy, birth, newborn care, and the development of the infant, as well as for offering counseling and education to the community. In 1990 ICM, which represents midwives in eighty-two countries, joined WHO to create a position statement on midwifery. This statement declared that when midwifery was utilized for pregnancy and childbirth, outcomes for mothers and babies were more favorable. These two organizations urged all countries to offer midwifery education, insisting that the increased availability of midwives would improve birth outcomes throughout the world by the year 2010. WHO and ICM believe that when midwives practice, birth is safer for mothers and babies.[22]

The midwives model of maternity care, as opposed to the medical model, offers considerable advantages, particularly for parents considering a gentle birth. Midwives have lower rates of interventions and higher rates of satisfaction. Midwives offer personalized prenatal care, respect for birth as a normal process, and encouragement for making informed choices. Qualified midwives offer competent maternity care for women seeking normal, natural, gentle births.

## MYTH: THE ELECTRONIC FETAL MONITOR WILL SAVE BABIES

The electronic fetal monitor (EFM) is one of the most widely used technological interventions in modern obstetrics. Fetal monitoring allows practitioners to listen to and evaluate the baby's heart rate throughout labor and birth. The idea is that if you could listen to every heartbeat and interpret early signs of fetal distress, you could save more babies from mental retardation, cerebral palsy, and even death. This initial premise has not been proved to be valid after systematic review of randomized controlled trials and almost forty years of clinical observation.

There are two types of EFMs. The external fetal monitor consists of two straps that are placed around the abdomen of the laboring woman. They are equipped with an ultrasound device that records the baby's heart rate and a sensor that detects the strength, duration, and frequency of the uterine contractions. The information is displayed on an oscilloscope and is captured on graph paper, which then becomes a permanent part of the mother's chart. Medical personnel are trained to interpret the graph or strip by comparing how the baby's heart rate responds to the contractions and how it varies during certain periods. The contractions are measured in length and strength and the intervals are timed. The internal fetal monitor gives the same information, but involves inserting an electrode into the skin layer of the baby's scalp while it is still in the womb in order to transmit the baby's heart rate.

In the past few years new attachments have been added to the external monitor that also record the mother's temperature, blood pressure, blood oxygen, heart rate, and sometimes even cervical dilation. The result: an all-in-one miracle machine that can, theoretically, take the place of a nurse at the bedside. Recent studies on the effectiveness of the EFM to diminish the risk of injury or death for the baby during childbirth show that the EFM is no more effective than a trained nurse who listens to and evaluates the baby's heartbeat intermittently.[23]

The first breakthrough in monitoring a baby's heart rate came in 1917 when a headband was added to the stethoscope. The headband allowed the doctor to listen to the baby's heartbeat while leaving his or her hands free to palpate the uterus and determine the intensity of uterine contractions. Many midwives still use this kind of stethoscope while monitoring women during labor. The ultrasound stethoscope, or doppler, developed in the 1960s, refined the art of what is termed "auscultation," or listening to the sound of the baby's heartbeat. The accepted way of evaluating the infant during labor was to auscultate the baby's heart rate periodically. How often and for how long depended entirely on the practitioner and his or her level of experience.

Fetal monitoring to determine the well-being of the baby during labor has always been a concern for midwives and physicians. The first EFM was available in

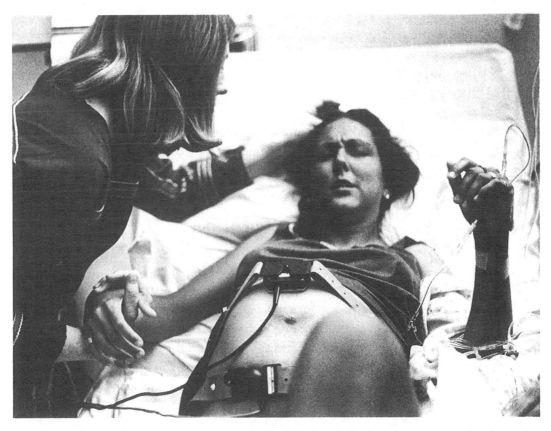

*Electronic fetal monitoring keeps a woman tied to the bed and usually on her back, the worst possible position for labor.*

1968 and was heralded as the greatest obstetrical advance since forceps. Doctors believed the EFM would eliminate the guesswork in labor. They could constantly observe the fetus with the EFM and more accurately monitor an infant whose mother had been given drugs. Physicians also believed that the EFM would reduce cesarean and infant mortality rates.

The large, cumbersome machine that housed the fetal monitor began showing up at the bedsides of laboring women in hospitals across the United States. As early as 1973, initial studies were released that supported the existence of a correlation between patterns of fetal heart rate and signs of fetal hypoxia, or oxygen deprivation. In the 1970s it was still believed that lack of oxygen during labor could cause epilepsy and cerebral palsy, as well as myriad problems ranging from mild learning disorders to criminal behavior.[24] Physicians believed that the EFM could detect early fetal distress caused by a lack of oxygen. Early detection would give them sufficient time to intervene, usually with an emergency cesarean, in order to prevent injury or death.

By 1978 nearly two-thirds of all births were electronically monitored. Nurses were trained to read the tracings of the EFM strip as a guide for intervention. The EFM strips were (and still are) used as legal protection against potential lawsuits. Medical literature was flooded with research on fetal heart-rate patterns, variations, and decelerations that gave credit to the fetal monitor in the detection of potential problems. The physicians' common response to questionable data from a fetal monitor was to perform a cesarean section. With the use of the EFM, cesarean rates throughout the United States gradually climbed. Interestingly enough, there has been no change in the number of cases of cerebral palsy, birth-related injuries, or neonatal mortality since use of the EFM was implemented.[25]

Could there have been something wrong with the initial reasoning? Did the EFM actually eliminate the guesswork in monitoring the fetus during labor and birth? By the 1980s some obstetricians were questioning the accuracy of the EFM readings. Physicians would perform an emergency cesarean based on an EFM reading that indicated probable fetal distress. When the surgery was completed, they would be surprised to find a perfectly normal, healthy infant. Many doctors have noted that they would do a cesarean for what appeared reasonable cause and out would come a baby with a high Apgar score (a visual rating system for determining a baby's health immediately after birth) and no distress. They looked for whatever could be causing the variation on the fetal monitor tracing strip. What many doctors and midwives have discovered is that often all that was needed to improve the apparent status of the baby was to change the mother's position in labor. Many other practitioners and childbirth reformers experienced the same unmistakable correlation between the rising cesarean rate and the widespread use of the EFM. As early as 1980 the National Institutes of Health cautioned against the use of the monitor for low-risk pregnancies, predicting that it would only contribute to more cesareans.[26]

In March 1987 Columbia University hosted a medical conference on controversies in the use of obstetrical technology entitled "Crisis in Obstetrics: The Management of Labor." Dr. Edward H. Hon, inventor of the EFM, asked his colleagues to consider the causes of the rising cesarean rate in the United States. He stated that he never intended the EFM to be used in routine obstetric management. "If you mess around with a process [birth] that works well 98 percent of the time, there is a potential for much harm."[27] Hon stressed that physicians lack patience with the childbirth process and subsequently use the monitor, which can wrongly determine fetal distress. He concluded, "The cesarean section is considered as a rescue mission of the baby by the white knight, but actually you've assaulted the mother."

Dr. Mortimer Rosen, who convened the conference, stated that the recent dramatic progress of technology has been accompanied by a change in patient expectations. Patients today expect a perfect outcome. This shift has caused physicians to be more cautious and to perform cesareans sooner rather than later. Unfortunately, the fear of litigation now plays a central role in physicians' decisions to intervene. Risk management has become a highly specialized medical specialty field in the past decade.

Even doctors with experience reading EFM tracings can be misled. In one study, reviewers were given two identical tracings along with the prenatal histories but were told that the outcome was good in one case and poor in the other. When the outcome was poor, the reviewers were more likely to disagree with the obstetrician's interpretation of the tracings and management of the labor.[28]

The EFM was thought to be a miracle technology that would wipe out cerebral palsy because it could alert doctors to early fetal distress. In actuality it is known to wrongly identify fetal distress 15 to 80 percent of the time. One 1982 study reported that EFMs had a 74 percent false-positive rate.[29] This means that 74 out of 100 times the monitor tracings indicated distress when there was none. Doctors have also found that sometimes the monitor indicates that there is no distress when in fact there has been severe oxygen deprivation or even infant death. In addition to the inconsistency of the EFM to accurately monitor fetal distress, researchers find that there is no relationship between fetal distress and certain disorders that have been associated with it. Dr. Karin Nelson and Dr. Jonas Ellenberg have written several books on cerebral palsy, in particular about its relationship to the events of labor and delivery and the origin of chronic neurologic disorders. They essentially ruled out fetal oxygen deprivation during labor and delivery as a cause of neurologic disorders. Their research also revealed a consistent cerebral palsy rate within the population since 1940. There has been no decrease in the number of children born with cerebral palsy since the introduction and widespread use of electronic fetal monitoring.

Mothers are also concerned about the use of the EFM, especially those who have experienced emergency cesareans because of apparent fetal distress. One mother related her experience:

I thought that everything was fine. I had just started pushing, the doctor had only been in to check me once in over six hours. He came in, looked at the monitor strip, and ordered the nurse to move me to the operating room for an immediate C-section. He didn't even tell us what was wrong. No one did. I'm happy about my baby, but it took me over a year to get past my anger and disappointment about my birth.

Of even greater concern than emergency cesareans caused by the false positives on the monitor is the fact that the monitor itself keeps a woman inactive and attached to the bed in the labor room. This can lead to the very fetal distress that the monitor so righteously interprets.

During the 1980s women organized groups such as the Cesarean Prevention Movement, now known as the International Cesarean Awareness Network (ICAN) and Cesareans/Support, Education and Concern (C/SEC) to offer education and support to other women who had had cesareans. These consumer groups sponsored educational conferences, gathered statistics, and networked with mothers throughout the United States. Both organizations support couples in finding information to make informed birth choices. They also encourage pregnant women to give birth vaginally after a cesarean.

Dr. Kenneth Leveno stated in 1986 in the *New England Journal of Medicine,* "Not all pregnancies, and particularly not those considered at low risk of perinatal complication, need continuous electronic fetal monitoring during labor."[30] In 1990 an even stronger statement came from Dr. Roger Freeman, who has written textbooks on the interpretation of the fetal monitor. Freeman published an editorial in the *New England Journal of Medicine* entitled "Intrapartum Fetal Monitoring: A Disappointing Story." He thoroughly reviewed previously published studies comparing the outcomes of labors that were continuously monitored and those that were monitored by nurses listening at regular intervals with fetoscopes. In all cases the outcomes were the same! Freeman's conclusion is that fetal monitors were adopted for surveillance before any conclusive studies indicated that they produced the results they were designed to achieve. Freeman suggests that before the fetal monitor is discarded a study should be undertaken comparing no monitoring at all during labor with either auscultation or EFMs. Freeman asserts that only then can we determine if monitoring makes a difference.[31]

Recent studies indicate that, at best, an EFM can only detect whether an infant is doing fine or whether it is in a "possible" state of distress. A low heart rate may indicate a sleeping baby, while a rapid heart rate may be a response to a stimulus or drug or may just indicate an active baby. If all the studies indicate that monitoring can be harmful, then why do we keep using it? One reason is that it is simply too easy to rely on the monitor to indicate how the labor is going. Too often the nurse will walk into a labor room and look at the monitor before turning her attention to the laboring woman. Everyone in the room tends to watch the monitor, including the mother.

Nurses have not been trained to listen to the baby's heartbeat with a Doppler or fetoscope. A technical bulletin from the American College of Obstetricians and Gynecologists states that either EFM or intermittent auscultation is acceptable for monitoring the condition of the baby and acknowledges the risk of increased intervention with continuous monitoring.[32]

Accurate monitoring of the baby with hand-held devices takes time and requires one-to-one nursing care. A university hospital attempted to use intermittent auscultation as the primary method of monitoring without increasing the number of staff. Auscultation was only successfully completed in thirty-one of 862 patients in labor.[33] If hospitals don't have enough staff to carry out safe auscultation of the baby's heartbeat, then we should inform women of the possibility that there are not enough nurses to watch over their labors. Intermittent monitoring is a "high-touch, low-tech" solution, which helps to reduce cesarean rates performed for fetal distress. The lack of nurses contributes to the continued use of a medical intervention that the literature deems totally unnecessary and dangerous. One can justifiably conclude that the hundreds of millions of health care dollars spent annually just on the use of Electronic Fetal Monitoring is a huge waste of money.[34]

## MYTH: ALL BABIES SHOULD BE BORN ON OR BEFORE THEIR DUE DATE

Every first-time mother I meet or speak with thinks that God should have designed pregnancy to last only thirty-eight weeks instead of a possible forty-two or more. Doctors would have you think the same thing by the numbers of healthy women entering hospitals for elective induction of labor. I reassure women every day that babies are born on their birthdays, not their due dates, and that the average first pregnancy lasts forty-one weeks and three days.[35] The "due date" is an arbitrary date, created by a German obstetrician in the 1800s.[36] It was based on taking the first day of the last menstrual period and then counting ahead by forty weeks. A great idea to "predict" when to start thinking about getting everything in order for baby, but never an accurate or dependable way of calculating when a baby will be born. Using ultrasound examination of the baby is not a completely accurate way of predicting due dates either, with reliability off by plus or minus two weeks.

In medical terms, a pregnancy is considered to be "full term" at thirty-seven weeks. Prior to thirty-seven weeks the pregnancy is labeled "pre-term." A pregnancy that goes past forty-two weeks is considered "post-term" or "post dates." Many women are not sure when they conceived or may not know the exact date of their menstrual period. Menstrual cycles also vary in length and this can be a determining factor in the length of the pregnancy.[37] There is nothing more frustrating for pregnant mothers than to go past their "due date" and then be labeled as overdue—as if their baby were a delayed package from FedEx!

Until recently, very little was known about how natural labors actually begin. Scientists knew that the release of oxytocin resulted in both uterine contractions and milk production. Pioneering research by scientists at Cornell University, Oxford in the United Kingdom, and the University of Auckland, New Zealand, confirms that a hormone is released from the baby's brain to initiate labor.[38] Two hormones, corticol and adrenocorticotropic hormone (ACTH), reach peak levels in the fetal bloodstream just before birth. Peter Nathanielsz, a medical doctor and researcher at Cornell University, suggests that the fetal brain may act as a tiny monitor, tracking its own development.[39] When the baby is ready for birth, a special part of the brain signals the fetal pituitary gland to increase ACTH secretion. The pituitary, in turn, tells the fetal adrenal gland to secrete more cortisol. These hormonal increases cause changes in the mother's hormones, including the release of oxytocin, which lead to uterine contractions. The common drugs used to induce labor interfere with the functioning of the fetal brain, causing this sequence to be short-circuited.

In the 1970s and 1980s it was rare to see an induction just for a pregnancy that was past forty-two weeks. In most cases a variety of non-invasive and unrestrictive methods were used to assess that the baby was doing well, and the mother was advised to take long walks and wait for the baby. Induction started to come into fashion in the late 1980s and is now the norm. Besides the mother being tired at the end of her pregnancy and ready for the baby to be born, are there valid medical reasons for induction of labor? The American College of Obstetricians and Gynecologists states that induction is "indicated when the benefits to either the mother or fetus outweigh those of continuing the pregnancy."[40] As with many of the areas of medicalized birth, the decision of whether continuing a pregnancy is dangerous or carries more risk than immediate birth is most often a completely subjective call. It is safe to presume that the interpretation of necessity is only accurate in 3 percent of cases.[41]

The majority of inductions are done to accommodate the mother's or the doctor's schedule, or what some would call "the seduction of induction." My mother fell prey to this tactic more than fifty years ago when her doctor announced that he was going out of town and if she wanted him to deliver her baby, she should just go and check into the hospital. It was two weeks prior to my "due date." My mother had a terrible reaction to the drug combination that they used and suffered for years with neurological problems, including episodes of blindness.

Another reason that doctors will induce labor is that they suspect the baby will be too large. The fear is that the baby will grow more in the next two or three weeks, so to avoid a possible cesarean or a shoulder dystocia (when the baby's shoulders get stuck) an elective induction is advised. We now have proof that elective inductions lead to twice as many cesareans as do labors that start on their own (including those with large babies).[42] A study at Swedish Medical Center in Seattle, Washington, reached the interesting conclusion that the individual physician influences the already elevated risk of cesarean delivery by his or her management of the labor. The more interventions, the higher the risk of cesarean.

Pitocin has been the drug of choice to induce labor, until very recently. Pitocin is a vile drug. The FDA removed its approval of Pitocin for the elective induction of labor in 1978. Common risks associated with the use of Pitocin for both induction and augmentation (speeding up the labor) include the following:

*For the mother:*
- higher rate of complicated labors and deliveries
- more use of analgesia or anesthesia because of the intensity of the contractions
- postpartum hemorrhage (only when used for induction; there has been no research to determine if hemorrhage is associated with augmentation of labor)
- higher rate of ruptured uterus and placental separation, which may lead to the death of the mother or baby

*For the baby:*
- fetal distress
- higher rate of jaundice in the newborn
- greater chance of a premature baby
- low Apgar scores at five minutes
- permanent central nervous system or brain damage
- fetal death

Now research is showing a possible link between the use of Pitocin and a higher incidence of autism. In a study at New York's Mount Sinai School of Medicine focusing on autistic patients, it was noted that 60 percent of them had been induced or their mothers had received pitocin in labor. National studies show that almost 50 percent of mothers are now induced, usually for non-medical reasons.[43] It is even common today for nurse-midwives in hospitals to use induction for all the same reasons that doctors give.[44]

Nurse-midwives tend to use what are commonly termed "ripening agents," referring to drugs that cause the cervix to soften and begin dilating. These include prostaglandin E2 (Cervidil or Prepidil), and misoprostol (Cytotec). There exists a huge controversy over the use of Cytotec, a drug developed to treat ulcers. The drug manufacturer even stated in a recent bulletin that use of this drug for labor has never been tested, approved, or recommended and they suggest complete discontinuance of its use.[45] They go on to explain that there has never been any testing on children whose mothers have received Cytotec to see if there are any long-term effects. Cytotec use for labor induction has been directly shown to increase the chances of uterine rupture. Women who were attempting a vaginal birth after a previous cesarean and were given Cytotec had an even greater risk of uterine rupture. Dr. Marsden Wagner, after a thorough review of available literature on induction and the use of Cytotec, concluded that "it is difficult for doctors to admit that they make mistakes. This [use of Cytotec] was a big mistake."[46] The American College of Obstetricians and Gynecologists is the only organization in the world that still justifies its use for induction of labor. All international maternal/child health organizations, as well as the manufacturer, endorse its withdrawal from use.

Are there any valid indications for using induction to begin labor? As I have previously stated, only if a medical condition in the mother or baby makes it riskier to stay pregnant. When Marianne was pregnant with her third baby, she called our office seeking a referral to a good home birth midwife. In the course of conversation she related her birth stories, as most women do.

> I'll never repeat the nightmare of my second birth. My doctor had suggested an ultrasound late in my pregnancy to determine the size of the baby. He told me he was concerned that the baby was getting too big and wanted to verify that with an ultrasound. I was 36 weeks at the time. Everything looked normal, or so I thought. He said that it was hard to tell and suggested another ultrasound in two weeks, if I had not gone into labor. Obedient, my husband and I went in at 38 weeks and this time he was very concerned. He stated that the baby was at least nine pounds and that if I didn't deliver right away I was risking complications, including birth injuries to the baby. He really made it sound dire.

Marianne recounted how she talked things over with her husband and then agreed to go to the hospital the following morning for an elective induction. Here is her description of what followed:

> That's when the nightmare really got started. My labor never really did, but boy they tried everything. First, the IV with Pitocin, then breaking my water, then upping the Pitocin until I was a mess. I had to have an epidural because the pain was so incredibly intense. My first birth had been long, but I hadn't taken any drugs. This time the contractions were right on top of each other. I couldn't even catch my breath. After about twelve hours of that I was only two centimeters dilated and then my doctor announced that the baby was showing signs of stress and he recommended a cesarean. This massively huge baby weighed seven pounds, nine ounces and I didn't even get to hold him for four hours.

I never recommend using an ultrasound to determine the size of the baby, as they are predominantly wrong. We found a home-birth midwife for Marianne who would help her have a vaginal birth, even after a cesarean.

With more women waiting longer to have their first babies, often negotiating complex work and childcare arrangements and brief maternity leaves, the temptation to induce may be very great. Women in high stress professions, accustomed to having a great deal of control over their lives and schedules, may be particularly susceptible to the seduction of induction. These conditions should not be exploited by birth practitioners who may, at times, have their own personal motives for encouraging induction. Patience is a virtue, especially when waiting for a baby.

## MYTH: DRUGS FOR PAIN RELIEF WON'T HURT THE BABY

Medical science originally believed that the placenta was a protective barrier between the mother and the baby, a filter that blocked the fetus from harmful substances ingested by the mother. However, in 1961 the shocking effects of thalidomide, a tranquilizer taken by pregnant women in Europe and Australia to relieve nausea, proved that the placental barrier theory was completely false. Babies were born without limbs, particularly arms, a condition produced by thalidomide's effect on the developing fetus.[47] Public outcry subsequently demanded more accurate testing of drugs prescribed by doctors for pregnancy and birth. Consumers pushed for truth in advertising, and for the first time pregnant women were routinely warned of potential hazards of over-the-counter and recreational drugs. These warnings now encompass the use of cigarettes and alcohol, as well as many environmental elements such as microwaves.

Childbirth advocates are now questioning the safety of drugs commonly given to women for pain relief, as well as the anesthetic agents administered during childbirth. Women need to be routinely and thoroughly warned by their health care providers about the possible effects of drugs on their babies and on themselves. Studies need to be done to chart the long-term effects on children whose mothers received drugs during childbirth.

The *Physicians' Desk Reference* lists all drugs manufactured in the United States and describes the possible side effects. Under each of the anesthetic agents commonly used for epidurals for women in labor, the *Physicians' Desk Reference* plainly states that there are no long-term studies on the effects of these drugs on the fetus. Nor have there been any long-term studies on the impact of these drugs on the child's life.

The epidural consists of an injection of an anesthetic agent (bupivacaine), sometimes coupled with a narcotic, into the epidural space near the spinal cord to numb the lower half of the body. When it works well women report that they still have some tingling sensation in their legs and they feel the "pressure" of the contractions, but not the pain. One of the rationales used by physicians to justify using an epidural is that it will protect the baby from the stress of labor. Good rationale, but not in the least backed up by scientific or empirical evidence.

A review of the medical literature will give you chills up and down your spine as you read about all the deleterious effects of epidural anesthesia. Epidurals can cause profound disturbances in the fetal heart rate.[48] It is often observed that a baby's heart rate will drop drastically within the first half-hour of administration of the epidural. Some babies will recover from the drugs, others remain susceptible, thus leading to emergency cesareans.[49] One of the effects that taking the epidural early in the labor has on the baby is "freezing" it into a position that leads to a dystocia or hold-up of the progress of descent. Generally, the baby's head gets stuck into an extended position and never becomes flexed allowing it to descend into the birth canal.[50] This can lead to an increase in the numbers of cesareans. There are several studies that indicate that when epidurals are given too early in labor, the chances of a cesarean are increased in some cases up to 50 percent.

Early administration of the epidural should be avoided. Some studies suggest that the side effects of an epidural cause the baby to become nervous and jittery, while other studies show that the baby is drowsy after birth. The varied results depend on which drug and how much was used. Babies whose mothers received epidurals are often observed as less alert after birth, crying more and having poorer visual skills.[51] These impairments often last for up to six weeks, making the early postpartum period more difficult for both mothers and babies.

Epidurals have been shown to:

- slow labor.
- lead to increased use of oxytocin (Pitocin).
- lead to increased use of forceps or vacuum.
- increase the likelihood of cesareans, especially in first-time mothers.
- increase the mother's temperature, resulting in her and the baby receiving antibiotics and invasive tests.
- cause a host of complications including long-term chronic problems and even maternal death.

Epidurals do cross through the placenta and cause these effects in the newborn:

- reduced muscle tone
- decreased sucking
- lowered neurobehavioral scores
- increased incidence of jaundice

Some women love the epidural choice but in most cases those women more than likely had uncomplicated vaginal births. The ones that contact my office with story after story of disappointment and frustration are the ones who felt that the epidural was the only thing offered for pain management and that they felt pressured both by medical staff and partners to have one. Most of their births became complicated, possibly a domino effect of the epidural, resulting in more forceps and vacuum extractions as well as lingering effects of the injection. "The epidural analgesia is associated with prolonged labor, an increase in uterine infection and more operative procedures such as cesarean sections or low-forceps deliveries," states Dr. Susan M. Ramin, assistant professor of obstetrics and gynecology at University of Texas Southwestern Medical Center in Dallas, which took on the largest study of epidural anesthesia to date.[52]

I have met women who have suffered for years after their birth experience with headaches and numbness from the epidural. There is really no way to know its effects on child development, and as one anesthesiologist put it, "An epidural is a very short-term solution, which may be creating long-term problems for our entire society." Much more research needs to be done before we can feel safe about the epidural for our children.

There are only a handful of researchers who are even looking into the correlation of drug use in childbirth and long-term effects on child development. Dr. Bertil Jacobson of Sweden's Karolinska Institute conducted a study on the long-term effects on children of morphine, Demerol, and phenobarbital taken by the mothers during labor. He examined whether babies whose mothers received barbiturates were born in a mood-altered state. Jacobson believes that as these children grow and reach puberty and their hormones shift, the imprinting that took place at the time of birth is restimulated. The subjects of the study, teenage drug users, have shown a high correlation between their drug abuse and the amount and timing of the drugs given to their mothers during labor.[53]

The developing brain of the baby is susceptible to insult from drugs because it continues to develop for up to two years after birth. In addition, drugs have a far greater impact on the baby than on the mother because of the baby's body size and the limited ability of a newborn's liver to excrete drugs. All drugs used in obstetrics are toxic for babies. Recent studies on babies whose mothers received obstetrical drugs for pain relief demonstrated a variety of adverse effects, including damage to the central nervous system; impaired sensory and motor responses; reduced ability to process and respond to incoming stimuli; interference with feeding, sucking, and rooting responses; lower scores on tests of infant development; and increased irritability. Narcotic withdrawal symptoms for a newborn can last up to two weeks and may include irritable crying and body tremors as the baby's body attempts to metabolize and excrete the drugs.[54] It is important to note that bonding with an infant who is motor or sensory impaired or suffering from drug withdrawal will be affected as well.

There is considerable evidence, both scientific and empirical, that narcotics cross the placenta in sufficient amounts to cause neonatal depression. For instance, studies have revealed that large amounts of Demerol can be found in a newborn if the mother received the drug within five hours of giving birth. Demerol can also contribute to a mother's feelings of depression after birth, since narcotics generally cause depression.

The narcotics that are offered today to women in labor are active for a shorter period of time, yet still affect the baby. Stadol and fentanyl, currently the two most commonly used narcotics, only last about an hour, thus not allowing them to be metabolized as much by the mother. A dose of Stadol given early in labor may still affect the baby right after birth, decreasing the baby's ability to nurse properly, but not as much as Demerol.

It is a woman's right to choose whether or not she wants drugs for pain relief; however, the general consensus in the United States is that most women need drugs to withstand the pain of childbirth. Unfortunately, many women have not been encouraged to experience their labor and birth without drugs but instead have been told that pain medication will make it bearable. It is not uncommon to hear women who may only be a few months pregnant already declaring that they will get an epidural as soon as they arrive at the hospital because they fear the pain of labor will be too great. In turn, out of a misguided sense of kindness, doctors and nurses who genuinely believe that drugs comfort a woman in labor and ease her pain are likely to encourage that woman to make use of the availability of drugs.

I have heard from childbirth educators in hospitals that they are often told not to dwell on or even discuss the harmful effects of the epidural, simply because too many women may begin questioning its benefits when they understand the incredible risks that are associated with it. In 2001, 54 percent of birthing women in America had an epidural.[55] While news reports focused on its benefits, not all women were happy with their epidural experiences. Women often don't realize the trade-offs that they will need to make when they get an epidural. The required intravenous line and the electronic monitor tie a woman to the bed. The inability to move or feel the lower half of the body frequently results in the insertion of a catheter to drain the urine from the bladder. Frequently the epidural is so effective that it eliminates uterine contractions. The nerves that tell the uterus to contract are all anesthetized and the uterus becomes quiet and must be stimulated artificially with Pitocin.

The drugs also take away a vital communication link with the baby. In a gentle birth mothers respond to position changes in the baby by moving and reacting with their bodies. With an epidural, the mother, not being able to feel where the baby is in relation to her own pelvis, is forced into positions and told when and how to push. I have even seen nurses lay across women's bellies in an effort to assist in pushing. Mechanical means of getting the baby out are often applied when women have epidurals. Forceps and vacuum extractors can be extremely harmful to the baby.

There are times when it is appropriate to use epidurals. I have witnessed an epidural work effectively for women who have been laboring for a very long time and were exhausted, and whose attendants placed the epidural perfectly. The instantaneous pain relief allowed them to rest and get a second wind in order to birth their babies.

A few simple measures applied during labor—such as moving about freely, changing positions, staying off her back, taking a shower or bath, and using non-pharmacological pain relief—can greatly reduce a woman's need for medication. Emotional support and encouragement from loved ones and childbirth attendants can also make a tremendous difference. When a laboring woman has a loving hand to hold, someone to rub her back, or the option of a warm tub of water to labor in, she may never need to consider drugs for pain relief. When a woman feels in charge of her labor and birth, is knowledgeable about the process and is confident of her ability to birth her baby, drugs and epidurals will become a little-used option.

## MYTH: ONCE A CESAREAN, ALWAYS A CESAREAN

The cesarean section has been the most commonly performed surgery in the United States since 1983, surpassing both the tonsillectomy and appendectomy. In 1970 only 5 percent of all births in the United States were by cesarean. By 1978 this figure had increased to 15 percent; by 1986, 25 percent of all women gave birth by major abdominal surgery. There was a slight decline in the numbers of cesarean births since 1990, with the lowest level of 20.8 percent occurring in 1997, due to the numbers of women successfully birthing vaginally after a previous cesarean.

But the rates are now at an all-time high. The cesarean birth rate rose to 27.6 percent of all births in 2003 (29.3 percent for non-Hispanic blacks). This is a 6 percent increase from the Centers for Disease Control's (CDC) 2002 data. In New York State, the CDC reports the 2003 cesarean section rate at 28.4 percent overall (29.1 percent for non-Hispanic blacks).[56] A state-by-state breakdown reveals cesarean birth rates in seven states at over 30 percent and for African-American women the number rose to sixteen states. Surveys of individual hospitals revealed cesarean rates at some hospitals were as high as 53 percent. There is a growing concern that women are starting to demand the right to a cesarean section for their birth and doctors are readily complying. An elective surgery for birth is seen by some as a reproductive right.

In April of 2000, a group of doctors met in Kansas City to discuss the viability and the ethics of recommending elective cesareans for all women.[57] In 2002, the question was posed again at a professional meeting of obstetricians, even citing the choice of elective plastic surgery as comparable to an elective cesarean.[58] Some of these preposterous ideas have actually been adopted in many large cities in Mexico, Argentina, and Brazil, where cesarean rates are extremely high, sometimes up to 90 percent in private hospitals.[59] The arguments in favor of elective birth surgery are thinly veiled as concern for women and the effects of childbearing.

There is little doubt that a scheduled cesarean is convenient, mostly for the doctor, who can plan his schedule accordingly. Mothers like the predictability of planning time off from work or school. They also like the idea of only a twenty-minute surgical procedure as opposed to hours and hours of labor. They appreciate the guarantee of not feeling anything at all during the surgery. But are these conveniences reason enough to risk the life of mother and baby? There is great hazard in assuming that there are fewer risks involved in a scheduled repeat or primary elective cesarean surgery than a vaginal birth. No evidence supports the idea that cesareans are as safe as vaginal birth for mother or baby. In fact, the increase in cesarean births risks the health and well-being of childbearing women and their babies.[60]

In 2003 close to one million women in the United States had cesareans for a variety of reasons.[61] Diony Young, editor of *Birth: Issues in Perinatal Care,* says that in the United States, a woman is likely to have a cesarean:

> [if] she's too big or too small; too early or too late; too old or too fearful; too tired of being pregnant or too tired of being in labor; if she's having twins, if she's breech, if she's previously had a cesarean; or if she's due and so is the weekend, Christmas, Thanksgiving, or New Year's Eve. Then again, she's also at risk if her doctor is in doubt, scared of a lawsuit, too busy, going out of town, or convinced that a cesarean is always safer . . . the reasons go on.[62]

Some of the reasons indicated on medical charts included fetal distress as indicated by the EFM; breech presentation of the baby; genital herpes in the mother; cephalo-pelvic disproportion (CPD), a condition in which the mother's pelvis is deemed too small for the baby to pass through; and dystocia, a term used for a labor that has not progressed along "normal" patterns. Within each of these "reasons" for a cesarean is a gray area that is left to the discretion of the attending physician. While no one questions that some cesareans are absolutely necessary, one must ask what has happened between 1970 and 2003 to increase the average cesarean rate in the United States from 5 percent to almost 30 percent.

The reason given by doctors today for approximately 40 percent of all cesareans is dystocia. A woman whose labor is not progressing "normally" may be advised to undergo a cesarean, although an exact definition of what it means to progress normally varies tremendously with each doctor. When a laboring woman's cervix does not efface and dilate, or when the baby does not descend during a prescribed number of hours, many physicians will diagnose dystocia and consider the diagnosis reasonable grounds for performing a cesarean.[63]

A typical hospital scenario during a slow labor is to administer Pitocin, a synthetic version of oxytocin, which a laboring woman's body produces naturally. Pitocin is given in order to speed up and intensify contractions. Natural oxytocin is accompanied by a panoply of pain-neutralizing endorphins, absent in the synthetic version. So Pitocin interferes with the body's ability to cope with pain. Thus, when women are given Pitocin, they are often offered a painkiller or an epidural as well.

While the Pitocin works to quicken the labor, the epidural or drugs for pain relief have the opposite effect. The epidural often "arrests" the downward progress of the baby. In addition, the administration of Pitocin effectively restricts the movements of the laboring woman because she is required to have an intravenous (IV) line and an internal fetal monitor. These restrictions can slow labor even further. In addition, the woman's bladder is no longer functioning, so she needs a catheter to take the urine away.

If the Pitocin does not work within a certain time limit, a laboring woman will often hear statements like, "We've tried everything; do you want to do this for another twelve hours?" or "You just weren't meant to have this baby vaginally." In this situation, a physician views a cesarean as an opportunity to save the mother from a "long and difficult" labor. Unfortunately, the mother will never know what the outcome might have been had there never been any interventions in the first place or if the clock had not run out.

The myth of always having to birth by cesarean after the first cesarean became a rule of thumb for physicians in the early part of the twentieth century. At that time, a diagnosis of CPD, or true dystocia, usually applied to women who had polio, rickets, or a small or deformed pelvis, conditions that prevented them from ever having a safe vaginal delivery. The reason given by physicians for about 300,000 of the 900,000 cesareans performed in the United States today is still dystocia.[64] Dystocia has become a diagnostic catch-all that gives doctors the latitude to translate "failure to wait" into a cesarean section.

From a childbirth reformer's perspective, a term such as "failure to progress" is really failure of the doctor to be patient. It is common knowledge that the longer a woman labors in the hospital, the greater the possibility for medical intervention. In addition, fear of a lawsuit will often motivate a physician to be excessively cautious and perform a cesarean rather than wait. As one doctor so aptly stated, "The only cesarean I have ever been sued for is the one I didn't do."

In the past, women were easily convinced by their physicians to schedule an elective cesarean for their next birth because the experience of a long labor ending in a cesarean the first time was so frustrating and painful. In the early 1980s cesarean consumer groups began to encourage women to attempt a vaginal birth after a cesarean (VBAC). Women organized cesarean support groups to work through their feelings about their previous cesarean births and to express their fear, anger, grief, or disappointment. After women "processed" their feelings, they were then supported in preparing for a vaginal birth and locating a physician who would assist them.

Deborah relates a typical VBAC success story:

I went through five doctors before I finally gave up my search to find a doctor who would let me give birth vaginally. For three months I didn't get any prenatal care. I didn't have any insurance anyway, so I called a lay midwife in the next town. She saw me reluctantly, but when I explained the circumstances of my first cesarean, she agreed to come to my home for the birth. You see, I had a cesarean for a foot-first breech baby, and this [second] baby seemed to be head down. The [vaginal] birth went just fine. My daughter watched the whole thing and held the baby with me just minutes after he was born. I'm so glad I stayed home.

In the early 1980s women who pursued a VBAC found the medical community resistant to their efforts. At that time, the American College of Obstetricians and Gynecologists (ACOG) had developed strict guidelines for VBACs. These guidelines allowed only for a short "trial labor" and ruled out any woman who had had a previous cesarean due to "failure to progress." Physicians feared that the intensity of strong contractions might stress the uterine incision and lead to sudden uterine rupture. This is a potentially dangerous situation for both mother and baby and can be difficult to detect. Between 1980 and 1985, only 5 percent of women with a previous cesarean gave birth vaginally. Over half a million cesarean births during this period could have been successful VBACs. ACOG revised its guidelines in 1985, suggesting that physicians could treat VBAC attempts almost like any normal births, with certain requirements: electronic fetal monitoring, IVs, and the presence of an anesthesiologist in case emergency surgery was required. Insurance companies and health care officials began to take note, realizing not only the enormous strain that cesarean births put on the immediate health care budget, but also the long-term implications. With pressure from the insurance industry, ACOG made the dramatic statement in 1988 that "routine repeat cesarean sections should be eliminated." VBAC was the new standard of practice, potentially eliminating one-third of all cesareans.[65] This shift was also due in part to consumer pressure, as well as to medical studies disproving the assumption that once a cesarean, always a cesarean. Through the efforts of the International Cesarean Awareness Network (ICAN) and other grassroots groups there was an increasing awareness of the safety of vaginal birth after cesarean and the numbers of VBACs increased 50 percent between 1989 and 1996, even though not all physicians agreed with the ACOG standard.

One woman who came from Alaska to a California birthing center had a water birth after two previous cesareans. Afterward she wrote, "I knew that I could do it. Once I got into the tub, I knew I couldn't get out. The other doctors quite literally destroyed my confidence in my ability to birth vaginally."

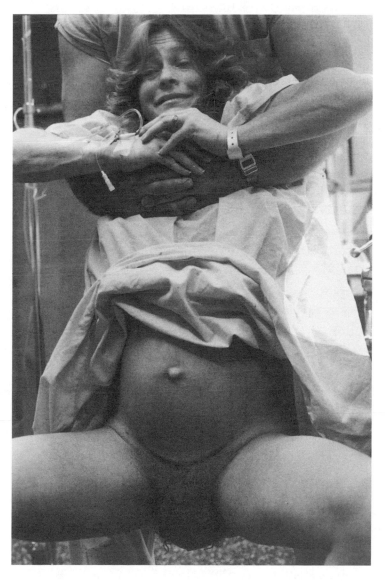

*Notice the cesarean scar on this woman's belly as she births her next baby vaginally*

Dr. Bruce Flamm has conducted a very comprehensive study on VBACs, focusing on ten southern California hospitals. Flamm correlated the experience of his own obstetrical practice with the study's findings in his book, *Birth After Cesarean: The Medical Facts.* Flamm emphatically stated, "Most women who attempt a natural birth after cesarean section will succeed. This has been proven beyond a shadow of a doubt."[66] A 1999 study in Switzerland revealed that 75 percent of women who waited for spontaneous onset of labor gave birth vaginally after a previous cesarean, concluding that there was no greater risk in attempting a vaginal birth.[67] The success rate was only 65 percent for those women who were induced to bring the onset of labor.

Doctors who encourage women to try to give birth vaginally after a cesarean often observe that women will give birth vaginally after they have had cesareans for a diagnosis of cephalopelvic disproportion, which means the baby's head is too big for the mother's pelvis. Yet, the babies these women gave birth to were bigger than the ones they were sectioned for. Commenting about VBACs at the Family Birth Center in Upland, California, where he practiced for nine years, retired obstetrician Michael Rosenthal stated that "of the several hundred VBACs, many of the women who came here gave birth to their biggest baby after previously being sectioned for what were considered large babies."[68]

For a time the number of VBAC births were up, the number of cesareans were down, and all looked quite good for women; and then the other shoe dropped. Managed care companies started mandating VBACs. Doctors, under pressure of not being paid for cesareans by some insurers, started offering VBACs without judicious screening. The number of VBACs rose and so did the complications, which were to be expected. An increase in uterine rupture made the headlines and all attention went to this horrific "side effect" of the original cesarean. In 1995, in Los Angeles County alone, there were twenty-four medical malpractice settlement claims relating to VBAC.[69] One very important point that the insurance industry failed to take into consideration was that if they truly wanted to reduce the cesarean birth rate in the United States, they should first tackle the *primary* cesarean rate. Looking at the core reasons of VBAC failure would mean that medicalized and interventional birth practices would have to be scrutinized. Making it easier for women to give birth, whether they had a previous cesarean or not, should have been the focus.

When malpractice cases started showing up in the press, doctors, insurance companies, and hospital risk managers started experiencing doubts about the wisdom of encouraging vaginal birth after a previous cesarean. A knee-jerk reaction from the insurance industry was to raise annual malpractice insurance premiums for doctors who offered VBACs or who provided medical coverage for midwives who offered VBACs. Insurance premiums were astronomical for some, causing birth center closures and forcing some doctors and midwives out of practice. The spiraling effects continued and in 1999 the American College of Obstetricians and Gynecologists sealed the fate of millions of women in this country to a repeat cesarean birth with the change of a single word.

The ACOG statement had previously read, "VBAC should be attempted in institutions equipped to respond to emergencies with physicians *readily* available."[70] "Readily" was changed to "immediately." That made all the difference to doctors who now had to be within the confines of the hospital or only a few minutes away throughout an entire labor. Doctors who could perform an emergency cesarean for midwife clients also had to be in the hospital during labor. Hospitals had to provide an operating room crew in the hospital for every woman attempting a vaginal birth after cesarean, just in case she experienced a uterine rupture.

The impact of this word was felt worldwide. By 2005 most rural hospitals, medium-sized city hospitals, and certified birth centers stopped offering the option of vaginal birth after cesarean, even for mothers who had experienced a VBAC already without complication. This was a financial decision by these hospitals who could not afford to keep surgery suites open around the clock and pay people to staff them. As indiscriminate as the 1989 policy in favor of VBAC, this exclusionary policy was even worse. From 1996 to 2003, the VBAC rate in the United States dropped by 63 percent.[71] Advocates of gentle birth reacted by compiling the evidence of the safety of VBAC, and they rallied together to help women understand what they had to do to prevent the first cesarean from happening. "Women still have the legal right to choose VBAC," stated Helen Bellanka, a family practice doctor from eastern Oregon. "There are no longer any hospitals on this side of the Cascades that will consent to a VBAC, so women are forced into traveling two or three hours to Portland. So, I tell women to refuse the repeat cesarean. The hospital cannot force you into it. If they did a surgery against your will, it would be considered physical assault."[72]

A few hospitals have decided to bite the bullet and provide anesthesia and obstetric coverage for those who decide on a VBAC. Tanja Johnson, CNM, clinical manager of the Family Birth Center of the Three Rivers Community Hospital in Grants Pass, Oregon, explained:

> We decided to honor a mom's choice to have a VBAC. We state on our consent form that we do not officially offer VBAC services due to limited medical personnel, as recommended by ACOG. However, a patient who refuses a cesarean and elects a trial of labor is supported in her decision. Our anesthesia is on-call for 12 hours and in-house for 12 hours. All of our providers have agreed to remain in the hospital for women attempting a vaginal birth after a cesarean while they are in active labor.[73]

Dr. Bruce Flamm agrees that this approach is a great way to comply with ACOG guidelines, also suggesting that in communities that have several hospitals with maternity units, the one that has in-house medical staff could do all the VBACs in that town.[74]

Given the controversy that has surrounded VBAC, women have to ask themselves, "How can I avoid a cesarean in the first place?"

Mothers face real risks when consenting to a cesarean or planning an elective one. Sadly, not every mother has the opportunity to receive this information before labor in order to make an informed rational decision and not be swayed in the throes of a medicalized birth. A comprehensive guide to understanding the impact of cesarean was developed from an exhaustive study of the available research by the Maternity Center Association. "What Every Pregnant Woman Needs to Know About Cesarean Section" was released in 2004 and contains a handy comparison chart of the risks of cesarean compared with the risks of vaginal birth. A copy can be viewed or ordered on their Web site. (See Appendix E, Resources)

According to the guide, following a cesarean mothers have an increased risk for:

Maternal death—risk is low
Emergency hysterectomy—risk is moderate
Blood clots and stroke—risk is low
Injuries from surgery—risk is very high
Longer time in hospital—risk is very high
Going back into the hospital—risk is moderate
Infection—risk is high
Bowel obstruction—risk is moderate
Pain, overall and at the incision site—risk is very high
Poor birth experience—risk is very high
Less early contact with the baby—risk is very high

The guide also lists other negative reactions that are experienced by women, but have not been conclusively researched:

Depression after birth
Psychological trauma
Poor overall mental health and self-esteem
Unfavorable reaction to the baby
Continued pelvic pain, sometimes even for years

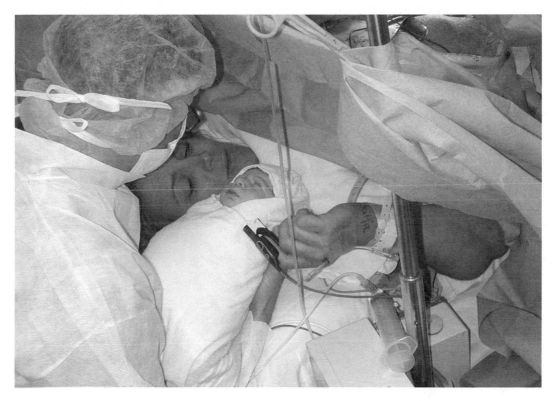

*Separation of mother and baby after a surgical birth is difficult for everyone.*

Women have to consider the risk to their future reproductive abilities as well. The evidence shows that mothers are at a much higher risk of not being able to conceive another baby after a cesarean. Some women even avoid having sex because they don't want to experience the same kind of birth.

The study also revealed other future reproductive complications and risks, including:

Ectopic pregnancy—risk is moderate
Placenta previa (the placenta attaches at or near the cervical opening)—risk is moderate for the first VBAC and high for any after that
Placenta accreta (the placenta grows into the wall of the uterus)—risk is moderate
Placental abruption (placenta comes off the wall of the uterus before the baby is born)—risk is moderate
Rupture of the uterus (wall of the uterus, especially at the site of previous cesarean scar, gives way)—risk is moderate

And what about the risks of surgery for the baby? The study found the following:

Accidental surgical cuts—risk is high

Respiratory problems—risk is high especially for a planned cesarean before 39 weeks

Not breastfeeding—risk is very high

Developing asthma—risk is high

Attachment disorders—risk is very high

There are also risks for a baby who is growing in a uterus that has one or more scars from a previous cesarean. Documentation and research show that those babies have a higher stillbirth and early infant death rate.[75] There are indications that those babies also have lower birth weights and are more often born prematurely. There are more central nervous system injuries noted as well as more malformations.

Women who give birth vaginally recover more quickly, sometimes by many months. Although some medical literature suggests that recovery from a cesarean should take only four weeks, not many women say that. They complain about pain, weakness and difficulties for many months. A postpartum follow-up study reported that six weeks after the birth, about two-thirds of the women who gave birth vaginally regained their usual energy, but only one-third of women who had cesareans had done so by that time.[76]

Cesarean birth can make taking care of a newborn very difficult. Fatigue and pain from the surgery make it difficult, if not impossible, for many of these mothers to hold and feed their babies as much as they would like, and illness can sometimes separate mothers and babies. The baby needs around-the-clock, on-call services and that is accomplished much more easily after a vaginal birth experience—a gentle one without surgical intervention.

Women who give birth vaginally feel more attached to their babies sooner. Research confirms that the first mother-baby contact and bond can begin right away after the birth. This bonding is in jeopardy after a cesarean birth. According to bonding researchers Marshall and Phyllis Klaus and John Kennell, a healthy newborn will stay awake and alert for forty minutes during his first hour of life and will experience 10 percent of his first week in this intense state.[77]

No one is happy over the increase in cesareans in the United States. Deanne Williams, executive director of the American College of Nurse-Midwives and Mary Ann Shah, president of ACNM's board of directors, state that the cesarean rates "are off the charts, and women are being duped into thinking that this is alright."[78] Tonya Jamois, president of International Cesarean Awareness Network, appeared on the Today Show in November of 2004, where she debated with a representative of the American College of Obstetricians and Gynecologists. Jamois, herself a practicing attorney in San Diego, California, stated plainly that there is no convincing evidence that a forced repeat cesarean section is better for mothers and babies. On the contrary, it has far worse implications. In an editorial Jamois stated, "Principles of law and ethics are settled. Pregnant women have the right to full disclosure of the risks and benefits of a recommended course of treatment, as well as alternatives to that treatment. They should be treated with respect and dignity and not manipulated and scared into a course preferred by the physician. Pregnant women have the right to make informed decisions on whether to consent to a cesarean."[79]

The cesarean controversy has had unintended consequences. Obstetricians are quitting over liability issues, nurse-midwives are being forced out of some hospitals because of lack of malpractice coverage, and families have to contend with having fewer and fewer options in the hospitals. The current situation is ripe for revolution—a revolution that can only come from the women themselves. Michel Odent points out that the quickest way to reduce the cesarean rate is to provide women with an environment conducive to an undisturbed birth. Women must take back their births and reclaim their right to birth in dignity and to protect their baby's right to a gentle birth.

## MYTH: AN EPISIOTOMY HEALS BETTER THAN A TEAR

The episiotomy, or cutting of the perineal tissue, is the most common obstetrical operation in the world, and in the United States the most common type of incision made on women.[80] The rates of episiotomy have been dropping, especially as the rates of cesarean births rise. The episiotomy is performed as the baby's head is crowning just before birth. The rationale used by obstetricians to justify the use of an episiotomy has included sparing the mother from perineal tears, saving the baby's head from damage, hastening the birth, and preventing serious damage to the woman's pelvic muscles.

Many midwives and childbirth reformers realize that an episiotomy is not necessary in most cases. When an episiotomy is performed, it carries the risks of any other surgical procedure: excessive blood loss, hematoma formation (a form of swelling or bruising), infection, or abscessing. Sometimes trauma from an episiotomy of the anal sphincter and rectal mucosa leads to loss of rectal tone and, in severe cases, a fistula, or hole, between the vagina and rectum. An episiotomy can complicate postpartum recovery.

There have been no conclusive studies that prove that an episiotomy would save the muscles from being stretched and losing tone or that it would yield a tighter vagina than one that is stretched naturally. On the contrary, an episiotomy and subsequent stitches can lead to less integrity of the perineum in later life. There is a current argument that a cesarean is a better choice for women who wish to preserve their perineums and prevent future problems with weak vaginal muscles and prolapse of vaginal or rectal tissue. The rationalization is that vaginal birth makes all the muscles in the vagina lax and they can never again be restored to a "virginal" state. What causes major problems with the musculature of the vaginal wall and perineum is primarily episiotomy and use of surgical instruments during a vaginal birth. Gentle birth advocates agree that it is important to abandon the routine use of episiotomy and only to use the procedure when a birth becomes difficult due to the baby's size or presentation.

Several important factors can prevent perineal tearing and the need for an episiotomy. One is for the mother to be in an upright position. Another is the ability to change positions while birthing her child. Most practitioners feel it is necessary to get the baby out as quickly as possible after the cervix has completely dilated. They ask women to strain, hold their breath, and bear down. These actions can lead to maternal hypotension (low blood pressure). If the vaginal tissues are distended too rapidly, the possibility of lacerations and the indication for episiotomy increases. The combination of birthing in the lithotomy position and strained pushing will cause the perineum to tear. If a woman is in a vertical squatting position or on her hands and knees when birthing, the pelvic area opens up. She is now working with the force of gravity instead of against it. Under these conditions there usually should be no need for an episiotomy. When a woman is allowed to move and change positions, she is in control of her birth.

A woman who is left alone while birthing will often place a hand on the perineum or on the baby's head as it is crowning. She can work with the contractions and slowly ease the baby out without tearing the perineum. If she has a strong urge to push, she can hold back by changing her breathing pattern to light pants or by vocalizing her energy, which will inhibit her from bearing down. In this way, the baby's head can slowly stretch the perineum.

Many midwives will apply hot compresses and warm oil to the perineal area between contractions to encourage relaxation. Sitting in a tub of warm water will help the perineum stretch, as will assisting the woman to relax her pelvic area. Midwives observe a "resting" phase toward the end of the first stage of labor. They report that some women often do not have the urge to push as soon as dilation is complete and that, in fact, the contractions slow down a bit. One California midwife described her experience:

> The mother asked me to check her while she was in the birthing tub. I told her that she was complete [fully dilated] and to listen to her body to know when she needed to push. She rested and moved slowly about for almost an hour. At one point she asked me if she should be pushing, and I told her only if she felt a strong urge. She didn't, so she continued to rest. All of a sudden her eyes widened and she said as she reached down, "The baby's here." Within four minutes the baby was in her arms. She hadn't pushed once. The baby had descended slowly and then, whoosh, was out in the water.

As long as the baby and mother are doing well there is no need to bear down in an effort to "rush" the baby out.

The use of water for labor has been linked with a significant decrease in episiotomies, almost eliminating them in hospitals where birth pools were used regularly. A funny thing started happening when the women in the water did not need an episiotomy. Providers realized they weren't necessary on women who weren't in the water, either. On one unit in England a few midwives started leaving the scissors out of the birth instrument packages on purpose or dropping them on the floor during a birth, so that none would be available. The episiotomy rate dropped significantly and women birthed without severe tearing.

On a 1993 trip to Russia I observed births taking place in a large hospital in the city of Nizhny Novgorod (formerly Gorky). The obstetrician would only walk into the room when it was time to cut the episiotomy. The doctor would stand at the foot of the delivery table and wait for the head to crown to a certain point, then reach in and, without an anesthetic, slice the perineum. It is hard for me to dispel the image of the doctor holding the scissors high in the air, poised and ready to cut on cue from the midwife. The episiotomy rate was 100 percent in all hospitals in Russia up to a few years ago. Natural childbirth is very slowly increasing in a few select hospitals where couples pay more for having no interventions.

In 1987 the episiotomy rate in the United States was 62 percent. By 1993, it had dropped to 50 percent of all vaginal births and in 1996 it had dropped again to 43 percent.[81] The Coalition for Improving Maternity Services recommends an episiotomy rate of no more than 20 percent with the ideal goal of 5 percent.[82]

There is a new device on the market which is touted as preventing episiotomies. The Epi-No is used by pregnant women in their last month of pregnancy to artificially stretch the perineal tissue. A balloonlike bulb is placed into the vagina and then inflated from zero to ten centimeters over a period of time. My initial reaction was one of distaste, thinking that a man must have invented this device. It may have some use in helping women practice vaginal exercises, known as Kegels. As far as stretching the perineal tissues, loving partners can do this for their wives or girl friends, or mothers can do it themselves. The perineal stretching also helps women by giving them the subliminal message that they can stretch and are willing to open to let the baby out. I usually suggest that women use a hot water bottle over a cloth soaked in castor oil or massage oil once a day, usually at bedtime, in the last two weeks of pregnancy. This brings blood supply to the tissues, feels good, and helps women practice visualizing the baby being born.

The best way to avoid an episiotomy is to hire a provider who doesn't do them; use a doula; give birth upright or in water; push with the contraction and breathe the baby down and out; apply warm compresses to the perineum during the second stage of labor and massage with oil; and definitely avoid having an epidural.

The work of Dr. Michel Odent and others have shown that the second stage of labor is not usually lengthened when it is allowed to proceed in an entirely instinctive manner. In a gentle birth, a woman does not need to be coached to push. Instead she needs to trust her instincts and open up to this wonderful process of letting go of the baby instead of pushing it out.

## MYTH: BIRTH NEEDS TO BE STERILE

During the past forty years of childbirth in the United States, there was a time when women were routinely strapped down to obstetric tables with their hands restrained in order to maintain a sterile field for the birth. The enema and shaving of a woman's pubic hair were ordered by doctors to avoid contamination of what physicians considered the "surgical site." In the process of creating a sterile field, the medical model separated the woman from her perineum. Doctors treated a sterile vaginal area as though it was devoid of any human element and inherent emotions.

When giving birth, a woman's instinct is often to reach down and feel the baby's head as it emerges. How unfortunate that women are often robbed of this experience in the name of sterility. A labor and delivery nurse from a hospital in Indiana wrote with the following observation. "One of our oldest physicians still to this day will slap the hand of mothers who reach down to touch their perineum, yelling at them that it's sterile down there." She went on to relate that the very same doctor later in the day performed circumcisions on two baby boys lying side by side and didn't bother changing scalpels. The truth is that birth cannot possibly be sterile, and there is no indication that nature ever intended it to be. When the baby emerges from the birth canal, he is covered with a film of the mother's vaginal bacteria. The baby is immune to these bacteria because he has shared the same ecosystem with the mother for the last nine months. While in the womb the baby receives the mother's antibodies through the placenta, and after birth he continues to receive these antibodies from the mother's colostrum during the first twenty-four hours of breastfeeding. There is no need to protect a newborn baby from healthy parents.

What is the purpose of these hospital procedures? Who are we protecting from infection, if not the baby? There are no elaborate sterile procedures in a home or birth-center birth. Sometimes gloves are not used by midwives because they consider human, skin-to-skin touch an important part of the emotional support they offer to women. However, because of the risk of AIDS and hepatitis, the use of gloves is generally recommended.*

---

*An important point to take into consideration regarding a sterile environment for birth is the risk of exposure to the HIV virus. All hospitals have instituted "universal precautions" that require midwives and physicians to wear goggles as well as other protective clothing during birth. This procedure is justified, especially when working with people in high-risk groups for HIV and hepatitis. It is done not to keep birth sterile but because the attendants need to protect themselves.

A few hospitals today still require anyone attending births to wear gowns, masks, and booties, or what are commonly referred to as "scrubs." Perhaps we have lessened our ability to be emotionally connected with the birth by requiring these clothes in the hospital. The drapes remove a woman from her body, her sensuality, and the experience of birth. The masks say, "I am keeping my distance." The emotional experience of a birth can be lost when it becomes a business transaction between the birthing couple and the doctor, garbed according to a dress code of green suits, masks, and gloves.

When women are free to wear whatever they want during labor and birth, and family and friends with them are not restricted with hospital gowns and masks, there seems to be greater verbal interaction and more emotional vulnerability. A woman who can remove her clothes to get into the shower or bath usually finds it easier to drop many of her inhibitions and surrender herself to the physical experience of her birth. She seems to be more willing to make noises, move around, and in general not conform to anyone else's ideas about how her birth should proceed. Fathers often join in more readily, willing to be physically close to their partners and sharing the emotional intensity of labor and birth. Sometimes fathers instinctively take off all their clothes and jump into the birthing tub at hospitals where birth pools are available. One midwife who had never experienced anything like that before thought to herself, "It is their birth—who am I to judge his behavior?" Some nurses will ask the father if he brought his swim trunks if the mother is intending to have a waterbirth. If not, they will provide him with a pair of surgical scrub pants.

When given enough privacy, some women will instinctively activate a sexual response in labor, rubbing or playfully stimulating their clitoris. At a midwifery conference in Vienna, Austria, Ina May Gaskin was scheduled to give a lecture on orgasm in labor. The small room that was scheduled to be used was bursting at the seams with midwives from all over the world who wanted to listen to Gaskin's experience of women being free to express their sexuality in labor. They also wanted to share their similar stories. When the barriers are taken down for women and birth is witnessed instead of controlled, anything is possible.

## MYTH: THE OLDER YOU ARE THE MORE DIFFICULT YOUR BIRTH WILL BE

Today many women are delaying childbearing until their late twenties, thirties, or even forties. Career moves, postponing marriage, and a desire for self-fulfillment are some of the reasons why women are having their first babies at an older age. The technology of infertility treatment has allowed older, sometimes infertile women to be able to either conceive using artificial means or have in vitro fertilization with viable embryos implanted. The National Center for Health Statistics reports that between 1975 and 1982 women who were between thirty and thirty-four years of age experienced a 23 percent increase in fertility.[83] During that same period, there was an 83 percent increase in women over the age of thirty-five having their first babies.

For a long time it was assumed that professional success, power, and full-time motherhood were mutually exclusive. For the first time in over twenty-five years, a growing number of women are choosing to take time out from the workforce to care for their children. The proportion of working mothers who also had infant children declined from a record high of 59 percent in 1998 to 55 percent in 2000—the first significant decline since 1976.[84] According to a recent Census Bureau paper, "Older mothers (age 30–34) and more educated women are increasingly likely to not work after their first child's birth."

Medicine and society have placed a great stigma on "older" women having babies. The current terminology is that these women are considered high risk for having gestational and birth-related complications. There are an infinite number of variables to be considered when looking at the overall health of a pregnant woman. The medical model of pregnancy wants each woman to fall within a certain set of arbitrary guidelines in order to be considered low risk: the woman should be twenty-two to twenty-four years old, she should be Rh positive with no history of a previous abortion or miscarriage, she should have had no abnormal Pap smears or childhood illnesses other than the measles, and she should have given birth within the last three years to a normal infant weighing between seven and nine pounds. Most pregnant women do not meet the standards laid out in these guidelines. Any factor that does not meet the medical model definition of a normal pregnancy can cause a woman to be labeled high risk. If she is thirty-five or older, she is considered obstetrically elderly.

Even if she is perfectly healthy and has a positive attitude about her pregnancy, an "older" woman will be subjected to a battery of tests, precautions, and careful screening throughout pregnancy, labor, and birth. Her history and physical exam might even read, "Elderly primipara with no apparent complications or abnormalities. High risk. AFP screening with follow-up amniocentesis recommended." Today women who are too old, too young, too fat, too poor, or who have had too many prior pregnancies—or who have had none—are all considered high risk.

Women who consult with physicians before arranging for a home birth are evaluated in the same manner. They are not judged healthy and suitable for a home birth but are merely considered low risk for possible complications. Risk is a tricky subject. We all walk around at some level of risk for accident, illness, or death. Do you tell your friends that they are at low risk for an automobile accident? The mere terminology suggests a disease process, not a normal state. The medical model only associates pregnancy with the possibility of complications, either high or low.

What are the factors that make an older woman high risk? The idea that older

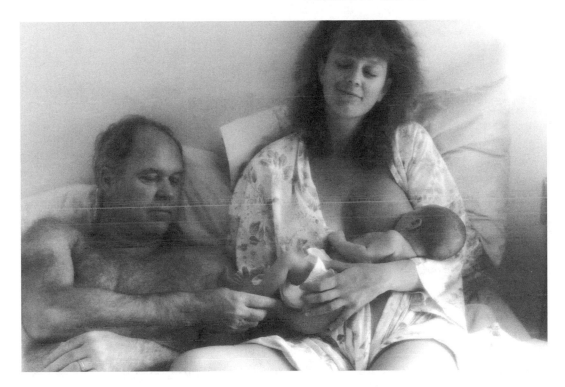

*An "older" couple feeling the intimacy of a beautiful birth experience in a birth center.*

women, especially first-time mothers, suffer more complications in pregnancy has been perpetuated for the last one hundred years. Medical texts have even stated that anyone between the ages of twenty-eight and forty is pushing the upper limit of youth. A number of seemingly conclusive studies indicated that advanced maternal age contributes to increased maternal mortality, infant mortality, perinatal mortality, pregnancy and labor complications, and a variety of birth defects, including Down's syndrome. It is possible that many studies were written in order to support the view of birth being an abnormal state, a disease state. By redefining what is normal, medicine has maintained more control. These studies have been accepted and handed down for the last two generations as being the measure of normalcy.

There are real genetic risks associated with age in both mothers and fathers. For women over thirty-five and men over fifty-five, the risk of having a baby with Down's syndrome increases every year. For a woman twenty years of age the risk is 1 in 2,000; at thirty-five, 1 in 365; and at forty-five, 1 in 32. It seemed perfectly logical that imperfections in genetics related to age would be reflected in birth statistics. In actuality, 80 percent of Down's syndrome babies in 1986 were born to women younger than thirty-five. This could mean that many Down's babies were aborted, thereby reducing the number of genetically imperfect babies born to women over thirty-five; or it could mean that Down's syndrome is not always relegated to obstetrically elderly women.[85]

With the average life span increasing, women today are not as old at thirty-five as our grandmothers were. Older women today are generally healthier and more health conscious. What used to be considered age-related complications such as diabetes, obesity, heart problems, and high blood pressure are experienced more on an individual basis than in the general population of older females. Women who consciously choose to delay pregnancy tend to be very physically and emotionally fit for motherhood.

A new and vocal movement is starting to address the problems faced by parents who leave successful careers or well-paying jobs to spend time with their children. Ann Crittenden, a Pulitzer Prize nominee and author of *The Price of Motherhood,* is one of the women leading the charge. In 2002, Crittenden joined forces with authors Naomi Wolf and Barbara Seaman, the National Association of Mothers Centers, and other grassroots women's organizations to launch Mothers Ought To Have Equal Rights (MOTHERS), a group that advocates improving the economic security of people who do caring work.

Crittenden suggests that while women have made significant gains in equality, mothers have been left behind. The economic hardships of motherhood are usually a much more devastating side effect of pregnancy and birth than the physical hardships. Crittenden finds that choosing to stay home with children has lasting financial consequences due to lost wages, unequal pay when re-entering the workforce, disparities in divorce law, and lost contributions to Social Security. "It's partly because people in positions of power have no idea how complex, subtle, and highly skilled the job of full-time parent is," says Crittenden. "People tend to think of it as babysitting, and that's only because they have never done it. If they had stayed home with children, they would know better."

Positive attitudes about pregnancy, birth, and becoming a mother are increasingly important for all women but especially for older women. It is important for them to know that they have had excellent prenatal care, will be supported emotionally, and will have adequate help after the birth. These women must consider all aspects of their family lives, including their relationships, possible career obligations, and the demands of a new baby.

## MYTH: IT'S BETTER NOT TO EAT OR DRINK DURING LABOR

If active labor lasts longer than twelve hours, a woman will probably get tired and hungry. A 1984 survey of U.S. and UK hospitals found that not one hospital allowed a woman to eat or drink what she wanted during labor.[86] About 50 percent allowed ice chips for a woman's thirst; some now allow clear liquids, such as water, iced tea, or popsicles. In either case, the calorie requirements and nutritional needs of the laboring woman have been virtually ignored. The rationale behind these restrictions is that if the woman were given general anesthesia or an epidural, she would be susceptible to vomiting. The anesthesia would keep her gag reflex from working, thus increasing her risk for aspiration pneumonia. In reality the risk of a mother dying from aspiration while under anesthesia is approximately seven in ten million births—hardly sufficient risk to justify placing restrictions on eating and drinking in labor.[87]

In reality the practice of withholding food or liquids increases the risk of dehydration and negative nitrogen balance in the laboring woman. There have been no scientific studies of the nutritional needs of laboring women; however, all women who have experienced labor know that it is a major aerobic event, burning up thousands of calories. A great deal of stamina is called for, not only physically but emotionally. What a time to tell a woman she can have "nothing by mouth"! Many women don't feel like eating during labor, but they should always have the option.

In an attempt to compensate for this lack of nutrition, an IV line is usually inserted into the mother's arm for continuous administration of fluid. Doctors view birth as a potential surgical operation and IVs are the norm for preparing for surgery. So, they require women to have one just in case. Although the dextrose or lactated ringers substance in the IV fluid does provide some calories, it is both insufficient and inappropriate to her needs.

The presence of the IV complicates the labor in many ways. Any puncture of the skin increases the risk of infection. It also immobilizes a woman in labor, encumbering her freedom to move. She can walk, but someone has to help her manage the IV pole, the tubing, and the bag or bottle. This is the last thing a woman in the midst of a contraction wants to be bothered with. Being hooked up to an IV also carries the psychological implication that birth is a state of illness. Many women just resign themselves to being patients in hospital beds instead of active birthing women.

The IV also makes it much easier to accept drugs. If a woman is faced with a painful shot, she may think twice about taking pain medication, but if it can be painlessly injected through the IV that has already been inserted, she finds it more difficult to object. Many women reach a point in their labor when they feel like they cannot take any more and are ready to throw in the towel. It is at these times that family, friends, or the birth assistant can make all the difference with reassuring words or encouragement. Unfortunately, at these times it's also the easiest to accept pain relief via the IV.

Given the option to eat, especially in early active labor, women at home and in birthing centers choose easily digested carbohydrates such as bread, cookies, toast, fruit, rice, or pasta, as well as light proteins such as cheese or yogurt. Some women like to sip milk shakes or protein shakes for strength.

During labor, dehydration shows up as dry lips, a racing pulse, and a lack of urination. A woman who needs protein will often become easily discouraged during labor and have a visible lack of energy. Her uterus may even get tired, in what is called uterine inertia. All of these situations can be remedied by asking her to eat and drink. By encouraging a woman to keep drinking fluids during labor and even offering spoonfuls of honey, midwives report that women often regain their strength and are able to accomplish a natural birth. If women in hospitals who were preparing for normal vaginal births ate and drank as they desired, the problem of food in the stomach could be dealt with by inserting a naso-gastric tube and suctioning out the contents of the stomach if an emergency occurred.

The prohibition of food and liquids during labor is an example of a cultural practice instituted for good reasons, but those reasons no longer exist with the knowledge we have today. Old habits are hard to break, though. In a February 2005 issue of *ePregnancy* magazine a small information tidbit reads, "most doctors will give the okay for popsicles, suckers, Jell-o and broths, but some doctors only allow ice chips and water. So ask your doctor before sending your partner to the cafeteria for a late-night nibble." It is time for this blanket policy to be abolished completely.

## MYTH: FAMILY AND FRIENDS INTERFERE DURING BIRTH

Some hospitals today still have policies that restrict the number of people a woman can have supporting her during her birth. A number of hospitals will only allow the father of the baby or perhaps one chosen birth support person. Birth rooms are often small and the mother is forced to choose who she wants to be with her during this life-changing experience. In some parts of the world bringing birth attendants and a support team into labor is not an option at all. In all of the former Soviet countries and in China women are delivered to the door of the hospital and not seen again until they are discharged.

Enforced separation of the birthing woman from her support system strongly contributes to a woman's level of anxiety or fear. Current research on hormones and their effect on the laboring woman points to the fact that fear adversely affects blood flow and uterine contractions. During a normal labor there is an increase in the flow of catecholamines, which activate the fight or flight response in both the mother and the baby. The stress of being alone during labor, separated from loved ones and surrounded by strangers, is enough to trigger an increased level of catecholamine release in the mother. This can produce weaker uterine contractions, prolonged labor, a decrease of blood flow to the uterus and placenta, and an increase in the amount of hormones released. The baby interprets these responses

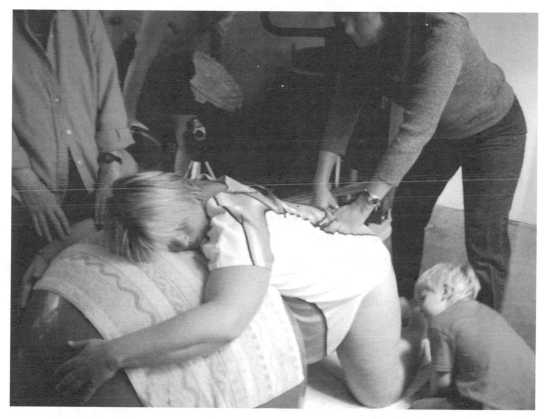

*Anticipation is sometimes hard, but gentle births happen in their own time and in their own way.*

in her mother as stress and her own hormone production increases, which in turn can cause distress, heart rate abnormalities, and even colitis and the release of meconium into the amniotic fluid.

Studies have shown that babies born by elective cesarean without active labor have absent or reduced levels of catecholamines, indicating that labor stimulates their release. For the baby the release of the catecholamines is vital because these hormones help regulate breathing efforts after birth. If they are not present, as in a baby who was born by cesarean that was not preceded by normal labor, the infant may experience respiratory distress. Niles Newton, one of the founding members of the International Childbirth Education Association, conducted interesting studies involving mice giving birth in different containers and contrivances. Her findings were significant. Mice whose labors were environmentally disturbed experienced significantly longer labors, as much as 72 percent longer under some conditions, and gave birth to 54 percent more dead pups than did the mice in the control group who birthed in a natural environment. Newton presented her data to colleagues at the 1974 National Congress on the Quality of Life, an American Medical Association conference. Newton emphasized that the human mammal (that is, the human mother), which has a more highly developed nervous system than that of the mouse, may be equally sensitive to environmental disturbances in labor.[88]

Marshall Klaus and John Kennell, the pediatricians who wrote about maternal-infant bonding, published a study in the *British Medical Journal* in 1986. The study randomly assigned more than four hundred laboring women either to continuous social support, which included back massage and verbal reassurance, or to routine hospital care with minimal support. Among women who received routine hospital care with minimal support, the rate of cesarean birth was more than twice that in the supported group. The women who were assigned labor companions and received massage, emotional encouragement, and support consistently experienced much shorter labors. The difference in actual labor time was approximately seven hours as compared to fifteen hours for those who did not receive help.[89]

This and other studies led to the formation of Doulas of North America in 1985. A doula is a woman who is experienced in giving one-to-one support in childbirth, concentrating on providing emotional and physical comfort. A woman can become a doula by attending one of many training courses throughout the United States. During these trainings the process of normal labor is emphasized and activities and actions that will assist a woman to achieve a natural childbirth experience are demonstrated and discussed.

> Medical studies have shown that having a doula present provides the following benefits:
> 50% reduction in cesarean rate
> 60% reduction in epidural requests
> 40% reduction in the use of Pitocin
> 25% shorter labor
> 30% reduction in use of analgesia
> 40% reduction in forceps use

A few simple measures can reassure a woman in labor and reduce her stress. Never leaving her alone in labor and providing strong emotional support, as the Klaus study points out, have been proved to decrease labor time and prevent distress in the fetus.

The American College of Obstetricians and Gynecologists has stated in a bulletin titled "Cesarean Evaluation" that "the continuous presence of nurses or other trained individuals who provide comfort and support to women in labor may lead to lower rates."[90] This is a landmark statement. It plainly recognizes the value of emotional support throughout the process of labor.

Newborn attachment is also enhanced when a woman is supported throughout the process. If she is feeling loved and nurtured, she is more available to nurture her baby. It is important for her to choose a person upon whom she can depend for emotional support. Many women want their husbands or partners present and choose an additional person as well to support them through the process of labor. Hospitals need to recognize how the rigid procedures, thoughtless routines, and unnecessary interventions that accompany hospital births increase stress, actually creating the problems that the interventions are trying to avoid. All women can plan for a supportive, undisturbed birth environment that includes continuous physical, emotional, and informational support.

## MYTH: THE BABY NEEDS TO BE OBSERVED IN A NEWBORN NURSERY

Most hospitals today allow newborns to room-in with their mothers. But the routine procedure is to separate babies from their mothers for some period of time immediately following the birth, reuniting the baby and mother only after observations, bath, measurements, and evaluations are done. The rationale behind forced separation is to prevent problems from developing in the newborns and to allow the mother to rest. Mothers who receive drugs or anesthesia during birth certainly do need time to "sober up" before they can care for their newborns, and the babies need time to let the effects of the drugs wear off. Most babies experience some form of respiratory depression when narcotic agents are used during labor and birth and do need more careful monitoring. But for the normal, unmedicated birth, separation interferes with some very vital functions.

In 1989 Dr. Marsden Wagner, an American-born pediatrician who is currently a consultant to the Maternal/Child Health division of the World Health Organization, lectured a group gathered in Jerusalem for an international symposium on pre- and perinatal psychology. Wagner stated emphatically, "I am convinced the procedure of placing all newborn babies in one room was the biggest mistake of modern medicine." He referred to the newborn nursery as "a cradle of germs, separating babies from their mothers at the most sensitive point of their relationship."[91] Dr. Wagner also cited several studies that link separation at birth with subsequent child abuse. The importance of the maternal-infant bond in the first few hours after birth has been the subject of many books in the past decade. Bonding is not a science, but there are identifiable characteristics that are associated with this process of emotional attachment.

The first few hours after birth are called the "maternal sensitive period."[92] The mother becomes deeply involved, on an emotional level, with her newborn. The first hour after birth is also a time of quiet alertness for the newborn. Later the baby goes into a deep resting stage for several hours, during which it is difficult to rouse him. The mother who holds and communicates with her baby immediately receives a sense of fulfillment and gratification. She lightly touches the baby with her fingertips and then gradually massages the baby's body. Her voice becomes high-pitched and she looks into the baby's face. They greet each other eye to eye. At birth the baby can see perfectly well from distances of about twelve to eighteen inches, just the distance from mother's to baby's face when he is cradled in her arms.

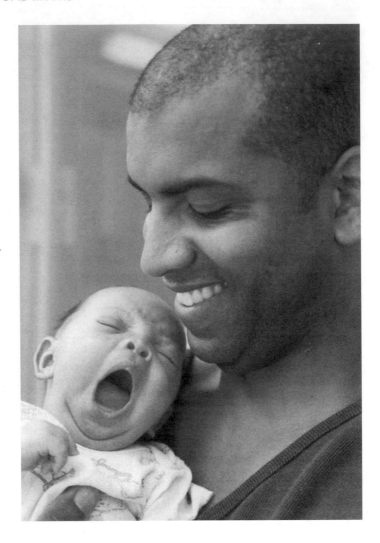

*Taking an active role in the birth of their babies lays the groundwork for fathers to enjoy the challenges of parenting.*

This period of heightened sensitivity is not restricted to mothers. Fathers and siblings bond emotionally during this period as well. Fathers of home-birth babies often talk about watching or assisting with the birth and holding the baby shortly afterward. Most men feel that this experience deepens their relationship with their partner. When siblings are included in the birth or in the first few hours after birth, they exhibit less sibling rivalry. Unfortunately, it is still a rare hospital that welcomes small children to experience the birth of their new baby brother or sister.

The procedures that are performed in the nursery can just as easily be done at the bedside, with the whole family participating. Heart rate, lung sounds, muscle tone, reflexes, and skin color can all be assessed while the baby is in her mother's arms. In healthy newborns with good respiratory function, these procedures do not need to be carried out immediately. Everything can be delayed for, at the very least, an hour. This quiet time can give the mother and father a chance to be intimate, initiate breast-feeding, and sense the new responsibilities this new creature brings.

Most parents love participating in the overall examination that takes place shortly after the birth. Siblings like to count fingers and toes. A great deal of teaching and information can be shared about this new person by including the parents in this process. A portable or sling-type scale to weigh the baby can be brought to the bedside. Many new fathers like to observe the scale and make the pronouncement of how much their baby weighs. Washing the baby is often not necessary, especially with a water-born infant. The Leboyer bath is still an available option, either in the delivery room or at the bedside. (Waterbirth and the Leboyer approach to birth are discussed in chapter 6.) The more responsibility the parents are encouraged to assume, the more confidence they exhibit. The nurse or midwife becomes a supportive assistant to the parents, offering gentle instruction only if it is called for. For the woman who truly needs to rest and have undisturbed sleep, the nursery provides an alternative, but it should remain an option for those who choose it and not something that is forced on all mothers.

Removing the baby to the nursery increases the risk of an infection. Every hospital is terrified of nursery staph infections. Newborns who become infected risk everything from aggressive antibiotic treatments to, in some cases, even death. Where do the babies get the infections? Simply from the noses and hands of hospital nursery personnel. When the mother keeps her baby with her, she cuddles him, kisses him, and massages him, showering his whole body with bacteria. But because the baby is familiar with her bacteria, it does not harm him and protects him from other foreign germs.

Taking the baby away from his parents also takes away their responsibilities. Caretaking of the baby starts immediately. For the woman who wants to assume this responsibility, taking the baby away from her is an insult to her abilities. She loses confidence and begins to wonder if she really is capable of taking care of a newborn. Perhaps those experienced nurses know something about babies that she doesn't. After all, while this may be her first experience with a newborn baby, they do this all the time. Nothing can shatter a mother's self-confidence more than to have a nurse breeze through bathing and diapering her baby. Even casually doubting her ability to mother impacts on her relationship with her child.

One of the strongest emotions to affect a woman at the time of birth is loss. The physical passage of the baby from intrauterine to extrauterine life means loss on many levels. Many women enjoy being pregnant, feeling their babies inside, and exulting in their increased self-awareness and sensitivity. A lot of attention is focused on the woman when she is pregnant. As soon as the baby is born, everything and everyone is focused on the baby's needs. Many women also feel a sense of loss when the actual birth does not match their expectations, especially if they were planning a gentle birth and ended up needing a cesarean section. Birth triggers a great range of feelings, and it is sometimes hard for a new mother to sort out just what is going on. She may be in shock over the birth and may display behaviors that resemble anything from denial and disbelief to fear, anxiety, guilt, hostility, crying, and lack of concentration. Physically she may exhibit sighing, weakness, shortness of breath, fatigue, and chest pain. All of these signs and symptoms are directly related to her grief over the loss, either real or imagined. In a hospital birth these manifestations are only complicated by the real loss of her baby to the newborn nursery. The easiest way to ease her emptiness is immediate and continuing contact with her baby. The physical closeness helps mitigate the sense of loss. If she is lovingly supported, she is also generally better able to process her feelings.

A single woman who had had a relatively easy home birth retained the placenta for a time that most doctors would consider abnormal. Instead of panicking, the midwife supported the mother through this period just as she had done during the birth. As they talked, the midwife asked the mother why she was not willing to let go of the pregnancy. The mother cried and admitted that as long as she was pregnant, she felt loved and nurtured. She had a fear that as a single mother she wouldn't get the support she needed to be a good mother. The midwife asked her to hold her baby and to tell him what a good mother she was. As she cradled her newborn in her arms, crying, she felt a huge contraction, stood up to go to the bathroom, and the placenta quite literally fell out. This is an example of the birth attendant helping the mother work through her feelings. Recognizing and dealing with these emotions, having maximum physical contact with the baby, and being supported by the entire family during and immediately after the birth will often prevent what medical experts have labeled postpartum depression.

## MYTH: BABY BOYS NEED TO BE CIRCUMCISED

For many years routine circumcision, the surgical removal of the foreskin of the penis, has been a medically and socially accepted convention in the United States. Today, however, increasing numbers of American parents are protecting their sons from routine circumcision at birth. Parents who read the growing body of literature and speak with educated and compassionate pediatricians and maternity care providers understand that the supposed medical reasons for circumcision are merely myths. The deepest and most pervasive myth, which made circumcision widely accepted in the United States, was that removal of the foreskin would deter or eliminate masturbation. In fact, no procedure in the history of medicine has been claimed to cure and prevent more diseases than circumcision. Claims were made by American physicians that circumcision could cure everything from mental illness to bed-wetting and a myriad of other common conditions.[93]

A belief has also been perpetuated that circumcision offered some protection against cancer or infection of the penis and cervical cancer in future female partners. Perhaps as influential was the often unspoken perception that an intact penis was somehow unhygienic. None of these "medical" reasons has ever been validated by research. In 1975 the American Academy of Pediatrics announced that there is no absolute medical indication for routine circumcision, yet it is still practiced today upon non-consenting and unwitting male babies.

Parents are not usually informed of the normal functions of an intact foreskin or of the risks of the operation. The foreskin is a perfectly normal part of the human body, and it has very definite purposes. The numbers of boys with their penises left intact have risen, as public awareness efforts increase, but the decline in circumcision rates has been slower than activists would desire. As with the medicalization of birth practices, circumcision became a universal practice in hospitals across America. It has become a billion-dollar practice, and at its core is a reluctance to give up a lucrative income source. An estimated 1.2 million newborn males are circumcised in the United States annually at a cost of between $150 and $275 million.[94] In 1949, when the National Health Service in the United Kingdom decided not to pay for circumcisions, the number performed dropped immediately to less than one-half of one percent of male newborns. The Canadian health system no longer reimburses for routine circumcision, and the number of circumcisions has steadily and dramatically dropped.

For years it was believed that the perception of pain in a newborn was much less than that of an adult.[95] Babies have always responded to painful stimuli, but it

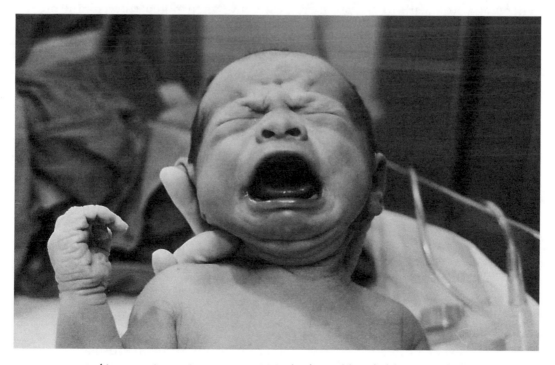

*Babies perceive pain more exquisitely than older children or adults.*

was thought that their responses were mere reflexes and that they were unaware of where the pain was and had no conscious thoughts about it. We now know that babies even perceive pain and respond to painful stimuli in the womb. As a nurse I watched newborn circumcision and witnessed the baby as he cried a helpless, panicky, breathless, high-pitched cry. Some babies even lapsed into a semi-coma. These newborns not only felt the pain, they felt it more exquisitely than any adult.[96]

Circumcision disrupts the baby's normal sleep patterns.[97] After the surgery, the baby is in pain and is in an exhausted, weakened, and debilitated condition. Most important, the circumcision procedure frequently causes the newborn to withdraw from his environment, thus interfering with his process of bonding and breast-feeding.[98]

Many people mistakenly believe that newborns do not have the capacity to remember painful experiences. People have also theorized that the newborn is protected from pain due to an innate adaptive mechanism that gives him a particularly high pain threshold, especially for the birth process. As a consequence of these misinformed beliefs, babies have suffered through excruciatingly painful procedures, the most common of which is circumcision.

In 1987 the *New England Journal of Medicine* published an extensively researched article, "Pain and Its Effects in the Human Neonate and Fetus." The authors, both from the department of anesthesia at Harvard Medical School and Boston Children's Hospital, write from the perspective that the risks of anesthesia, both general and local, are to be considered carefully when potentially painful procedures are to be performed on neonates as well as premature infants. They believe, based on their research, that the experience of pain can be more devastating than the risks associated with anesthesia.[99] All the current research indicates that babies are cognizant not only at birth but also within the womb. Mechanisms are present for interpreting pain as early as the twentieth to thirtieth weeks of gestation.

Parents must be aware of the potential pain and trauma—both physical and emotional—the procedure entails when considering this unnecessary procedure. Even with anesthesia of some kind, circumcision is painful and may produce psychological scarring on a very deep level. Noted psychiatrists now believe that a newborn's birth experience, whether it be painful or pleasant, will profoundly influence his behavior for the rest of his life. Psychiatrist Stanislav Grof states, "How one is born seems to be closely related to one's general attitude toward life, the ratio of optimism to pessimism, how one relates to other people, and one's ability to confront challenges."[100] The infant experiences the procedure as an attack and may conceptualize that his mother, the only person with whom he shares a psychological bond, has abandoned him and has willingly allowed him to be harmed. This perceived lack of protection by the mother could interrupt the formation of the baby's trust, a necessary ingredient for healthy attachment and bonding.[101]

When couples are looking at the circumcision debate, it is best to start with an understanding of the function of the normal foreskin. The small piece of skin that is cut from the infant penis would normally grow into a large protective covering of the adult male penis. Look at the palm of your hand, fingers stretched out, and measure from the tip of your index finger down to the top of the wrist. The entire surface of the hand, with fingers included, is equal to the amount of skin that is missing on the adult penis when a circumcision is performed on an infant.

The foreskin is a uniquely specialized, sensitive, functional organ of touch. No other part of the body serves the same purpose. As a modified extension of the penile shaft skin, the foreskin covers and usually extends beyond the glans before folding under itself and finding its circumferential point of attachment just behind the corona (the rim of the glans).[102] It protects the glans from abrasion and contact with clothes. The foreskin also increases sexual pleasure by sliding up and down on the shaft, stimulating the glans by alternately covering and exposing it. Like the undersurface of the eyelids or the inside of the cheek, the undersurface of the foreskin consists of mucous membrane. The tissue which lies against the penis contains glands which secrete emollients, lubricants, and protective antibodies. Similar glands are found in the eyelids and mouth. The muscle fibers of the foreskin are whirled, forming a kind of sphincter that ensures optimum protection of the urinary tract from contaminants of all kinds.

At birth, the foreskin is usually attached to the glans, very much as a fingernail is attached to a finger. By puberty, the penis will usually have completed its development, and the foreskin will have separated from the glans. This separation occurs in its own time; there is no set age by which the foreskin and glans must be separated. One wise doctor described the process thus, "The foreskin therefore can be likened to a rosebud which remains closed and muzzled. Like a rosebud, it will only blossom when the time is right. No one opens a rosebud to make it blossom."[103] All boys eventually discover that the foreskin retracts, much to their delight. There is no reason for parents or physicians to ever manipulate or retract the foreskin. It will separate and roll back only when it is ready, sometime later in childhood.

The risks associated with anesthesia are usually explained, but hemorrhage, infection, mutilation, and death are additional concerns that new parents should be informed about before they consent to removing their new son's sensitive foreskin. Babies have been permanently damaged by the procedure, sometimes even requiring a sex-change operation. The child's future sexual response should also be considered.

One of the foreskin's functions is to facilitate smooth, gentle movement between the mucosal surfaces of the two partners during intercourse. The foreskin enables the penis to slip in and out of the vagina nonabrasively inside its own slick sheath of self-lubricating, movable skin. The female is thus stimulated by moving pressure rather than by friction only, as when the male's foreskin is missing.[104] Women who have had sex with intact partners and those without foreskins state the experience is vastly different, most often indicating a preference for natural intact penises.[105]

Unfortunately, even after reading all the medical literature and knowing that 80 percent of the male population of the world is intact, some parents use the excuse that they want their baby to look like their daddy or brother.[106] All children are unique and deserve to be viewed uniquely. No child will ever feel slighted or damaged if their penis is not exactly like their father's. In fact, the opposite is true. When my intact four-year-old son asked why other boys on the beach looked different, I explained what caused the difference. With shock, horror, and tears, he grabbed his penis and begged me to never let anyone do that to him. Many mothers report the very same reaction in their intact sons. When faced with the choice of not circumcising a younger son, mothers and fathers may feel a sense of guilt about the damage that they may have done with their first son and they may not want to admit their mistake. It is always best to be truthful with a child, even if it means swallowing your pride and admitting you didn't know how damaging a circumcision really was when you first allowed it.

Some parents choose to circumcise their sons as part of a religious ritual and have strong feelings about the issue. There is a growing movement among non-Orthodox Jewish parents to eliminate this ritual. Several national organizations, including Jews Against Circumcision, counsel families on making this important decision. Whether done by a physician in the hospital, or a *mohel* in a ritual *brit milah*, the procedure has significant complication rates. Mortality may actually be higher than previously thought since some of these deaths have not been attributed to circumcision, but listed only under their secondary causes, such as hemorrhage or infection. But many parents, perhaps most, make the decision to circumcise for social reasons.

There are a number of advocacy organizations against newborn circumcision whose members are physicians and nurses. Mark Reiss, a member of Doctors Opposing Circumcision, is a retired Jewish physician. Reiss speaks especially to Jewish couples not only about the dangers of circumcision, but about the change in Jewish attitude. He states, "Growing numbers of American Jews are now leaving their sons intact as they view circumcision as a part of Jewish law that they can no longer accept."[107] Sympathetic doctors like Reiss and nurses are making a difference. In 1992 a group of twenty-two nurses at a hospital in Santa Fe issued a proclamation that they could no longer participate in newborn circumcisions. They considered themselves to be conscientious objectors. This concrete action is a step that more medical practitioners can take to protect the rights of the newborn. The Alliance for Transforming the Lives of Children (ATLC) along with the

Coalition for Improving Maternity Services (CIMS) both support an elimination of non-medically indicated circumcision. When asked how many circumcisions are done today that are medically indicated or of benefit to the child, ATLC founder, doctor John Travis, responds with a great big "zero."[108]

In the opening address at the 1989 Pre- and Perinatal Psychology Association of North America conference held at the University of Massachusetts, Dr. Lee Salk, respected pediatric psychiatrist from Columbia University, implored the audience to consider the feelings of the newly born child when caring for and handling these tiny people. He cited studies about the influence of the experience of birth and the neonatal period on a person's later behavior. Dr. Salk also noted his own research with babies who are born prematurely and who spend time in neonatal intensive care units. His work focuses on the subsequent behavior of individuals who experience multiple invasive and painful procedures and endure consistent deprivation of human touch. What he found was an extremely high rate of behavior problems with this group as compared to a similar group of children born in the same hospital during the same time period. There was even a high rate of five- to ten-year-olds with severe psychotic behavior.[109] He concluded that we must rethink how we handle babies at birth. This knowledge strongly suggests that humane considerations should apply as forcefully to the care of newborns and young nonverbal infants as they do to children and adults in similar painful and stressful situations. There should be no remaining doubt that circumcision wounds and harms the baby and the person the baby will become. Parents who respect their son's wholeness grant him his birthright—his body, perfect and beautiful and whole.

# CHAPTER FOUR

# A Gentle Revolution

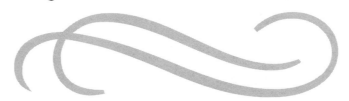

Throughout the world, more and more people are joining the parents and practitioners who are calling for changes in maternity care. There have always been individual complaints against the increased medicalization of childbirth. Voices of protest were raised over fifty years ago and have continued steadily to this day. Every mother, childbirth educator, physician, or midwife who has spoken out about the normalcy of birth or written about the need for change has contributed to what has become a gentle birth revolution.

The expanding social consciousness of women has had a profound effect on the gentle birth revolution. Women are demanding to be in control of their bodies and to fully participate in their birthing process. This change parallels women's change of status in the workplace and in the home. Economic necessity forced many mothers to enter the workforce even with small children at home. In 1950 women made up only 30 percent of the workforce. By 1970 an interesting trend began with close to 60 percent of women working until age twenty-four. There was a visible drop in the female workforce until age thirty-five, reflecting that women stayed at home with children during those critical ten years. A steady rise in workplace figures shows that after staying home women then went back to work until age fifty-five.

In 2003, women were no longer staying home full time to be with their children. The rates for women in the workplace now mirror those of men, with over 60 percent working at least part-time. More women than men work part-time trying to balance family, children and work obligations.[1]

With their role no longer confined to simply that of homemaker, women started choosing when they were going to bear children. It naturally followed that some would choose how they would give birth. This choice, however, remains primarily a middle-class phenomenon. Many segments of society have never had the opportunity to choose when, where, or how to have their babies. Conditions such as poverty, poor nutrition, language barriers, single and early motherhood, and lack of insurance coverage or available services create circumstances that cause women to feel that they have no choices.

Alicia was seventeen when she became pregnant with her first baby. Neither her mother nor the baby's father could provide financial support for her, so she applied for welfare and Medicaid health care. Out of over twenty obstetricians in her home town, only one would take Medicaid patients. The prenatal treatment she received was average. She had no complaints until she began reading about natural childbirth, and voiced her interest in pursuing that option. Her physician flatly refused to acknowledge any of Alicia's desires, telling her she was lucky that she had a doctor who would see her.

Alicia's labor began early one morning three weeks before her due date. She immediately called her doctor to give him a progress report, then went about her usual activities. She felt very confident that everything was fine, and she knew from the reading she had done that her labor was still very mild and did not require her to be in the hospital. Late in the afternoon she received a phone call from the labor nurse at the hospital. Alicia was told in no uncertain terms that she must come to the hospital to be admitted or the sheriff would come over to pick her up and bring her in. From then on Alicia felt as if she were no more than a pregnant body. No one consulted her, informed her, or respected her feelings during the course of her labor. She wanted a completely natural birth but was given drugs to stimulate her labor and drugs to control the pain, and she was never once encouraged to be in charge. She said, "It was as if they were punishing me for getting pregnant in the first place. They acted like I wasn't even there and it was their job to get the baby out of me as quickly as possible." Alicia and her son were separated right after birth due to his low birth weight (just over five pounds) even though he was healthy.

Alicia's lack of choice for that baby led her to seek alternative care just fifteen months later. This time she contacted midwives, came to childbirth education classes, and arranged to give birth at a freestanding birth center about thirty minutes from her home. She birthed her second baby in warm water at the center, empowered by being totally in charge. She said, "I can't believe the difference between the two births, not even two years apart. In the hospital I felt like it wasn't my birth or my baby. It was theirs. There is just no comparison—none!"

As more physicians and midwives embrace a perspective that views childbirth as a normal event, the gentle birth experience becomes a feasible option for all women. Birth can be experienced as an uncomplicated, natural event in which a woman can express her power, her emotions, and her sexuality and be supported

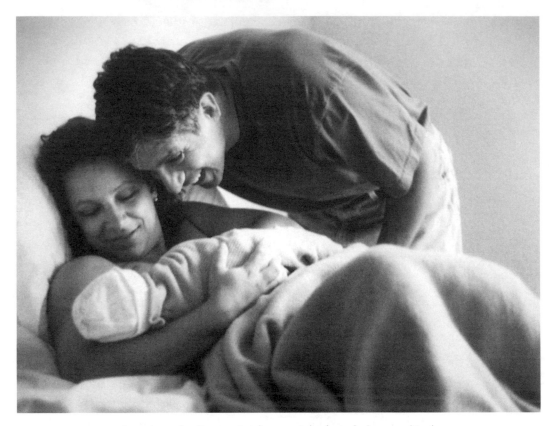

*A couple enjoys the first quiet hour with their baby at a birth center.*

by those people she loves. Her child can enter the world calmly, serenely, and joyously and can immediately become part of the family into which he has been born, being with his parents in the moments after birth and during the bonding period that follows. Childbirth can be child-centered, mother-friendly, family-centered; above all, it can be gentle while still being safe.

Some of the most influential reformers of childbirth practices over the last fifty years have been a handful of physicians who demonstrated the validity and safety of gentle birth practices. In more recent years, hundreds of childbirth educators, nurses, midwives, and doulas have begun to influence change on a global scale. Consumers who seek changes in hospital policy have seen that the joint cooperation of doctors, midwives, and nurses has been an essential ingredient in implementing these changes.

## BIRTH WITHOUT FEAR

One of the first proponents of "natural birth" was English obstetrician Grantly Dick-Read. He was outspoken about women's ability to birth normally and without pain. In his book *Childbirth without Fear: The Principles and Practices of Natural*

*Childbirth,* Dick-Read proposed that fear produces tension and tension produces pain. This was a radical theory in the 1930s, when anesthesia and painkillers were routinely administered for all normal births in the hospital. Read's book met strong opposition in England. He was even accused by some of his English colleagues of abusing women by refusing to medicate them. Though it was written in the 1930s, the book wasn't published in the United States until 1944.

Dick-Read's "radical" ideas asked women to view their bodies as healthy and to see pregnancy and birth as a natural process. He developed his theory of painless childbirth by watching women give birth normally, without assistance of any kind. He then analyzed the situations and noted what had helped each woman through her labor. Early in his career Dick-Read attended a home birth where the woman refused the chloroform he offered. Surprised by this, he asked the woman why she was so stoic. She turned to him, almost apologetic for her refusal of drugs, and said, "It didn't hurt, doctor. It wasn't meant to, was it?" This now-famous quote became Dick-Read's standard and was used by the women who began the "natural childbirth movement" in the United States. Dick-Read placed great emphasis on the role of birth attendants who were supportive of women. He felt that a woman should be educated about the process of labor and participate fully in her birth, and he instructed women in a series of breathing exercises that were designed to relax them and remove stress and fear during labor.

Dick-Read emphasized that even though a woman had the ability to birth normally, her doctor ultimately knew the best way to manage her labor and birth. Dick-Read's teachings were never given the opportunity to prove themselves on a wide scale because obstetricians objected strongly to the time-consuming "natural" birth. Hospitals and birthing practices in the United States during the 1940s and 1950s made it difficult, if not impossible, for women to achieve a purely "natural" birth. When American women were discovered on labor wards with Dick-Read's book tucked into their labor beds, doctors and nurses would ridicule them for wanting to participate in the birth of their babies.

At this time, however, a few childbirth educators, like pioneer Margaret Gamper of Chicago, started classes using Dick-Read's book as a natural childbirth guide. Gamper combined Dick-Read's methods of relaxation with her own massage techniques. She began teaching Chicago-area couples in 1947 and taught childbirth education for over thirty years. She influenced many birth practitioners, including Dr. Robert Bradley of Denver, who, with his nurse Rhondda Hartman, developed the Bradley method of "Husband-Coached Childbirth."[2] Even though Gamper's teachings, based on Dick-Read's book, were successful, the rules and regulations of hospital confinement stood in the way of many women who wanted to achieve a "natural birth."

## BIRTH WITHOUT PAIN

A new method of preparing for birth evolved in the 1950s in France. Ironically, the French phrase for labor is "entrer en douleurs," which loosely translated means, "enter the period of pain." Ferdinand Lamaze and Pierre Vellay, two French obstetricians, traveled to Russia in 1951 to observe methods of childbirth that utilized concentration and mind control. The Lamaze method of conditioning techniques was originally developed from Ivan Petrovich Pavlov's behavioral research. The Soviet government had adopted techniques based on Pavlovian principles as the official method of childbirth. The Russians believed that the fear and pain that women experienced during labor and birth was a learned response. The conditioning techniques replaced the fear responses with active breathing techniques to "recondition" a woman during labor. When a contraction came, instead of tightening with fear, a woman was trained to breathe, to massage her abdomen lightly, and to focus on an external point in the room. The two French physicians took this information back to Paris where they began to train women to use these techniques in hospital births.[3]

An American woman, Marjorie Karmel, who had come to France seeking support for a natural birth experience, met Dr. Lamaze by chance. She told him that the Dick-Read method could offer childbirth without fear; Lamaze responded by assuring her that he could help her have childbirth without pain. Karmel trained with Lamaze and his nurse and gave birth to her first child in a French hospital in 1956. That same year, the Pope sanctioned the use of the Lamaze, or psychoprophylactic, techniques for childbirth. Charged by the experience, Karmel began to write about it as soon as she returned to the United States. Her article was refused for publication on the grounds that it was too controversial—perhaps because the technique came from behind the Iron Curtain. *Harper's Bazaar* finally published Karmel's article in 1957. In 1959, after giving birth a second time using the Lamaze techniques, Karmel published the stories of her birth experiences in the now-famous book *Thank You, Dr. Lamaze.*[4]

Childbirth reformer Elizabeth Bing joined with Karmel and obstetrician Benjamin Segal to begin the American Society for Psychoprophylaxis in Obstetrics in 1960. They began to introduce the idea of Lamaze training to small groups of doctors and nurses. The two women felt it would be more effective to work within the hospital system in order to introduce the method. The organization encouraged couples to work with their physicians but never to question the physicians' ultimate authority. In Bing's book *Six Practical Lessons for an Easier Childbirth,* published in 1967, she states, "If he himself [the doctor] suggests medication, accept it willingly even though you don't feel the need for it. He undoubtedly has good reasons for his decision." *Six Practical Lessons* became the bible for parents and professionals involved in studying and teaching Lamaze. The book has had twenty printings and has been published in many foreign languages.[5]

At no point in the early development of the Lamaze techniques were women encouraged to work with their bodies, feelings, or emotions. Many women who studied the techniques felt that the methods actually served to separate women from their bodies. By focusing on something outside of herself, the birthing mother simply replaced the drugs with mind-control techniques, which limited conscious participation. The birth was still conducted the way her doctor felt was appropriate. The judgment of the doctor was considered infallible, and the mother was rarely included in decisions about her own labor and birth. Most hospitals today offer courses that have the name Lamaze but in actuality prepare women more for the experience of birth in that particular hospital than does the original French method of pain control. When Marjorie Karmel wrote the first edition of her book, psychoprophylaxis was the only nondrug alternative to complete narcosis. Today Lamaze courses often teach women about additional pain-control options, including the appropriate time to request an epidural or other medication. Hospital rules about fetal monitoring and other procedures are also stressed. The content of the courses is changing, but the physician and hospital maintain control of the birth experience.

One of the keys to Lamaze preparation was the training of the support person who would "coach" the mother throughout her labor and delivery. In France this person was usually the midwife. In the United States the midwife was replaced by the husband for several reasons. The number of hospital personnel needed to instruct and support the mothers on a one-to-one basis would be too great for the hospital to justify. So the husbands, who wanted to be with their wives in most cases anyway, were converted into labor-room attendants. Unfortunately, this new role changed the husband from a loving, emotionally supportive partner to an active member of the birthing "team." The doctor now depended on the husband to keep the "little woman" under control during her labor and birth.

Lamaze instructors today are a diverse group. The medical requirements to become an instructor were dropped, opening the program to motivated mothers, as well as nurses. The programs which prepare future childbirth educators very thoroughly cover all aspects of normal birth and require a preceptor to watch new instructors teach classes to pregnant couples. Attending births is also a critical part of the course.

Lamaze as it was originally taught is no longer promoted. A new approach which supports mother-friendly childbirth and standards for normal birth may have had its roots in France a half-century ago, but it is now focused on helping women to be in charge of their experience. Teachers today are often doulas, as well as childbirth educators. They work within the system to bring about changes.

There is still resistance from physicians as more couples understand what it means to receive mother-friendly care. When certified nurse-midwife Linda

Church, the mother of six children, began teaching Lamaze preparation for child-birth, she drew on her own experiences, including the frustrations that she had encountered as a patient in the hospital at which she taught. Church encouraged women to take control of their births and to ask for what they wanted. Some doctors called Church to complain about the fact that their patients had to be "rein-structed" about the proper way to give birth after they had taken her class; others admired the strength and courage that these educated couples displayed.

In the face of growing evidence doctors proceed to monitor, give epidurals, perform episiotomies, and use forceps and perform cesareans as they see necessary. The new hospital childbirth educator has a tough job ahead of her to "prepare" the couple for the rigors of the hospital childbirth experience.

## BIRTH WITHOUT VIOLENCE

With the introduction of medical interventions in childbirth, the bulk of midwife knowledge, based on thousands of years of tradition, was either lost or cast aside as nothing more than old wives' tales. French physician Frederick Leboyer was the first doctor to express what many women know instinctively: A newborn is a complete being with feelings, one who possesses the ability to perceive his or her environment and to interact with it. Leboyer had attended the birth of more than nine thousand babies when he wrote *Birth without Violence,* published in 1975. He suspected that conventional hospital births were actually causing damage to new-born children. Leboyer noted that in France, a nation of fifty million people, there were more than one million dysfunctional children. Leboyer wanted to know if this was related in some way to the manner in which the children were handled at birth.[6] As part of his research, Leboyer retired from his obstetrical practice and studied so-called primitive childbirth practices in a remote area of India for several years.

Leboyer's premise of birth without violence was considered revolutionary at the time. He considered the birth process from the infant's point of view and sug-gested measures that would greatly reduce trauma for the newborn child. Leboyer instituted practices that reduced the noise and lights in the delivery room and encouraged relaxation for the woman. As soon after the birth as possible, the baby was immersed in a basin filled with warm water that closely approximated the con-ditions of the womb. Leboyer felt that this helped the infant recover from the stress of its birth.

Couples who read and believed in Leboyer's work often met resistance from their physicians when they requested a Leboyer-style birth. The dim lights and warm baths were not welcome additions to the routines of doctors and hospitals. Many couples began to see birth from the baby's perspective, but Leboyer's theories virtually ignored the mother's participation in the birth of her baby. They considered the baby a victim of birth, the survivor of the "crushing" effects of the mother's uterine contractions. Women strived to have the best birth possible for the sake of the baby, but if the birth didn't go as planned or intervention became necessary, the couple was burdened with blame and guilt.

Despite this drawback, the impact of Leboyer's methods was extremely beneficial. Many midwives and couples used Leboyer's book as a reason to create alternatives for giving birth outside the hospital system. *Birth without Violence* became a best-seller in France, the United States, England, Germany, Sweden, Brazil, Italy, Holland, and other countries, indicating that the world was ready for a new understanding of birth. Today there is a much deeper understanding and awareness of just how vital it is to keep the birth gentle for the baby's sake, but it took other pioneers to lead the way.

## BIRTH REBORN

In 1962 Dr. Michel Odent went to Pithiviers, a small town near Paris, to take charge of surgery at the public hospital. His surgical responsibilities included overseeing the hospital's small maternity clinic, which served the women of Pithiviers and nearby villages. Odent had a special advantage in being a surgeon and not an obstetrician because he was not conditioned to use the obstetric rituals of the day. Odent depended on the six midwives who worked with him and learned obstetrics from their practical experience. He also talked with women and observed them giving birth. Odent and the midwives read and discussed books such as Leboyer's *Birth without Violence* and medical anthropologist Ivan Illich's *Medical Nemesis,* which examined what Illich described as the "disease of medical progress." Illich coined the term iatrogenic for "medically caused" illness, asserting that the medical establishment had become a major threat to health throughout the world.[7]

Illich's indictment of medical practices spoke strongly to the question Odent and the midwives at Pithiviers were asking themselves about childbirth: Are medical procedures and interventions necessary in a normal labor and birth? The doctor and midwives were further inspired by their own sense of discovery while working with and observing women in labor. Odent gradually developed birthing practices based on the simplification or elimination of unnecessary medical procedures like shaving, enemas, gowning, gloving, draping, and the lithotomy position. His clinic began to view childbirth not as a medically controlled event but as an integral part of the sexual and emotional life of a mother and her baby. Odent and the midwives saw themselves as "facilitators" whose task was to intervene as little as possible in this natural event, allowing the birth of a child to occur in an instinctual and gentle way.

In 1976, after gentle birth practices were implemented at Pithiviers, Odent saw the perinatal mortality rate at the hospital drop to 10 deaths per 1,000 live births. The overall perinatal mortality rate in France at that time was about 20 deaths per 1,000 live births.[8]

In 1984 Odent wrote *Birth Reborn,* which recounts his experiences in the Pithiviers clinic. Doris Haire, president of the American Foundation for Maternal and Child Health, stated in the foreword, "There have been very few milestones in the worldwide movement to reform and humanize the birth experience. *Birth Reborn* is one of them. Every life has but one beginning." Just as Leboyer's *Birth without Violence* raised the public's awareness concerning gentle birth for the baby, Odent's *Birth Reborn* offered a new perspective in gentle birth for the woman.

Odent left France in 1985 and began a private practice in London, where he founded the Primal Health Research Centre. Odent describes the "primal period" as encompassing fetal life, birth, and the year following birth. The research center has established a data bank with hundreds of articles published in authoritative medical and scientific journals, all of which explore the links between the "primal

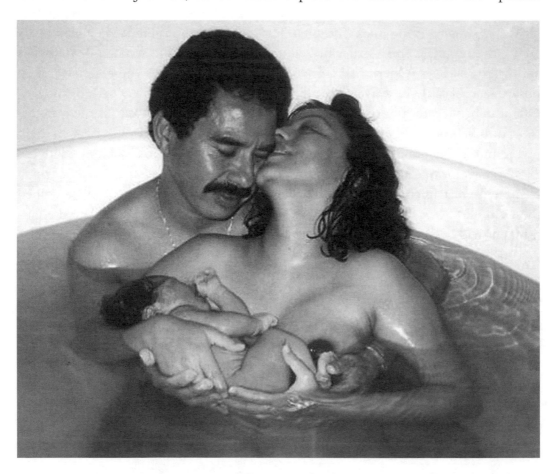

*Cradled in a circle of love*

period" and the health and behavior of children and adults.[9] He continues to publish books and numerous articles on this undeniable connection.

His work also became a catalyst for midwives and physicians all over the world
who read *Birth Reborn* and incorporated the idea, which they had instinctively
known for years: Birth is not a medical event, and the less intervention the better
the outcome.

## BIRTH WITHOUT RULES

Over the past twenty years there has been a rediscovery by midwives, hundreds of
physicians, and concerned couples of just what the cost has been for the mothers
and children who have experienced medically controlled births. Neither doctors
nor women have been able to distinguish between iatrogenic complications and
complications that would have developed had there not been medical interventions. Troublesome outcomes perpetuated the impression in women that their bodies were not trustworthy, so women yielded even more control to medical
management. Practitioners of gentle birth advocate that the medical establishment
trust women in childbirth, that they step back and respect what is natural, and that
they only apply technology when it is called for.

A young American mother living in Guatemala took these ideas to heart when
she read them in *Birth Reborn*. Jennifer Gallardo had attended births as a Spanish-
speaking doula in San Diego before moving to Guatemala, and she had heard that
the hospitals in her newly adopted country could be treacherous for women. She
was bound and determined to make a difference for women in Guatemala City.
Latin American women are taught to be compliant with those in authority, much
more so than women in the United States. Horror is the word she uses to describe
the conditions in Guatemala in 1994. Here she heard about the worst possible treatment of women: forced separation from their families, let alone their babies, after
birth; episiotomies performed in 100 percent of births; Pitocin used for every
woman; and babies being held upside down and slapped, just like in the movies.
She felt guided to assist the women with whom she shared stories of birth experiences that were anything but gentle. With the goal of becoming a midwife one day,
she sought to attend births in the city she now called home.

Gallardo gained permission to come in at night in one of the two public hospitals. Fluent in Spanish, she would coach women through the experience and try
to protect them from injury. On one of these occasions she was working with a
woman who was close to giving birth when the doctor came in to do the
"required" episiotomy. She suggested that she be allowed to show him how the
birth could be done without one. The midwife on duty and the doctor agreed to
let Gallardo put on gloves and show them how a natural birth was done. She had

read books and watched films, and attended many births as an assistant, but had never been responsible for catching the baby. All went exceedingly well and the mother's perineum remained intact even with one of the baby's hands presenting with the head. Gallardo was invited back. The doctor, it turns out, was intrigued and interested in learning more about gentle birth.[10]

Not long after this Gallardo started attending births in her home, where she would eventually open the Centro de Parto Natural Andaluz in 1994. The name *Andaluz* had a special meaning for the young midwife. In Spanish, *luz* means light and it is also the verb for birth. *Anda* means "to go to." Loosely translated it has the meaning, "to go into the light." Looking back, Gallardo relates that her calling to serve women came from a higher power:

> I knew that God wanted me to be there for those women in Guatemala and so many to follow. My family, though very supportive, sometimes worried about me going about in the streets of Guatemala City at all hours, but I felt not only guided, but protected. Everyone was happy when I started a birth center where women could come, instead of me going out to them.

While in Guatemala Gallardo gave birth to her next two babies at the birth center, as did four of her sisters, and all of the births were waterbirths. She was the midwife for the births of all of her sisters' children. The birth center ran successfully for four years before Gallardo and her husband decided to come back to the United States with their four children and establish a similar center here.

They chose to locate their facility in the Portland, Oregon area because the laws in Oregon were favorable for midwifery and birth centers. As soon as they arrived in the States, Gallardo became a Certified Professional Midwife and obtained a license to practice in Oregon. Searching for an ideal location, they found a new medical building being built overlooking a natural wetland and within a short driving distance of a university medical center. Andaluz Waterbirth Center opened in June of 1999, boasting three birth rooms, two with built-in deep baths for water labor and waterbirth. Gallardo had an expectation when the birth center opened that if she provided the Portland area with a place where women could feel loved, nurtured, and protected, they would come and birth without technology and drugs. A few women who came for tours decided that not having the option of an epidural or any pain medication was not right for them, but the majority of women came there seeking an alternative to the standard hospital practices of the area. Those women were seeking safe midwifery care that supported their choices.

A large winding carpeted staircase greets visitors as they enter the birth center building. Gallardo joked about having a birth center on the second floor. "If a woman comes to the center and can make it all the way up the stairs without stopping for a contraction, we know that her labor is not in full swing." A tour of the center conducted by one of the apprentice midwives on a busy Saturday morning reveals a richly decorated interior with large four-poster beds, couches in the birth rooms, and windows overlooking the wetlands. The bathtubs, which are built right into the room design rather than in separate bathrooms, are arrayed with vases of flowers in the corner and large and small candles along the ledge. One room has paintings and pictures of angels on three walls. The family room also serves as a classroom for weekly free birth preparation classes. Gallardo states, "I like couples to come to the birth center for their classes. They get used to the space and when babies are born here during a class, they all feel so much more a part of the birthing process."

The kitchen is abundantly stocked with all kinds of drinks, snacks, and breakfast foods—the most requested type of food following a birth. A small laundry facility and supply room is busy as last night's birth laundry is being processed. There is a play-house built into the walls of the family/waiting room full of building toys. Everything is immaculately clean and fresh, with colors that are harmonious, warm, and restful. Large black-and-white photographs of pregnant women and mothers with nursing babies decorate the walls. There are photo albums full of images of the previous six hundred client births—almost entirely waterbirths—taken by the midwives at the center, who are all now amateur photographers. In the reception area an older woman is anxiously waiting to enter one of the birthing rooms. Her daughter-in-law has just given birth to her first grandchild. The sounds of a newborn baby and the happy murmurings of his loving family could be faintly heard down the hall.

Gallardo insists that all clients take a birth class at the center so that the midwives can reinforce the normalcy of birth and give couples with similar due dates the opportunity to form support groups outside of class. Gallardo explains,

> The classes evolved to our own style of teaching about childbirth, which includes an exploration of all the issues that are important to a family. We like to work with the couples so that they know what to expect during labor, all the while reassuring them that their bodies know how to give birth. We always have mothers who have already given birth here come into class and share their experience. It is very good to let the expectant mothers know what their lives will be like the week after the baby is born, too.

The importance of having a relaxed relationship to the birthplace and the midwives cannot be underestimated. Each time a mother drops by or has a prenatal visit the birth center becomes more familiar. When she eventually arrives to have her baby, she does not have to cope with adjusting to a strange place.

When the laboring woman arrives at the birth center, she and her partner have notified the midwives and know which room they will use for their labor and birth. The women voice their preference of rooms prenatally and the midwife on call makes sure the temperature is right, the candles are lit, and the bath is ready for the mother as she arrives. The woman may have as many companions as she wants, but the midwives avoid treating the birth as a party. They try to selectively reduce the number of spectators to ensure the mother's privacy. The woman is expected to wear her own comfortable clothing, or she may choose to not wear anything. She can decorate the room with personal possessions. She is also encouraged to eat lightly whenever she is hungry, and fluids are made readily available.

Women may move freely about during all stages of labor. They can walk in the halls, go outside, climb up and down the entrance stairway and can give birth in whatever position they choose. Infants are never separated from their mothers after the birth except for valid medical reasons. All of these choices allow women to focus on the process of giving birth. After the birth, the midwives request that mother and baby stay for a designated period, usually six to twelve hours, to be evaluated. If complications are going to develop with the baby, they will usually occur within the first few hours. Couples don't seem to mind staying in the comfort of the birth center after the birth. The mother and father relax and explore the presence of their new little being, enjoy a catered meal, bathe in the deep bath and accept visitors before going home. Some couples even stay a full twenty-four hours, sleeping at the center that first night.

Birth centers just like Andaluz are in all parts of the United States and North America. Most have been built within the past ten to fifteen years. Some are operated by physicians, but the majority were established by midwives, both certified nurse-midwives and certified professional midwives. National Association of Childbearing Centers founder Kitty Ernst, CNM, states, "Every community ideally should have a birthing center—a place where women of childbearing age can receive a wide array of services, including classes, moral support, and companionship." Indeed, many cultures throughout history have had the tradition of central locations for giving birth.

At a birth center a woman is not left alone during her labor unless she requests privacy. The same nurse or midwife is there with the laboring mother from the moment she enters the door until she leaves with her new baby. Once women experience a birth-center birth, the continuity of care brings them back for all of their babies. Ernst states emphatically, "We must move normal birth out of the hospital. Birth needs to remain a private and personal matter."[11] The birth center will continue to play a big part in the future of gentle birth.

## BIRTH WITH CONSCIOUSNESS

As we learn and understand more about the seeds of human consciousness and brain development we begin to see how much our lives are influenced by our prenatal experiences of life and the birth event. Looking at the experience of birth from the perspective of the baby who is being born, or looking back at how we ourselves were born, gives us an entirely new consciousness about conception, pregnancy, birth, and early parenting. The pre- and perinatal psychology movement is revealing more and more about the roots of the human psyche.

Author and birth activist Jeannine Parvati Baker introduced the concept of conscious conception two decades ago when she shared her insights regarding birth and parenting as a spiritual path. Baker strongly believed that a conscious communication was happening between the spirit of the child and the couple who wanted to become pregnant. She encouraged couples to approach sex thoughtfully with a focus on the creative energy that would enhance conception. She believed this mindfulness was a path that would lead to the healing of parent, child, and planet.[12] What Baker wrote from intuition and inspiration in the 1980s has now been proven in scientific and medical literature.

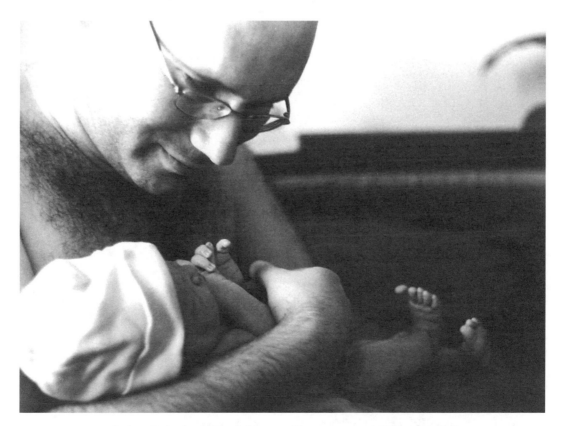

*A father feels the bliss of skin-to-skin contact with his new baby.*

Michel Odent presents an effective case in several of his books and journal articles about how infants develop the capacity to love prenatally and through the birth experience.[13] The secretion of oxytocin, known as "the love hormone," and its presence in mothers and newborns sheds new light on why some people turn out the way they do. Births involving the use of drugs prevent the normal production of this crucial hormone. Studies have been published that link drug-managed births to different forms of impaired capacity to love, such as autism, sociopathic and criminal behavior, and even schizophrenia.[14]

The effect of bonding or attachment between mother and newborn has been the subject of much research. Animal studies showed us over twenty-five years ago that mammals that were separated from their newborns at birth later rejected their babies at an alarming rate.[15] Dr. Niles Newton revealed that newborn mammals whose births were interrupted through disturbing the privacy of the birth environment, interventions, or cesarean, or whose mothers were unconscious, had a much more difficult time establishing a bond with their mothers.[16] Sometimes those mothers totally rejected their offspring.

Keeping the baby and mother together as an intact dyad should be the ultimate goal of every birth provider, but more often than not this is not the case. Hospital routines and birth practices that interfere with the bonding of a mother and baby have been associated with the development of chronic childhood health problems. Researcher and psychotherapist Antonio Madrid, Ph.D., relates how he first was introduced to the possibility that there was a connection between a traumatic birth experience with interruption of bonding and the development of asthma in the child:

> The first time this issue was drawn forcibly to our attention involved the case of a severely asthmatic eight year old girl. She was on several kinds of medication and was placed on steroids several times each year. She was frequently taken to the emergency room—in the two months before we saw her, she had been to the emergency room four times. Our staff tried to help this girl with an array of hypnotic techniques, but we eventually concluded that we could not relieve her symptoms.
>
> The mother, however, wanted to continue counseling herself, and we worked with her for eight more months. In the fifth month of therapy, while talking about her daughter, she said that much to her shame she did not feel any love for her daughter. She then went on to describe the conditions of her pregnancy and delivery. It was a birth nightmare. The child's father had left her three months before the birth, totally devastating her. Her own mother had been in the labor room and berated her throughout the entire process. The medical staff greatly disappointed her. She was harangued and insulted by a labor room nurse. Her own physician was not there and her baby was delivered by a stranger.

Because the baby girl was born jaundiced, she was immediately taken away for treatment, and the mother did not see her baby for eight hours. When the baby was allowed to come home she became ill again and had to return to the hospital for almost a week. When the baby recovered and finally returned home, the mother reported that the baby felt so strange that she felt like telling the nurses to keep it. We asked her to change the birth in her imagination with the help of hypnosis. We walked the mother through a perfect birth—this time there was no sadness about the separation from the father of her child, her own mother was not in the room, a good nurse was present, the correct doctor was in attendance, and a healthy baby was born who stayed with her. We asked the mother to keep this history as a new psychological birth history to use whenever she wanted. This whole procedure took about 20 minutes.

At the end of three more months of counseling, without again returning to this birth scene whatsoever, she reported that she was leaving the state. At the end of her final session, she stopped in the office doorway, came back in, and said: "Oh, remember that session where we did that hospital thing? Well, my daughter's asthma went away after that and it hasn't returned except for one time, when she was away from home; and it got better as soon as she got back home. She has not been to an emergency room since that session. And she does not need any medicine. And remember how I never felt any love for her? Well, I do now."[17]

This startling revelation sparked Madrid's interest in the possible connections between failed bonding and episodes of moderate to severe childhood asthma. He has found that removal of the infant alone is not usually enough to cause irreparable damage, but when coupled with a mother who is emotionally unavailable or unresponsive due to her own emotional trauma, the stage is set for problems. Madrid and his group of psychotherapists went on to further study childhood asthma and possible treatments.

The first results of the Madrid study reveal a definite correlation between lack of attachment, emotional difficulties in the mother, and the presence of childhood asthma. As a result of treating the mothers with regressive therapy and having them "correct" the emotional trauma and script a new gentle birth experience, the children not only improved, but some of them were totally free of asthma, even without being treated psychologically themselves.[18]

Doctors Marshall Klaus and John Kennell pointed out the strong connections between a mother's emotions and the baby's behavior in their work on bonding back in the 1970s. They suggested that a mother's ability to bond with her child can be impeded if she is experiencing a competing emotion. The competing emotion must be so intense that it could block out the bonding emotions. Such emotions include grief: grief for the death or loss of someone close, grief following a previous miscarriage or baby death, or the shock of a divorce or separation.[19]

Other competing emotions include intense fear, severe depression, and serious marital problems. Drug addiction can act as a competing emotion, as the mother is powerfully bonded to the drug and emotionally unavailable to her baby. Ambivalence about being pregnant in the first place, or not wanting the baby during pregnancy or at birth, inevitably results in a lack of bonding.

All the studies agree that the ingredients of a gentle birth serve to support the mother so that she falls completely and inexorably in love with the baby. When the lights are low; when the mother is supported, not observed; when her body rhythms are not interrupted; when she is not stimulated with artificial hormones or numbed with drugs; when she is allowed complete and uninterrupted access to her newborn, both mother and baby experience the start of life with a sensitive aware-ness. As the child grows into adulthood, she will have more vibrant health, be more intelligent, display empathy, be well adjusted and more confident, and overall will be a better citizen of the world.

Joseph Chilton Pearce summed it up beautifully when he stated, "We either understand the psychology of birth and its impact on the evolution of human life or we can choose to continue defending ourselves."[20]

## WOMEN TAKE BACK THEIR BIRTHS

Since the early 1950s, consumers, the recipients of maternity care, have voiced strong opinions about the necessity for a gentler, more humane system of maternity care. Entire organizations have evolved to deal with the results of women's birth experiences in the hospital system. In 1958 an anonymous nurse wrote a letter to the *Ladies' Home Journal* detailing the cruelty she saw in the maternity practices of the day. For well over a year the magazine was flooded with letters from mothers writing to confirm these allegations. Stories abounded of women who were left alone, tied to delivery tables, manipulated with drugs to either delay or hasten delivery (depending on the doctor's schedule), and kept from giving birth because their doctors had not yet arrived. Mothers wrote that their children had been brain-damaged as a direct result of the hospital personnel's violent treatment, even abuse, inflicted on the women during labor and delivery. During this same time, parent education groups were developing across the country in an effort to remove some of the fear surrounding the birth process and to improve birth management in local hospitals.

One such group was led by Lester Hazel and her husband Bill in the Washington, D.C., area. They traveled to the Maternity Center Association (MCA) in New York, which was founded in 1915, to learn about childbirth education and the Dick-Read method of childbirth. Like other parent groups, they sought to improve obstetrical medical management through the addition of services such as childbirth education, breast-feeding instruction, family participation, and rooming-in, without alienating anyone within the existing medical system.

In 1959 the MCA sponsored a gathering of all those who were interested in childbirth reform. Many of the parent childbirth education groups across the country attended. The International Childbirth Education Association (ICEA) emerged from this gathering, joining thirty parent groups together for their first national meeting in 1960.[21] The beliefs held by this organization were not radical or revolutionary, but maintained that birth belonged to the parents and not to the hospital. The members of the organization felt that each couple had the right to choose the kind of birth experience that was right for them and safe for their baby.

The ICEA brought together not only parents but professionals who desired change. Consultants for the group included anthropologists Margaret Mead and Ashley Montagu, who were both outspoken advocates for revision of maternity care in the United States. The ICEA, which has remained primarily a consumer organization, today has over 11,000 members worldwide and publishes an array of educational books, tapes, and videos. They continue to support their original beliefs that birth belongs to each individual family and that parents have the right to make informed choices.

The founding of La Leche League International (LLLI) in 1956 by a group of concerned women from the Chicago area is an example of a strong consumer-led coalition. The seven women cofounders had breast-fed their babies without the support or encouragement of their doctors or the nurses in the hospital. One of the founders, Marian Tompson, thought that it was strange that mothers who bottle-fed their babies were given much support, but women who wanted to breast-feed their babies were consistently advised to give up. The plan of the founding members was to offer encouragement and information about breast-feeding to their friends and neighbors through small support-group classes.

Doctors initially objected to these women giving out "professional medical information," but LLLI members held fast and increased their efforts in researching the effects of formula and early solids on the infant, as well as the emotional aspects of breast-feeding. League members resolved that they were, after all, the ones who were breast-feeding, not the doctors. LLLI today prints materials, sponsors seminars and support groups, trains facilitators, and encourages breast-feeding worldwide.

LLLI, though singular in its focus on breast-feeding, has provided a tangible network of support for women who seek alternative birth options. Referrals to sympathetic doctors and home-birth midwives are easily found at local LLLI meetings. Women tell of their experiences in finding supportive practitioners, as well as sharing their birth and breast-feeding stories. LLLI has been responsible for the demedicalization of breast-feeding and continues to have a strong influence on the humanization of childbirth practices.

The women's movement in the 1960s and 1970s created an atmosphere that led women to question medical practices concerning their bodies. The feminist movement spent much more time claiming the right to abortion than it did in claiming the right to natural childbirth; burning bras was not necessarily an effort to make breast-feeding easier. But some feminists took up the call for reform, claiming that the right to choice in childbirth is the right to ultimately control their bodies.

In 1971 the Boston Women's Health Collective produced a book titled *Our Bodies, Ourselves* that stressed the importance of women reclaiming responsibility for their bodies. The authors felt it was essential for women to know how their bodies functioned, especially during pregnancy, labor, and birth. The book contained pictures of home births in the Boston area and encouraged women to accept the responsibility for their birth outcomes by becoming educated in all areas of reproductive health. The Boston Women's Health Collective introduced women to the idea of the transforming power of birth, and to midwives who could assist them as opposed to physicians who would try to control the physiology of the birth process.

During the 1970s many counterculture groups emerged and began using *Our Bodies, Ourselves* as a guide for women's health care. These groups were most prevalent on the West Coast, but there were others sprinkled throughout the United States. One such group started The Farm in Tennessee, an intentional community of originally three hundred like-minded vegetarians and would-be farmers. In the early 1970s founders Ina May Gaskin and her husband Stephen attended the births of women in this alternative community and began teaching what Ina May called "spiritual midwifery" in her 1975 book of the same name. This couple saw themselves as traditionalists, yet at the same time they felt strongly that women had the right to choose where and how they were to give birth. In Ina May's words, "We feel that returning the major responsibility for normal childbirth to well-trained midwives rather than have it rest with a predominantly male and profit-oriented medical establishment is a major advance in self-determination for women."[22]

This rise of home-birth activism in the 1970s, fueled by freedom of choice, sparked the reemergence of the midwife all across the United States. The gentle birth revolution has spread from places like The Farm to middle America. Other grassroots organizations have formed to educate both consumers and professionals. The International Association of Parents and Professionals for Safe Alternatives in Childbirth (NAPSAC) has been working toward maternity care reform since 1975. Founded by Lee and David Stewart after the births of their five children, all born at home into the hands of their father, NAPSAC worked throughout the 1970s and 1980s to support couples and provide legal aid for midwives and doctors who found themselves battling the system. Sometimes couples would use litigation to achieve their rights to an out-of-hospital birth, relying on organizations like NAPSAC for support. NAPSAC is active to this day in the reform movement.

One voice of protest that has made a significant contribution to making birth more humane is that of Esther Booth Zorn, founder of the Cesarean Prevention Movement (CPM). In 1982, Zorn and Liz Belden Handler were sitting at Zorn's dining room table discussing, among other things, the rising rates of cesarean births and how impossible it was for women to give birth again vaginally after even one cesarean. Armed with Nancy Wainer Cohen's historic book, *Silent Knife,** published in 1983, Zorn and a small group of women sparked a movement toward the prevention of primary cesareans, as well as motivating mothers to give birth vaginally after a cesarean. They also helped mothers recover from the debilitating effects of cesarean births.

Just two years after the founding of CPM, the American College of Obstetricians and Gynecologists issued guidelines promoting vaginal births after previous cesareans. Those guidelines were revised in 1988 and a flurry of research and controversy was sparked. CPM changed its name to International Cesarean Awareness Network (ICAN) in 1992 to reflect a more positive stance. ICAN works today to battle the stigma that cesarean birth carries with regard to a woman's reproductive capabilities and its negative effects on her own thinking. Beginning with grassroots networking, and ultimately establishing chapters in cities in every state in the United States and many in Canada and Mexico, ICAN is a great example of what women can accomplish when they are motivated to take back their births.

In 2004 mothers with small babies in slings and strollers, and fathers with babies and toddlers in backpacks, staged multiple protests around the country. They were marching in defense of choice—the right to choose to give birth vaginally after a previous, possibly unnecessary, cesarean. Hundreds of families in multiple cities took placards to the streets in front of hospitals that had ended VBAC possibilities because of fear of liability and litigation. The pendulum swings perpetually and ICAN is helping it swing back in favor of families.

In 1996 a group of mothers, who actually met through the Internet, founded a grassroots organization to promote the midwives model of care and to bring awareness to the public about midwifery in the United States. Citizens for Midwifery provides information and support to consumers and advises mothers in all geographical areas on how to use activism to change not only attitudes but policy. Mother and activist Susan Hodges, one of the original founders, originally worked as a liaison between Midwives Alliance of North America and consumer groups in her home state of Georgia. With her guidance many states have now formed or

---

*The term VBAC—vaginal birth after cesarean—was coined by Nancy Wainer Cohen.

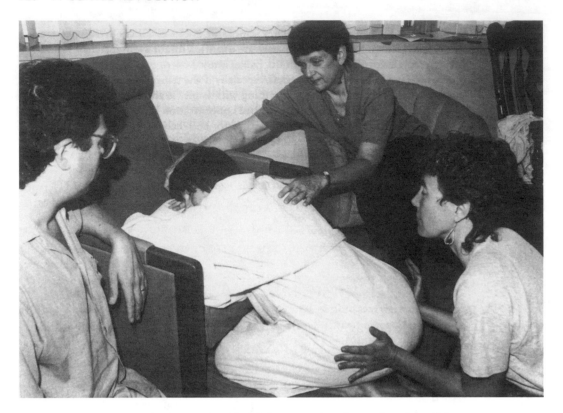

*Partner, doula, and midwife keep mother focused and confident.*

reenergized "friends of midwives" organizations. These groups aid parents in understanding the applicable laws and licensing in their individual states and they communicate the desire for the midwives model of care to be accepted as the standard of practice in all birth settings. Citizens for Midwifery raises consumer awareness and "how to" activism into an art form through its exceptionally informative Web site.

A 1995 Lamaze International conference in Chicago was the backdrop for meetings of individuals and heads of other maternity organizations around the United States, as well as the Lamaze leadership. The common thread in that meeting was the acknowledgment that the medical establishment was not heeding the overwhelming body of scientific evidence which demonstrated over and over the detrimental effects of interfering with normal childbirth. The question was posed, "How can we, as a group of concerned birth professionals, join together to effect change?" The answer did not come from that meeting. Instead, it generated more questions and more meetings until the Coalition for Improving Maternity Services (CIMS) was born later that year.

It was no easy task getting a group of powerful opinionated individuals, many of whom were representing membership organizations, to come to a consensus on one of the most powerful documents created about birth in the last century. The

Mother-Friendly Childbirth Initiative was ratified by this core group in July of 1996. It not only states the problems with maternity care, but provides the expectation of normalcy when it is used as a guideline for providers and hospitals to follow. The Coalition has begun the process of "grading" hospitals that want to become designated as mother-friendly.[23]

To be considered mother-friendly the hospital must first abide by the precepts of UNICEF and the World Health Organization's recommendations for being baby-friendly. Very clear and precise instructions are given on achieving baby-friendly status in any hospital: All women need to hear about the benefits and management of breast-feeding. Nurses need to be able to help mothers initiate breast-feeding soon after birth. Newborns should only be fed breast milk—no water or artificial baby milk (formula), no artificial nipples or pacifiers. This recommendation is difficult to follow when drug companies load up maternity units with sample bottles of formula, which end up going home with new mothers—against WHO and UNICEF guidelines. I was shocked to find when I was researching the new edition of this book that in the United States only forty-two hospitals out of almost four thousand are designated as baby-friendly.

Other prerequisites to become recognized as mother-friendly include reducing the cesarean birth rate to no more than 15 percent; supporting vaginal birth after cesarean at a rate of at least 60 percent; eliminating routine interventions that are not supported by the medical evidence; and educating maternity staff on ways to manage pain without the use of drugs. In other words, hospitals must show evidence of practicing gentle birth. [For a reprint of both the Baby-Friendly Hospital Initiative (BFHI) and the Mother-Friendly Childbirth Initiative (MFCI), go to the Web site: www.motherfriendly.org]

The MFCI mission is to promote a wellness model of maternity care that will improve birth outcomes and substantially reduce costs. This evidence-based mother-, baby-, and family-friendly model focuses on prevention and wellness as the alternatives to high-cost screening, diagnosis, and treatment programs. It is the hope of the coalition founders that the Mother-Friendly Childbirth Initiative will be the standard to which all maternity care practices will aspire.

The dividing lines have been drawn, setting the stage for revolutionary or adversarial activity. The consumer remains the last to be consulted when decisions concerning maternity care are made. Yet birthing women do have the power—the consumer power—to change the current system. Thousands of letters in support of midwifery-based maternity services poured into the White House during the health care reform committee discussions in 1993. Consumers can and are changing the face of maternity care.

There are many individual revolutionaries—thousands upon thousands of mothers, fathers, midwives, doctors, psychologists, social workers, and legislators, all of whom want to advance toward an integration of holistic and humanistic principles in the birth place. Anthropologist Robbie Davis-Floyd, along with childbirth reformer Michel Odent, share the belief that we will quickly move into a "post-electronic age of childbirth" when women are again in control of birth, and technology takes its rightful place as a tool for special circumstances.[24]

Odent stresses that if we care about the well-being of the human race, we must urgently attend to finding ways of ensuring that pregnancy and birth are allowed to proceed undisturbed, as nature has designed.[25] Gentle birth holds the keys that are essential if we are to ensure our capacity both to love and be loved, and thus our long-term mental health and well-being and that of our planet.

## CHAPTER FIVE

# Midwifery in America: A Growing Tradition

The term midwife (meaning literally "with woman") is often used to describe anyone, other than a doctor, who helps a woman through her pregnancy, labor, and birth. As we saw in chapter 3, women traditionally have attended other women in childbirth, drawing on the strength of their own experiences of giving birth to support and empower them. The knowledge of birthing was passed from generation to generation. This continuity of tradition was interrupted by the development of obstetrics as a profession and the institutionalization of childbirth.

The traditions of childbirth are now being restored by the women who are educating other women to reclaim mastery over their bodies and their ability to give birth. Traditions of prevention rather than cure, as well as respect for intimacy, privacy, family integrity, responsibility, patience, and the understanding of what it means to be a woman, are some of the "tools" a midwife uses during a labor and birth. It is the consumer, the birthing woman and her family, who has led this resurgence, for ultimately she is the one who gives birth; the midwife or obstetrician simply attends her. Thanks to these women the profession of midwifery, virtually eliminated by the American Medical Association (AMA) in the 1920s and 1930s, is reemerging in the United States. During the past decade the number of women choosing care by midwives has doubled.[1]

When midwifery statistics were first recorded in 1975, less than one percent of the babies in the United States were welcomed by midwives. In 2002, that percentage had risen to 10.[2] The path has been an uphill climb, but women now want their midwives and are requesting them with greater and greater frequency. A 2003 survey in *American Baby* magazine revealed that mothers who received midwifery care had more satisfying births, spent more time with their providers, and didn't ask for as much medication as the women who were attended by physicians.[3] Outside of the United States and Canada, the entire industrialized world uses the services of midwives as the gatekeepers for pregnant and birthing women.

Pediatrician Marsden Wagner, former European head of the World Health Organization (WHO), Women's and Children's Health Division, has appeared before numerous legislative committees and explained the policy that WHO has maintained a for thirty years: "[C]are during normal pregnancy, birth and following birth should be the duty of the midwifery profession."[4] Here in the United States the midwife continues to struggle to find her rightful place.

## THE MIDWIVES MODEL OF MATERNITY CARE

Midwifery and medicine are two distinct disciplines, based on different approaches to pregnancy and birth. The midwives model recognizes that pregnancy and birth are natural processes. It focuses on the intimate relationship between mother and child during pregnancy, birth, and breast-feeding. It better understands the needs of mother and baby as a finely tuned, integrated system. The midwives model encourages women to be in charge of their lives and their experiences. When a mother cooperates with her environment and a balance is established between herself and her relationships, she shares this balance with her child. All organisms on earth constantly seek a balanced state. The midwives model of care recognizes the dynamics of the mind-body connection. Midwives often encourage women to see pregnancy as an opportunity to heal imbalances in self and relationship. A midwife's role is not to manage, but to support, encourage, and guide. A midwife does not empower women; she assists women as they empower themselves.

The medical model, on the other hand, views pregnancy and the birth process on a very physical level. Doctors see the potential for physical problems that could occur for the mother and baby, focusing on the uterus and the fetus, and dealing with them from a technological perspective. The medical model seeks to manage each pregnancy and birth as if it were already something impaired or broken. The midwives model of care sees pregnancy as part of a life continuum incorporating all of life's experiences, including childbirth. The midwives model also recognizes and acknowledges the influence of many factors on the outcome of pregnancy and birth. Midwives honor and support a woman's right to make her own decisions, giving her the tools to make informed choices. The medical model of care requires mothers to obediently follow all of the recommendations of the doctor and labor nurses without the benefit of fully informed consent.

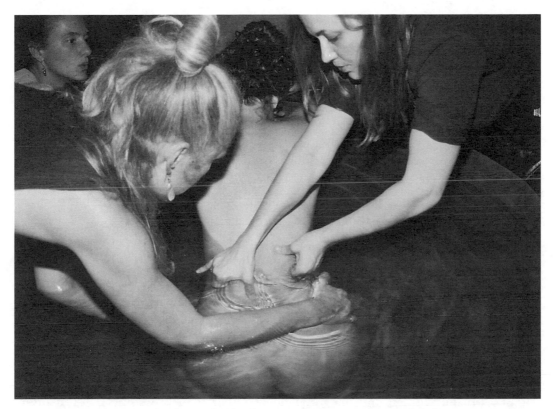

*A midwife and doula work together to provide a mother with a hip squeeze and sacral pressure.*

There is a saying that simplifies the difference between the midwives model of care and the medical model: "Midwives see birth as a miracle, and only mess with it if there's trouble. Obstetricians see birth as trouble, and if they don't mess with it, it's a miracle."

There are physicians who practice the midwives model of care and there are, unfortunately, midwives who don't practice it. Physicians and midwives who do follow the midwives model of care embrace a noninterventionist approach to childbearing that lets nature take its course during labor and birth. When they remove themselves from actively managing a birth, the practitioners experience labor and birth from a special vantage point. They can watch, listen, and observe each woman as she gives birth in a way that is powerful, life-affirming, and joyful. They become more conscious of the connections between attitude and outcome, between fear and failure, between trust and surrender. Midwives have become very adept at recognizing energy blocks that can influence the outcome of a birth. Midwives often draw upon their intuitive skills more than their acquired knowledge, blending art and skill to make decisions and to facilitate normal birth. Medical anthropologist Robbie Davis-Floyd describes this art and skill in interviews that she conducted with midwives for the book *Childbirth and Authoritative Knowledge: Cross-Cultural Perspectives.*[5] Inner knowing constitutes a primary source of authoritative knowledge for the midwife. She relies upon her intuition to guide her, often setting aside the medical model protocol or requirement to assess other reasons for circumstances.

When certified nurse-midwife Mary Jackson observed a client's labor slow down and stall for an unusually long time, she sensed that there was something holding the mother back that was not physical. Her intuition told her that there was something keeping the mother from opening up. Following her intuition, Jackson decided to sensitively discuss her feelings with the woman, who reacted by telling her midwife that there was indeed something holding her back.

She said she had had an abortion when she was younger, and had never told her husband. She said she was afraid that he would think less of her for having had one. Jackson encouraged her to share her secret with her husband. So she left the couple alone, and the woman was able to discuss her fears with her husband. Many tears were shed by both husband and wife, and they soon called for their midwife. The woman's contractions had intensified, and within the hour their baby son was born. Trusting her intuition, Jackson had recognized the blocked energy and helped the woman get in touch with it by turning inward. The midwife had focused on the woman and her inner needs rather than providing medical intervention for a stalled labor.

## Putting Normal into Perspective

While being experts in normal birth, midwives are also experienced in identifying, and are prepared to deal with, the minor complications that sometimes arise during birth. When midwives come together, whether locally in support groups and peer review meetings or nationally at midwifery conventions, they share their best or their scariest birth stories. They use these sessions to educate themselves and to receive support from other practicing midwives. Actually, whenever two or more midwives meet, birth stories naturally abound. I have experienced many of these sessions and have heard hundreds of firsthand accounts of midwives dealing successfully with problem births.

*Midwifery Today* magazine, founded to support the growth of the midwifery profession, sponsors sessions like this and has published a series of books entitled *Tricks of the Trade.*[6] Each one of the books contains specific advice, usually based on experience, for dealing with the concerns of pregnancy, birth, and postpartum care.

A common concern of couples contemplating a home birth is how midwives handle emergencies or complications during labor and birth. Remember that midwives see only healthy women and screen for problems during pregnancy. A midwife will automatically refer women with pregnancy-related problems to an obstetrician. She will continually check and observe a woman's physical and emotional state during regular prenatal visits. Midwives do not hesitate to refuse to attend a home birth if they are even slightly suspicious of serious complications that may require a hospital setting.

Some conditions that most providers assume are complications of pregnancy are actually reactions of the normal physiology of the placenta. For example, all women experience a lower level of hemoglobin in the blood during the last months of pregnancy. Commonly thought to be anemia, it is actually a normal reaction to an increase in blood volume, which dilutes the concentration of iron in the blood.[7] Giving iron supplements and requiring women to be "risked out" of home births is unfortunately not based on science, but superstition. Likewise, higher blood pressure can sometimes be an indication for transfer of care to an obstetrician, but most often it indicates a normal function.[8] A midwife will evaluate all conditions which may be influencing the blood pressure reading.

A midwife's primary objective during pregnancy is to assist the mother in growing a very healthy placenta. By counseling the mother about nutrition, stress, and exercise, the midwife knows that complications in labor can usually be avoided. A common diagnosis in pregnancy that may cause a woman to be deemed high risk is termed "gestational diabetes." The commonsense nutritional advice that midwives give women, which includes avoiding sugary drinks and foods and eating plenty of complex carbohydrates, is quite effective at controlling what has been called by some physiologists a "diagnosis looking for a disease."[9]

Of course, even when mothers do all the right things to prepare for childbirth, some births will present problems. Traditionally, midwives try "every trick in the book" when dealing with a slow or difficult labor before calling in a physician or transporting a laboring woman to the hospital. The "tricks" that midwives use include simple techniques for relaxation and breathing but may also include complementary therapies including energetic bodywork, massage, herbs, homeopathy, and acupuncture. These techniques, which some midwives study in depth for years, are utilized with the understanding that childbirth is a physical, mental, emotional, and spiritual process that needs to occur in a balanced and integrated way.

The midwife at a home birth will have all her instruments laid out, readily accessible, and the oxygen tank turned on, ready for an emergency should one arise. Many couples worry that the umbilical cord may be wrapped around the baby's neck, a very common occurrence that can be easily handled by a midwife in a home birth. About 25 percent of all babies have the cord wrapped around their necks. A midwife feels the tautness of the cord and slips it over the baby's head or down over the shoulder. If it is too tight to move, the midwife clamps and cuts it, knowing that the rest of the baby must be born as quickly as possible. Such babies may also need a little help getting their breathing started.

Some babies get stuck, a situation called shoulder dystocia. They are gently eased out with position changes by the mother, manipulations of the baby, and, very rarely, emergency episiotomies. I experienced a dystocia situation during the birth of my own third child. Labor had been progressing very quickly and smoothly. I spent early labor walking up and down a quiet street, occasionally hugging a tree during a strong contraction. After only two hours I climbed into our outdoor spa. There I labored for another two hours and then started to push. The midwife had climbed into the water with me and my partner, and just after the baby's head emerged, she checked to determine whether the cord was around the baby's neck. It was not, but she did find that the cord had partially emerged with the head and was being pinched between the baby's shoulder and my pubic bone. In addition, the baby was stuck. His heartbeat decreased rapidly. The midwife acted quickly to rotate the baby's shoulders and bring him out of me, through the water, and up into my arms. Abraham was limp and blue, but he pinked up right away and nursed within the first three minutes after his birth.

When a situation needs more than the midwife can offer, she has the mother transported to the hospital. Midwives transport laboring women to hospitals for a variety of reasons. The most common reason for transports are labors that progress slowly. Women with slow labors often get tired and need assistance with fluid administration and possible augmentation of labor with synthetic oxytocin. If the midwife has good rapport with the backup doctor and the hospital, the birth can often proceed as if the mother and midwife were still at home. When Jill Cohen, an Oregon midwife, takes a client to the hospital, her consulting physician listens carefully, asks Jill her opinion, makes suggestions, and sometimes allows her to "catch" the baby.

Not every hospital is that welcoming or accommodating. In the past, midwives have had to drop women off at the door in fear of going into the medical environment. Most midwives today must have a relationship with a supervising physician so that better transfer of care happens for the mothers. It is possible to have a smooth system of transfer of care from home to hospital, but more education needs to take place for both midwives and hospital doctors and nurses.

## THE EVOLUTION OF MIDWIFERY

For the consumer, the different types of midwives and the terminology describing them may be extremely confusing. There are lay midwives, direct-entry midwives, certified midwives, certified professional midwives, certified nurse-midwives, and spiritual midwives. No wonder some people ask, "What is a midwife?"

There are two main categories of midwives in the United States—certified nurse-midwives (CNM), who are trained in both nursing and midwifery, and direct-entry midwives (DEM), who trained as midwives without being nurses first. CNMs, are those with formal medical education. In order to become a CNM in the United States, a person must attend an accredited school of nursing and receive either an associate's degree or a bachelor's degree in the applied science of nursing. The individual must pass the licensing examination in his or her state and usually must complete one year of work in a hospital labor and delivery area before being admitted to one of forty-six nurse-midwifery training programs in the country.

Within the category of direct-entry midwives are several subcategories reflecting the varying legal status of these midwives in different states and the fact that until recently there was no nationally recognized credential available for direct-entry midwives. (For an updated chart showing the legality of midwifery in all states, visit Citizens for Midwifery at their website: www.cfmidwifery.org) Direct-entry midwives include highly trained and very competent midwives. However, anyone may call him- or herself a midwife at this time, so it is up to you to find out if a midwife is qualified and has sufficient experience to satisfy your needs. For assistance in evaluating a midwife's credentials, refer to Appendix B, Questions to Ask a Midwife.

Most industrialized countries have programs that are specifically designed to teach midwifery. The practitioners trained in these programs are referred to as direct-entry midwives because they bypass nursing education and enter directly into midwifery from a training program. The United States currently has more than a dozen midwifery education programs, accredited to provide training in anatomy, physiology, biology, chemistry, psychology, and nutrition, as well as care during pregnancy, labor, birth, and postpartum, and care of the newborn.

Around the world, especially in developing countries, empirically trained midwives attend three-quarters of all births. These women often have no formal education and may simply be women who have given birth themselves. Their familiarity with the birth process is experiential, and their customs tell them that childbirth is normal. These midwives are usually called lay midwives. The International Confederation of Midwives and the World Health Organization are making a concerted effort to recognize and formally educate these midwives, whom they term Traditional Birth Attendants (TBAs).

Lay midwives here in the United States have often begun practicing after their own disappointing birth experiences in hospitals. The lay midwives who responded to the home-birth movement of the 1970s were usually young mothers who had an awareness of the need for alternative birth choices. Many couples could not find physicians or CNMs in their area so they turned to nurses, childbirth educators, or neighbors for assistance and support. A great many couples ignored their fear of and warnings by the medical establishment and gave birth at home by themselves.

The women who stepped forth to help these couples learned by doing, and they developed their own styles of care that were similar to the styles of CNMs but were

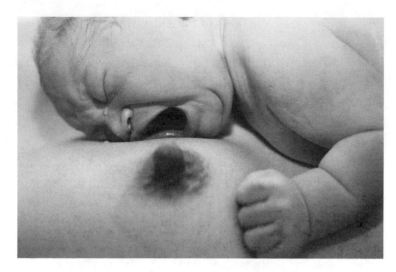

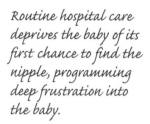

*Routine hospital care deprives the baby of its first chance to find the nipple, programming deep frustration into the baby.*

not limited by legal and hospital restrictions. These providers instantly received the title of "midwife." Other couples came to these "midwives" as the word spread through the community's grapevine. The holistic health movement of the early 1980s emphasized the interrelatedness of the emotional, social, psychological, and spiritual aspects of healing and resulted in more couples seeking alternative care for pregnancy. Midwives viewed themselves as protectors of women and children and of normal birth. Many times a midwife was the birthing mother's friend and was never seen as an authority figure. Midwives did not "deliver" babies; they taught women how to care for themselves during pregnancy, how to acknowledge their ability to give birth, and how to care for their babies after they were born.

One such midwife is Ina May Gaskin, often referred to in America as the "mother of the midwifery movement." Not long after becoming a mother, and awakened by her own horrendous hospital childbirth experience, twenty-seven-year-old Ina May and her then husband and daughter packed up and left for California to, as she delightfully puts it, "become hippies." There Ina May's transformation from mother to midwifery guru commenced in earnest as she was exposed for the first time to a variety of women relating tales of their own unmedicated, out-of-hospital births. A frequent guest speaker at midwifery conferences today, she recalls with amazing detail those stories that show how life-affirming and beautiful women's births can be when supported in the right place with the right people.

In 1970, a pregnant Ina May set off with approximately 250 other followers of Stephen Gaskin, a counterculture and peace protagonist, on what came to be known as "the Caravan"—a five-month-long speaking tour across the United States. Ina May would eventually marry Stephen Gaskin. Traveling in colorful converted school buses, the group stopped in towns and cities and on college campuses so that Stephen could lecture on topics as diverse as the Vietnam War, politics, and sex. One evening, while the buses were parked at Northwestern University, a pregnant woman from among the Caravan group went into labor. Having no money to pay doctors and not believing in accepting welfare, the woman's own husband caught the healthy baby boy. This would be the first of eleven babies born on the buses during the Caravan.[10] "When each birth took place," writes Gaskin in *Spiritual Midwifery,* "we all parked in a sort of protective formation around the bus in which the birth would take place, and everyone waited for the baby's first cry."

By the third birth within the group, Ina May found she was a natural at attending births. Mothers began to request her presence during their labors and births. She knew she was experiencing a calling to become a midwife. But Ina May still had had no medical training, until an obstetrician, having read in the local newspaper about the visiting hippies' bus births, took the trouble to visit the Caravan and offer her and a few other women some training in the essentials of midwifery. Gaskin remembers that

> [h]e took the time to educate us on how to recognize any complications we might encounter, and what to do if we did. He showed us how to stimulate a baby to breathe, what to do if the umbilical cord was wrapped tightly around the baby's neck and what to do if the mother hemorrhaged. He taught us sterile technique and provided us with some necessary medications and instruments. My very first obstetrics textbook came from this doctor from Rhode Island. He gave us instructions on how to provide good prenatal care.

With this rudimentary start to her education as a midwife, Ina May was present for each of the next births that took place on the Caravan. Sadly, the tenth birth, that of her own child, ended with the death of her two-months-premature son, born on a bus in Grand Platte, Nebraska. At only three pounds, the baby lived a mere twelve hours and died in Gaskin's arms. Her grief over her loss only strengthened her resolve to continue helping other women to achieve empowering births with healthy babies.

The group of 250 young people decided to establish an intentional community in rolling farmland in the middle of Tennessee. Named The Farm, the community flourished during the 1970s, eventually reaching a population peak of 1,500 in 1980. Since the early 1980s the Farm population has held steady at more than 200 residents.

With a thriving community of men and women of childbearing age living on the Farm, pregnancy and childbirth became common occurrences. Soon after the community's founding, and with the support of a sympathetic local doctor, Ina May and several other women established an on-site midwifery clinic to which Farm residents could come for prenatal and childbirth care. Births took place wherever the mother wished to be, usually in her home. Women from outside the community were also able to hire the Farm's midwives as birth attendants at a cost of less

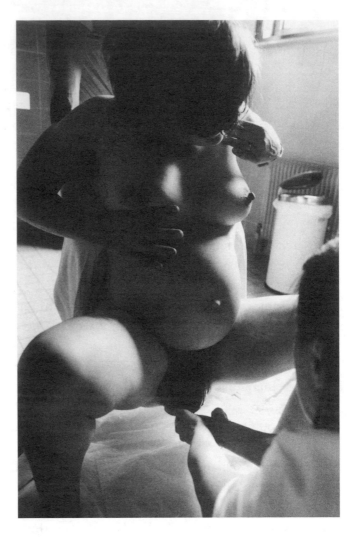

*A midwife simply watches and waits as the baby's head emerges.*

than half that for local obstetric care. Today, the majority of the one hundred births a year the Farm midwives handle are for women living outside the community.

With the publication of *Spiritual Midwifery* in 1976, Ina May Gaskin's work on The Farm began to receive wider notice. A mix of first-person homebirth stories, black-and-white birth photography, and information on caring for women in pregnancy and childbirth, the book laid out Gaskin's philosophy that birth is a spiritual event akin to making love, and that women could take back the power to give birth without excessive and unnecessary medical intervention. These were revolutionary ideas at a time when the ancient profession of direct-entry or "lay" midwifery had all but died out in the United States.

Today lay midwives have grown up, so to speak. Early on, there was a growing concern that direct-entry midwives needed a uniform educational standard and a way to be recognized as professionals. After attending several hundred births, some women sought formal education and even longer and more difficult apprenticeships from accredited schools or foreign programs. Some even went on to nursing school and became certified nurse-midwives. These early midwives were often leaders in their states, pushing for licensing and third-party reimbursement. Some started midwifery schools to train and certify others. Oregon midwife Holly Scholles began a home study group for an eager group of Portland lay midwives and apprentices in 1993. This six-month structured program eventually grew into the College of Midwifery, licensed and authorized by the U.S. Board of Higher Education and the Midwifery Education Accreditation Council, with a three-year Bachelor of Science in Midwifery degree. Midwives increasingly viewed themselves as true professionals.

With the founding of the Midwives Alliance of North America (MANA) in 1982, the profession of midwifery began to have a new voice. Traditionalists concerned with preserving the integrity of the family joined with feminists who were concerned with women's right to control their reproductive capacities. Both welcomed diverse cultural groups that had remained virtually hidden from public view: Native American, Amish, Mexican American, Mormon, Jewish, Muslim, and Asian women came together as midwives, but more importantly as women, in a show of solidarity. It was and is the hope of MANA that this union of midwives will not only support the work efforts of a group of dedicated women but also demonstrate that the midwives model of maternity care is mother-centered, thus focused on human need.

Ina May Gaskin, respected for her lay midwifery roots and revered by many for her unfailing determination to provide quality prenatal and birth care for the women of her community, was on the founding board of this new organization. Continuously active in the organization, she was president of MANA from 1996 until 2002, during which time she completed a very popular new book, *Ina May's Guide to Childbirth*.

MANA created a body to govern education and to provide for uniform testing of core competencies, thus validating other avenues of education, including the time-honored apprenticeship model. In 1987 educators, program directors, and experienced midwives in the field of direct-entry midwifery decided it was time to begin developing a national credential, the Certified Professional Midwife (CPM) designation, which is administered through the North American Registry of Midwives (NARM) and has rigorous standards for knowledge, skills, and experience. Today's Certified Professional Midwife represents the dedication of hundreds of women within the midwifery profession who, despite in many cases being prosecuted, discriminated against, or ignored, worked diligently to provide a reliable standard of care for birthing families. As of January 2005, there have been just under 1,000 CPM credentials issued to midwives in the United States, Mexico, and Canada.[11]

Canadian midwives have made excellent progress in the past decade with establishing midwifery education programs, licensing provisions, and midwifery organizations in almost all the provinces. All of the schools bypass the nursing requirement, following the European model of a direct path to a degree in midwifery.[12]

Statistically, direct-entry midwives have an excellent record for safe and healthy home-birth practices. In New Mexico, direct-entry midwives have been legally recognized since 1980, after practicing midwifery openly since 1921. Statistics have been kept on the outcomes of home births in New Mexico. To no one's surprise, statistics for midwife-attended births are much better than those for physician-attended births in the areas of infant and maternal death, necessity for transport to the hospital, episiotomy, and cesarean section.

CPMs usually practice independently of physician supervision but refer those patients with high-risk conditions to appropriate care by a medical doctor. Some states require a supervisory relationship with a physician before the midwife can obtain a license to practice in that state.

Yet the license to practice in one state does not ensure the ability to practice in another, due to the lack of common legislation governing the practice of midwifery. The United States has no federal legislation that defines the educational requirements for licensing or the parameters in which a midwife will practice. The legal status of direct-entry midwives has been dependent on individual state laws. Strong lobbying from state medical associations kept states like California and Colorado from adopting bills that would legalize direct-entry midwifery for several decades.[13]

## MIDWIFERY REVOLUTION

Nurse midwifery has been in existence since the 1920s. The first program for the training of CNMs was the Frontier Nursing Service, founded in 1925 by Mary Breckenridge in Leslie County, Kentucky, serving families in the isolated and remote Appalachian Mountains. The second school of nurse-midwifery was started in 1932 through the Maternity Center Association (MCA) in New York. Both programs, revolutionary for their time, were begun in an effort to provide quality care for the poor and underprivileged in America. The MCA gave entrance priority to public health nurses or practicing midwives from states with high infant mortality rates. It was expected that these CNMs would return to their states and establish public health programs for the training and supervising of lay midwives. In 1955 the American College of Nurse-Midwives, the professional organization for nurse-midwives, was founded, and celebrated its fiftieth anniversary in 2005. It was created to assure safety and quality of nurse-midwifery education. National accreditation of educational programs wasn't begun until 1970.[14]

The CNM plays a special role in health care because she can work within the established system with obstetricians or be directly hired by a hospital. CNMs are

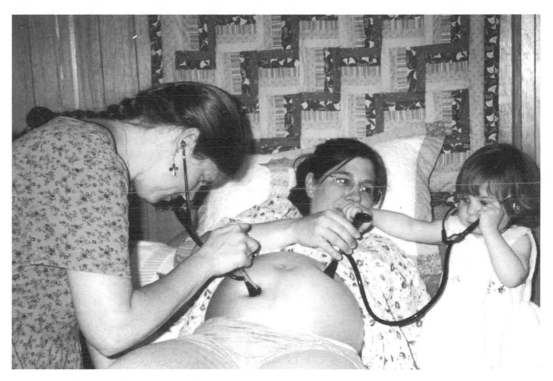

*A midwife uses each prenatal visit as an educational opportunity,
even for the youngest members of the family.*

the only midwives who are allowed to attend births in hospitals. Working in this capacity, the CNM is no longer seen as the competitor that the traditional or direct-entry midwife had been. CNMs introduce the vital practice of the midwives model of care into the hospital setting.

Midwife-attended hospital births doubled in the years between 1970 and 1980 to an all-time high of 1 percent of all births in the United States. By the end of 2002 the number of nurse-midwife-attended births had increased again to over 10 percent. Many of the changes that have been made in obstetric practices in hospitals are directly attributable to the presence of nurse-midwives. Waterbirth practices in hospitals would never have spread into three hundred hospitals if nurse-midwives had not been there to lead the way.

Despite the steady rise and presence of the nurse-midwife in hospitals, it appears she is sometimes caught in the middle. CNMs in all states encounter difficulty in getting jobs, hospital privileges, prescriptive privileges, and reimbursement, says CNM Deanne Williams, executive director of ACNM. Doctors sometimes refuse to support the granting of hospital privileges to independent CNMs. Establishing a collaborative relationship with an obstetrician also poses difficulties for some independent nurse-midwives. Obstetricians sometimes claim that their malpractice insurance coverage would not allow them to share a practice with midwives. There is some truth to this as insurance companies create barriers to access to midwifery care in many ways. The lack of affordable or even available malpractice insurance is a huge area of concern for many nurse-midwives, especially those who own and operate freestanding birth centers.

Lonnie Morris is a busy nurse-midwife in New Jersey. She operated a successful freestanding birth center for more than a decade. Without advance notice, in 2002 the malpractice insurance premiums for her birth center rose by 300 percent, causing her to close her doors. Within a year the very same insurance dilemma occurred for the Elizabeth Seton Childbearing Center in Manhattan. Operating continuously since the early 1970s, this birth center, begun by the Maternity Center Association, was forced to close its doors in August 2003, when insurance premiums rose 400 percent. Mothers, midwives, and community activists protested and rallied for both birth centers without success. The more than four hundred families that these birth centers attended each year now find that they must go into the hospital. Morris stated after her center closed, "If I can't get women into my birth center, I'll just have to put the birth center into the hospital." She continues to advocate for women's rights and for change of hospital policy.

American College of Nurse-Midwives has a very busy lobbyist in Washington and members are active in advising state legislators on matters affecting the licensing of midwives and insurance reimbursement Though technically legal in every state, widespread use of nurse-midwifery care has been hampered by some outdated legislation. The Northwest and Northeast regions of the United States have more CNMs because their laws are less restrictive regarding nurse-midwifery practice, particularly with regard to reimbursement and prescription-writing privileges.

Nurse-midwives are sensitive practitioners and in the facilities where they work they often foster the type of family-centered care that couples began demanding in the 1970s. Yet as she continues to seek change, the CNM is often criticized by the physicians or hospital that hire her. CNMs are often targets for animosity all the way around. In the United States some direct-entry midwives have accused CNMs of catering to the physicians—of becoming handmaidens to the doctors, or worse, being mini-doctors themselves. The 1990s saw a concerted effort to bridge the two groups in terms of understanding each other's roles, establishing educational expectations, and ultimately providing better outcomes for all women. The development of the Certified Midwife (CM) credential is an outgrowth of the effort by the ACNM to recognize that a direct path to midwifery is an accepted educational route.

Certified Midwives have completed a program of midwifery training for nurses, without first becoming a nurse. The entry requirement is a bachelor's degree in some other field of study besides nursing. It is a fast track for midwifery, and issues a certificate from The American College of Nurse-Midwives Certification Council (ACC). CMs are held to the same standards for practice, philosophy, and code of ethics as certified nurse-midwives. The certification examination is the same as for certified nurse-midwives. CMs practice independently, at medical clinics, or at hospitals as physician assistants. As a relatively new profession, CMs are not yet recognized by every state.

## THE POLITICS OF MIDWIFERY

Malpractice insurance premiums, obtaining hospital privileges, and making licensure available for all midwives are not the only problems that face the growing profession of midwifery. Midwives are discriminated against in many ways. Unfair prosecutions of midwives continue today in many states, even those where they are authorized to practice. For example, if a baby dies or is stillborn in the hospital, it is considered by health officials to be the will of God. But if a baby dies or is stillborn at home, the midwife may be charged with felony manslaughter, which is subject to the death penalty in some states and life imprisonment in others. Many of these cases have gone to trial, and midwives have been imprisoned, but fortunately no one has received more than a sentence of a few years. Nevertheless, midwives must still endure the stress of court appearances, attorney fees, and loss of income, all of which can amount to hundreds of thousands of dollars.

Charging midwives with practicing medicine or midwifery without a license goes back to the 1970s, when the public and the county medical societies first became aware of the home birth movement. A highly publicized court case in Santa Cruz county in 1974 brought attention to a group of lay midwives who started out teaching childbirth education classes and providing labor support for women in the hospital during birth. Gradually they began to help couples give birth at home. In 1971 Raven Lang and seven other lay midwives opened the Birth Center in Santa Cruz in an effort to provide adequate prenatal care for women who wanted to have home births. The doctors of the county had earlier met and voted to refuse care to any woman who intended to give birth at home.

The women running the Birth Center met regularly and brought knowledgeable practitioners into the area for workshops. They learned to assess fetal condition, take blood pressures, handle hemorrhages, and repair lacerations. They learned about the importance of nutrition, and they learned newborn resuscitation procedures. As the Birth Center became successful, more women in and around the Santa Cruz area began to use the services of the midwives.

In 1974 a couple used the Birth Center for prenatal care. What this couple failed to tell the midwives, who had felt uneasy about the way the couple acted, was that they were undercover agents for the state of California. When two midwives were summoned to the home of the undercover agent for a supposedly premature labor, money was forced into their hands as soon as they entered the door and they were arrested. Raven Lang, who was no longer living in the area but happened to be visiting that day, was notified about the event by one of the other midwives. Lang arrived at the Birth Center after notifying the press. She was just in time to see the police removing everything from the house as evidence of the "midwifery ring."[15]

Three midwives were charged with treating a physical condition and practicing medicine without a license. The court case went on for several years and ended up in the Supreme Court of California. The district attorney of Santa Cruz eventually dropped the case because the Birth Center had closed and the midwives were no longer practicing. Some of the midwives went on to become certified nurse-midwives and are still practicing today. Even though the Supreme Court finally ruled against the midwives, saying that they were practicing medicine without a license, the midwives felt that they had won a small victory. The publicity helped the cause of home birth by exposing the injustice of a medical monopoly over childbirth.[16] However, the arrest and prosecution of midwives for home birth did not end in 1978 with this case.

In 1979 Arkansas made it illegal for lay midwives to attend births, leaving many long-practicing midwives out of work and many poor rural families without access to maternity care. After ten years of court cases and vague and confusing legislation, Bill Clinton, then governor of Arkansas, finally approved a uniform midwifery law and midwifery once again became legal in 1989.[17] Between 1974 and 1994 there were at least forty-five investigations and/or court cases involving direct-entry midwives in California alone. One California attorney, Stephen Keller, who has defended many of these midwives, has compared these investigations to a modern-day witch hunt.[18] Fearing prosecution, many midwives worked covertly in states where practice was either illegal or where midwives were targeted for investigation. When you hear about a midwifery investigation or case, most people assume that there must have been something terribly wrong to warrant the charges. This is rarely, if ever, the case.

As a registered nurse practicing as an unlicensed midwife in California, I was charged with "practicing midwifery without a license" in December of 1991. Stephen Keller was my attorney and I worked closely with him during the next four years as the State of California diligently tried to remove my nursing license. Even after I left California in 1992 and moved to Oregon, where midwifery is legal, the assistant attorney general of California was assigned to continue prosecuting the case. The amount of money that was spent by California taxpayers on my case alone was close to $700,000. At the end of 1996, the attorney general's office dropped all the charges and sent me a letter stating that I could keep my license, but if I practiced again in California, they could reopen the case. This was a typical prosecution.

Activists in the California Association of Midwives (CAM), worked hard with twenty years of bill introductions, revisions, defeats, and reintroductions before the very first bill recognizing midwives was passed in 1993. The midwives and political supporters continue to improve the regulation of midwifery in California to the benefit of all families.

Even after the passage of midwifery legislation the prosecutions in California continued. In 1994 the California Board of Medical Quality Assurance sent armed agents to the home of a southern California midwife, holding her thirteen-year-old daughter on the floor at gunpoint, while they searched her home in order to build a case against her for the practice of midwifery. The same year, Lynn Amin, the licensed owner of an out-of-hospital birth center in Riverside, California, was arrested and chained to a wall in a jail cell with her hands cuffed behind her back for many hours. Amin's partner, Lorri Walker, a registered nurse-practitioner, was entrapped by undercover officers posing as a pregnant couple. When she started to take the woman's blood pressure, she was arrested and handcuffed. Walker fought the system and was vindicated, continuing on to become a certified nurse-midwife and run a very successful Orange Country freestanding birth center.

California is not the only state where prosecutions have continued. Cases have been reported in 36 states involving at least 145 midwives who have been subjected to legal action instigated by the medical authorities.[19] An Ohio Mennonite midwife was jailed, not for harming anyone, but for saving a woman's life with a shot of Pitocin when the woman hemorrhaged. She was jailed for contempt when she refused to reveal where she obtained her supply of Pitocin. When over one hundred people showed up in front of the court house to pray for her release, the judge decided to make an example of her.[20]

Ironically, there is a bill waiting for approval in the Ohio general assembly that would have spared her from prosecution. State bill HB 477, sponsored by Rep. Diana Fessler, a former lay midwife, fulfills the 1998 recommendation of a special study council set up by Ohio's general assembly that "the practice of midwifery be legal in Ohio and that any ambiguity in the law on this issue be resolved to prevent prosecution of either direct-entry midwives or parents who choose to use direct-entry midwives." Rep. Fessler reflects that the silence of the law with regard to direct-entry midwives is dangerous. "Although current state law includes a provision governing certified nurse-midwives, the law does not address the practice of midwifery by non-nurse midwives. As a result, non-nurse midwives continue to be concerned that an overzealous prosecutor could charge them with practicing medicine without a license."[21]

The devastation that random prosecution brings upon the midwives and their families is obvious. The health departments and licensing systems throughout the United States in which all of these cases are fought imply that the midwives are guilty until someone proves them innocent. The burden of proof is always on the midwives even if there is no procedure in place for them to become licensed. This is a veritable "catch-22" which causes financial hardship and discouragement for many innocent women. Concerned about this injustice and about preserving their rights to home birth, hundreds of women have come together to push midwifery licensing bills through state legislatures in many states.

Even in states that issue midwifery licenses, however, many midwives refuse to be governed by them. In Florida, which had a long history of licensed midwives dating back to the 1920s, licensing was changed in 1984 to recognize only those who were currently enrolled in new educational programs. This quickly reduced the number of licensed midwives; others practiced illegally. On the one hand it is good for midwives to be licensed, recognized, and regulated: It assures a rigorous standard of education and provides for peer review, and confers the respect and prestige midwives deserve. On the other hand, licensing limits a midwife's scope of practice to whatever a state committee judges to be "normal."

Many direct-entry midwives are still forced to practice in ambiguous legal territory. In some states midwifery is legal but no licensing is available. In other states there is simply no legislation making it almost impossible for the consumer to judge the credentials of midwives in their state. (Refer to www.cfmidwifery.org for a complete state-by-state listing.) The nineteen states that do license direct-entry midwives to attend births out of the hospital use the NARM exam or the CPM process as the basis for licensure. States that are seeking licensure for direct-entry midwives are planning legislation which requires the CPM credential for licensure.

As of early 2005, twenty-three states recognize and regulate direct-entry midwives; although in two of the states, New York and Rhode Island, only the CM credential is acceptable. Regulation varies from state to state, including requirements and procedures for licensure, certification, registration, and documentation. Only nine states and the District of Columbia actually prohibit the practice of direct-entry midwives, but in five more states licensure is required but unavailable. In the remaining states direct-entry midwives practice without any kind of state regulation, and in a few their legal status in not entirely clear. So it can be said that essentially direct-entry midwives are practicing legally in about thirty-four states, but are considered unlawful in fourteen states. However, these figures are subject to change as new legislation is enacted or new legal opinions are established that can change status in the legal states where direct-entry midwives are neither specifically regulated nor specifically prohibited.

All fifty states license CNMs. Almost all states regulate nurse-midwifery through the Registered Nurses Board of each state. To inquire whether a particular practitioner is licensed or registered with your state, call the state offices that govern med-

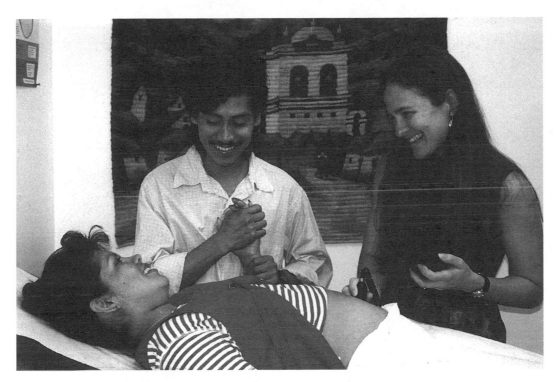

*Midwives strive to provide care that is culturally sensitive.*

ical, nursing, or midwifery practices. To find a midwife you may also call or visit the Web sites of the American College of Nurse-Midwives (ACNM) or the Midwives Alliance of North America (MANA) (see Appendix E, Resources).

## A MIDWIFE FOR EVERY MOTHER

The midwifery profession continues to fight to have the right to provide a midwives model of care to a growing number of couples who seek alternatives. More and more, midwives are being seen by both the medical profession and consumers as viable providers of safe, natural maternity care. This realization leads to a new problem—the lack of enough midwives in the United States to provide this care to those who desire it.

Kitty Ernst, CNM and founder of the National Association of Childbearing Centers (NACC), states that there just aren't enough midwives to fill the demand of concerned couples seeking choices in childbirth. A collaboration between the Maternity Center Association and midwifery educators across the country created the Community-Based Nurse-Midwifery Education Program (CNEP) in 1989. The program, originally funded by PEW Charitable Trust, allows qualified registered nurses to obtain a graduate degree in nurse-midwifery while studying at home under the guidance of an experienced CNM mentor. The student midwife can stay in her own community, maintain her family life, and graduate in less than four years. Upon completion of the program, each student agrees to become a mentor, ensuring that the numbers of students will continue to increase exponentially. The program has graduated over 900 new CNMs, adding to the total of 6,600 already practicing in the United States, according to ACNM's 2003 Annual Report.

There have been and still exist sharp divisions and disagreements between ACNM and MANA over the nature of midwifery and the definition of what constitutes appropriate midwifery education and competent midwifery care. Nevertheless, both these organizations place high value on coexistence and cooperation. CNMs and CPMs have learned to put aside their differences, to respect one another's educational processes, and to work together so that more women and families can benefit from their services. Professional midwives and consumer advocates throughout North America believe that midwifery care should be available as a choice for all women who experience uncomplicated pregnancies. The numbers of midwives will increase as more educational programs are created that bypass the requirement for a nursing degree before studying midwifery.

Above all, midwives recognize birth as a life event that brings women together, especially when that event is not invaded by the use of technology and institutional rituals. Midwives respect and value all women regardless of geographic location, socioeconomic status, age, cultural and ethnic background, gender orientation, or religion. Elizabeth Davis, midwife, author, and cofounder of The National Midwifery Institute, writes, "A strong motive for becoming a midwife is the common desire of women to come closer to one another—not just emotionally as friends but in the powerful sense of working together and establishing support systems for one another."[22] It is this point of view that sustains midwives and motivates them to maintain their professional practice despite serious and draining legal and certification issues.

# CHAPTER SIX

# *Waterbirth*

The thought of birthing a baby into water seems startling to many people until they hear the rationale and reasons behind such an interesting approach to birth. People usually listen with curiosity, and almost everyone finally draws the same conclusion: "Waterbirth certainly makes sense."

Most people feel relaxed and find great comfort in water. Perhaps because we begin our lives in the womb surrounded by liquid, this basic familiarity stays with us. Human beings are composed primarily of water, and many special characteristics we have link us to aquatic mammals; perhaps we carry the memory of a time when the human species had an "aquatic interlude." A three-day-old fetus is 97 percent water; at eight months the fetus is 81 percent water. By the time a human has grown to adulthood, the adult body is still 50 to 70 percent water, depending on the amount of fatty tissue.[1]

Human beings' natural alliance with water is best witnessed by observing babies who can swim naturally and easily long before they learn to sit up or crawl. During their first year of life, babies will calmly and happily paddle under water, gazing around with eyes wide open. Babies instinctively know not to breathe while their heads are submerged under water.

## WHY WATERBIRTH?

For thousands of years women have been using water to ease labor and facilitate birth. Wherever there has been even slightly warm water, there have been women bathing in it, using it ritually, and finding great comfort in it, especially in labor. Soaking in a tub of water to ease labor sounds inviting to most women. If the water is where a woman wants to be and there are no complications, then in the water is where she will feel the most comfortable. When it is time to birth the baby, there is no reason to ask the mother to get out of the water.

When a woman in labor relaxes in a warm deep bath, free from gravity's pull on her body, with sensory stimulation reduced, her body is less likely to secrete stress-related hormones. This allows her body to produce the pain inhibitors—endorphins—that complement labor. Noradrenaline and catecholamines, the hormones that are released during stress, actually raise the blood pressure and can inhibit or slow labor.[2] A laboring woman who is able to relax physically is able to relax mentally as well. Many women, midwives, and doctors acknowledge the analgesic effect of water. Thousands of these mothers state they would never be able to consider laboring without water again.

Women achieve a level of comfort in water that in turn reduces their levels of fear and stress. Women's perception of pain is greatly influenced by their level of anxiety. When labor becomes physically easier, a woman's ability to concentrate calmly is improved and she is able to focus inward on the birth processes. Water helps some women reach a state of consciousness in which their fear and resistance are diminished or removed completely; their bodies then relax, and their babies are born in the easiest way possible.

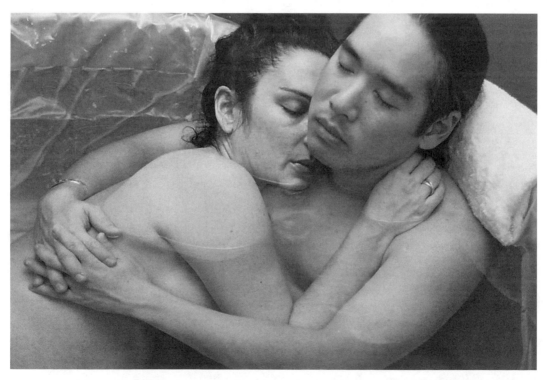

*The water provides a safe place for complete surrender to the power of birth.*

Many women report being better able to concentrate once they get into the water. Doctors and midwives who attend waterbirths find that the mere sound of water pouring into the birth pool or bathtub helps some women release whatever inhibitions were slowing the birth, at times so quickly that the birth occurs even before the birth pool is filled. Oftentimes women climb into the birth pool to labor and the birth happens before they can get out.

Another benefit of laboring in water is the elasticity that water imparts to the tissues of the perineum, reducing the incidence and severity of tearing and eliminating the need for episiotomies.[3] Dr. Michel Odent, the first physician to keep waterbirth statistics, reported that in one hundred waterbirths he had attended, no episiotomies were performed and there were only twenty-nine cases of tearing, all of which were minor surface tears.[4] An initial 1989 nationwide survey published in the *Journal of Nurse-Midwifery* produced statistics indicating that the use of water for labor and birth results in fewer incidents of perineal tearing with less severity.[5] More recent studies, especially a review of 2,000 births in the United Kingdom, published in 2002, report the same conclusions.[6]

The body responses of mother and baby are intricately linked. The ease of the mother who labors and gives birth in water is transferred to the child who is born in the water. The emotions the mother feels can also be felt by the child because the hormones her body secretes in response to her emotions are absorbed by the child. In a medically controlled birth, drugs or synthetic hormones the mother receives are also received by the child. If the mother's delivery is easy and smooth, so, too, is the baby's birth. The baby spends less time in the cramped birth canal and is free from fear, frustration, or other painful emotions a long and difficult labor might arouse in the mother. The mother is more emotionally available to immediately receive and attach to her child.

The baby emerges into the water and is "caught" either by the mother, father, or birth attendant. While in the water the child has freedom of movement in familiar fluid surroundings. A baby's limbs can also unfold with greater ease during those first moments when he leaves the mother's body and enters the water. The water offers a familiar comfort after the stress of the birth, reassuring the child and allowing his bodily systems time to organize. During the birth, babies often open their eyes, move in all directions, and use their limbs. Water mitigates the shock and sensory overload that are so often an inextricable part of birth. Lights and sounds are softer when perceived from under the water, and even the touch of his mother's skin to his own tender skin is softened by the presence of water. The same element, familiar and secure for the baby, is comforting and relaxing for the mother. Together, the mother and baby are profoundly affected by this gentlest of gentle births.

# WATERBIRTH HISTORY

In the sixth century B.C., Aristotle concluded that water was the first principle of life. He observed that the seeds of everything had a "moist nature." However, it was not until the 1700s that scientists began to understand and identify the properties of water, including its value as a form of hydrotherapy. An obscure book called *Water Cures,* printed in London in 1723, describes the benefits of water used for all kinds of conditions, including bathing during pregnancy and labor.[7] Intuitively, human beings have always been drawn to the soothing comfort of water.

Historically, there is little concrete evidence that ancient cultures practiced waterbirth on a large scale, but it has been used by cultures all over the world. There are legends that the ancient Egyptians birthed selected babies under water. These babies became priests and priestesses. The ancient Minoans on the island of Crete are said to have used a sacred temple for waterbirth. Art on frescoes in the Minoan ruins depict dolphins and their special connection with humans and water. One can only speculate about the connection between these pictures and their creators.

The Chumash Indians of the central California coast tell stories about their women laboring in tide pools and shallow inlets along the beach while the men of the tribe drummed and chanted. Chumash elder Grandfather Semu, before his death in 2004 at close to one hundred years old, recalled that when he was a boy, women would often go to the beach and labor in the shallow water. He also remembers that on many of these occasions, dolphins would appear nearby in the water, staying close to the woman until the baby was born. He even recounts watching a pregnant woman enter the water and come out onto the beach to enter her "birth hut" with a baby in her arms and a white cord hanging down. His presence as a child was accepted but men were usually not part of the birth process. Their role on the beach during birth times was only to aid in the building of fires and birth huts and to drum traditional songs of celebration and welcoming as the babies were born.[8]

Other Indian tribes in North, Central, and South America, as well as the Maoris of New Zealand and the Samoan people of the Pacific, may have given birth in shallow ocean or river environments. Traditions from the Hawaiian Islands maintain that certain families on the islands have been born in water for many thousands of generations.

Many midwives suspect that waterbirth was taking place before the advent of physicians and hospitals, even though it has not been documented. Where there was water, especially warm water, women used it to relieve labor pains. The first recorded modern waterbirth took place in France in 1803. The case, which was detailed in a French medical society journal, reports that a woman who had been laboring for forty-eight hours sought temporary relief from her nonprogressing labor in a warm bath. After just moments in the bath, the baby came out so quickly that she didn't have time to leave the water to deliver her child.[9]

Subsequent reports of waterbirth were scattered until the 1960s, when documentation of waterbirths began in the Soviet Union. Interesting stories emerged about the work of Igor Charcovsky, a primarily self-educated Russian scientist and healer who conducted research on animals laboring and birthing in water. He also observed human babies' behavior in water, including that of his daughter Veta, who was born prematurely in 1963. Charcovsky placed his newborn daughter in a pool of warm water for several weeks, theorizing that she would not have to combat gravity and subsequently would not waste as much energy to survive as she would struggling in the hospital incubator. Charcovsky's daughter survived, and he continued experimenting with water, newborns, and the effects of gravity on all aspects of human labor.[10]

## BEYOND THE LEBOYER BATH

During the same time period as the discoveries in Russia, Dr. Frederick Leboyer introduced the concept of the warm bath for the baby after birth. Through his search for ways to bring babies less violently into the world, Leboyer discovered the beneficial effects of warm water on newborns.[11]

The Leboyer bath consists simply of placing the infant, immediately following birth, into a basin of water heated to body temperature. The baby then can experience the comforting return to the pleasure of the fluid world it has just left behind. During Leboyer baths, babies are often wide-eyed and attentive and smile serenely as they move their arms and legs playfully in the water. They can even swim and propel themselves in the water.

Leboyer practiced in a hospital just outside Paris in the small suburb of Les Lilas. I had the opportunity to tour the hospital's maternity and labor wards in 1984. A large round birth pool stood in a separate room adjacent to the traditional delivery room. When asked if women ever gave birth in this birth pool, the midwife just threw back her head and laughed. "Of course, babies come in the water. Women just don't want to get out once they get comfortable in the water." When I asked how the birth pool had become a permanent fixture in this maternity hospital, it was related that Leboyer had become friends with Michel Odent in Pithiviers in the early 1970s. Odent was the first physician to recognize the beneficial effects of warm water for labor and birth.[12] Leboyer agreed with Odent's philosophy and incorporated the option of using birthing pools into his hospital practice.

The midwives at the Les Lilas hospital spoke about the differences they observed in the babies born in water. "We can tell which babies have been born in water. They are like little grown-ups. You know that they understand you. It is very special to be with them."

Through his poetic writing and compelling photographs, Leboyer presented the world of the newborn infant as it had never been seen before. His contribution was a giant step toward sensitizing the world to the birth experience from the baby's perspective. Leboyer's vision, which was to eliminate the violence and trauma of birth, has more than anything else influenced the adoption of gentle birthing techniques throughout the world.

## LABOR POOLS IN FRANCE

One of the first publicly outspoken proponents of waterbirth was French physician Michel Odent, former head of surgery at a state hospital in Pithiviers, France. By providing women with a warm bath for labor and birth, Odent offered them more comfort and freedom than they had ever known before. "My question was how not to disturb the physiological processes of birth; and when you weigh this question, of course, it makes things different—a different kind of birthing room, water to help some women, darkness, and so on."[13]

The main focus of Odent's work has been to assist each woman to give birth in her own way using her instincts. According to Odent, understanding this principle transforms birth, making it an intensely rewarding emotional and physical

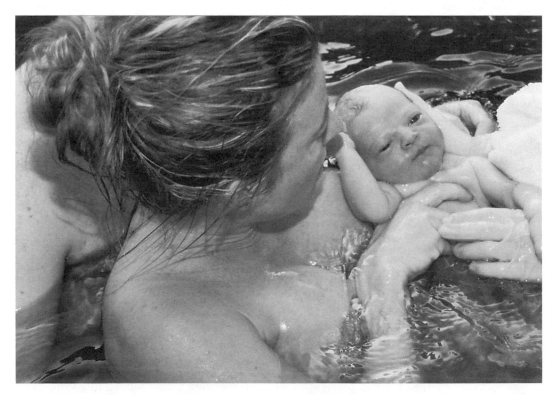

*Parents delight in receiving their water-born baby.*

experience. Warm-water baths to rest in during labor—and, for some, to give birth in—were an option for women at Pithiviers. Although he claims waterbirths were never promoted, Odent would say smilingly to a woman in labor, "Waterbirth is a possibility." This stressed the idea that she should not consciously plan to have a waterbirth but should follow her instincts during labor and birth, knowing it was an option.

Many women who arrived at Pithiviers to give birth had never heard of waterbirth, but when they saw the large, circular blue pool full of warm water, many felt a great attraction to it. In his book *Birth Reborn,* Odent writes, "Some women who are strongly drawn to water throughout pregnancy are even more attracted to it during labor. Still others tell us that they don't like the water or can't swim. Yet as labor begins, these same women will suddenly move toward the pool, enter eagerly and not want to leave."[14] The pool, which was seven feet in diameter and two feet deep, was large enough to easily accommodate two people. The pool was filled with ordinary tap water at 98 degrees Fahrenheit and did not contain any added salts or chemicals.

Odent found that when a woman's contractions become more painful and less efficient, resting in a warm bath often provides relief, especially for women whose dilation has not progressed beyond five centimeters. In the pool, labor almost immediately becomes easier and more efficient. In a similar situation in the hospital doctors would, without hesitation, resort to the use of interventions, including drugs.

Women who choose to leave the water before the birth occurs discover what Odent calls the "fetal ejection response." These women suddenly have an urge to leave the water. As they enter the cooler temperature of the air, the change of environment triggers an adrenaline release, and the baby comes very quickly.[15] Odent believes that a woman who has no preconceptions about how her birth should be will know whether it is appropriate to remain in the water for the birth or whether she should birth the baby out of the pool.

While in Pithiviers I watched a young woman climb out of the pool and squat, supported by her husband, close to the floor where a white sheet had been spread. The midwife, Dominique Pourre, sat in front of her in complete silence. She had asked me to remain silent as well, telling me that I could better "feel" the birth with my whole self. The only sounds in that darkened room were the beautiful, primal sounds emanating from the mother as she birthed her baby. That experience of normal birth eventually influenced and changed my life.

On the occasion of his one hundredth waterbirth, Odent published an article summarizing his waterbirth experiences for the British medical journal *The Lancet.* In the article he states, "We have found no risk attached either to labor or to birth underwater. The use of warm water during labor requires further research, but we hope that other experience would confirm that immersion in warm water is an efficient, easy and economical way to reduce the use of drugs and the rate of intervention in parturition."[16]

Odent now lives in London and is actively involved with writing and research on what he calls "primal health." Primal health is dependent on the interconnected functioning of many organ systems in the body, which together form what he calls the primary adaptive system. Odent believes that the conditions for optimal maturation and functioning of the primary adaptive system are largely dependent on the conditions before, during, and after birth. According to Odent, medicine needs to acknowledge the profound influence of pre- and perinatal conditions on health throughout the individual's life span. He has dedicated the past decade to research substantiating this hypothesis.

For Odent, waterbirth itself has never been a goal. Through his work at Pithiviers, Odent strove to enable all women to give birth with confidence in whatever birthing position they chose. This new freedom naturally led to the use of water as a labor and birthing option. It wasn't long before word of Odent's work spread to open-minded parents, physicians, and midwives throughout the world.

## MAKING WAVES IN THE UNITED STATES

By 1981, a small group of midwives in the United states had heard about Dr. Odent's success and the pioneering research of Igor Charcovsky in the Soviet Union. At the same time, many parents wanted to give their children a vastly different entrance into the world, one that was different from their own births, experienced in the era of "twilight sleep" and heavy sedation. Many of these concerned couples had experienced rebirthing, a regression technique developed in the 1970s for tapping into repressed emotions and memories, including memories of their own births. A rebirthing session involves deep, nonstop breathing, often while sitting in a tub of water, and can result in the spontaneous release of deeply buried emotions.[17] There are many types of regressive therapies today, but this was one of the first to recognize that memories of the pre-birth, birth, and early childhood experience affect your present life and possibly how you birth and parent your own children.

During the early 1980s, when these young couples began birthing their own babies in water, most of the births were uncomplicated and fulfilling experiences. Unfortunately, some couples attempted to birth their babies by themselves, without the necessary education or an experienced midwife or doctor in attendance. There were a few accidental newborn deaths, presumably from leaving the baby under the water too long. Parents sometimes left their newborn babies submerged under water for as long as twenty minutes, believing that doing so gave the babies time to completely unfold, relax, and recuperate from the stress of birth. This shocked the parents and midwives who had been strong proponents of waterbirth, and they began to doubt its safety. The parents whose babies had died subsequently learned that the placenta can separate before the umbilical cord stops pulsating, thus leaving the baby without a source of oxygen. Today every waterbirth practitioner recognizes the fact that a newborn baby needs to be brought to the surface of the water very soon after birth.

In late 1988 the Waterbirth International project of the Global Maternal/Child Health Association (GMCHA) was begun to meet the need for accurate information on the use of water for labor and birth. My personal experience with waterbirth helped me decide to create Waterbirth International keeping one goal in mind—to make waterbirth an available option for all women. Option is the key word in knowing that this method of birth is not right for every woman, but every woman should be given an informed choice of whether it makes sense for her. The gathering of statistical data, publication of research articles, and communication with providers around the world who were actively providing waterbirth were the first tasks that Waterbirth International tackled.

As more physicians and childbirth practitioners were willing to work with women who wanted to birth in water, more information on waterbirth became available. Dr. Odent's book, *Birth Reborn*, was published in the United States in 1984, and the following year the first U.S. birth center to offer waterbirth as an option was opened by an obstetrician.

In 1985 there was one birth center in the United States, owned and operated by a physician, that offered women the same atmosphere that Dr. Odent had created in France. The Family Birthing Center of Upland, in southern California, was operated from 1985 until 1995 by Dr. Michael Rosenthal.[18] Inspired by the philosophy and work of Odent, Rosenthal transformed his practice from traditional obstetrics to a noninterventionist approach. The evolution of Rosenthal's obstetrical practice was also affected by his own observations of women giving birth naturally. Rosenthal felt that there was a big difference between parents' level of satisfaction after hospital births and the level of satisfaction of the obstetricians who attended the births. The traditional obstetrical view of a positive birth experience is a safe delivery. To obstetricians survival of the newborn was the only objective. However, when Rosenthal talked with parents about their hospital births, they often expressed dissatisfaction. Parents wanted more options and control over giving birth.

Rosenthal's philosophical changes inspired him to open his own birth center. He and a team of midwives provided an environment that supported women's choices in birth, enriching the birth experience for the entire family. In his former days as a traditional obstetrician, Rosenthal viewed the birth process as a medical event to be controlled on a timeline. He successfully learned to step back and empower the woman to give birth. "When women control the birth process and actively participate free of traditional interventions, they derive emotional strength and a great sense of achievement," states Rosenthal. "At the Family Birthing Center, we felt strongly that women were giving birth. They weren't coming here to have their babies delivered. Part of our effort was to restore control of birth back to women. We took the term 'nonintervention' in a very literal sense. It often meant that women gave birth without me using my hands."[19]

Rosenthal and Linda Church, the certified nurse-midwife who worked at the Family Birthing Center for its first five years, accumulated extensive experience with waterbirth. By the time Rosenthal sold the birth center, almost one thousand women had birthed their babies in water at the center. There were no complications or infections in either the mothers or the babies.

Because of the success rate at the Family Birthing Center, both Rosenthal and Church published articles on waterbirth in professional journals, receiving attention among their colleagues.[20] In turn, women who sought this kind of birth experience during the years of the center's operation traveled great distances—from as far away as Alaska—to have their babies there. Providers came from many places around the world to witness the ease of incorporating water into the maternity care environment. "Waterbirth is a reasonable option for reasonable people," states Rosenthal. "All their lives women have gotten into baths when they were uncomfortable. They use a warm bath for menstrual cramps or when they've had a bad day. Women expect a warm bath to relax them, and it works." He adds,

> The use of warm water for labor and birth might be viewed as radical and new in the human experience; however, from a historical perspective, the use of most obstetric interventions, such as spinal or epidural anesthesia, narcotics, and forceps, are comparatively recent. The use of water should be considered one of the most risk-free interventions. If the bath had been used earlier in this century, we might never have passed through the era of "twilight sleep" sedation that depressed babies and removed mothers from conscious participation in birth.
>
> I believe that the benefits to the baby derive primarily from being born to a relaxed mother who is conscious and free of drugs. A significant observable fact of a waterbirth is that the experience is joyful and devoid of fear. The child who shares this experience with its mother reaps the benefits of her positive birth experience for a lifetime. Subsequently the child begins to fit its parents' belief that water babies are somehow special.

In reflecting on his experience with waterbirth and on its future, Rosenthal believes that parents hold the key to making waterbirth accessible everywhere. "Waterbirth is a reasonable thing to do, and there is only one way it's going to happen. It will not come from universities; it will not come from doctors; it will come from consumers, that is, mothers and fathers who demand it. As more birthing places offer waterbirth as an option, women will walk away from doctors who say no. The establishment will be forced to change because the consumer demands it."

Parents have been asking for waterbirth and providers have been responding. Here in the United States, waterbirth is now an option in almost all of the freestanding birth centers and in close to 10 percent of all hospitals.

When Dr. Lisa Stolper, an obstetrician in Keene, New Hampshire, wanted to incorporate a noninterventionist approach to birth at the Cheshire Medical Center, she immediately thought about the benefits of water immersion in labor. The waterbirth program began in the fall of 1998, with one of the labor and delivery nurses anticipating being the first client to use the new spa that was installed in a converted labor room.

Using water in labor was not the only change that Stolper and the staff decided to introduce. Even before the introduction of water they conducted a series of investigations and appointed an obstetrics task force to look at all birth practices in this medium-sized rural hospital where about five hundred babies are born each year. Stolper was introduced to Michel Odent's book, *Birth Reborn,* and experienced an epiphany; she then patiently sought to change the paradigm of obstetric care at her hospital.

Stolper and her staff firmly believed in the power of continuous labor support and the difference a trained doula could make in the labor room. A volunteer doula program was introduced in 1999 with great success. Presenting their statistics at the International Waterbirth Congress in 2004, Dr. Stolper, Carmen Carignan, one of the labor nurses, and Sarah Ellsworth, a certified nurse-midwife, illustrated that a combined approach of baths and doulas for women resulted in a remarkable drop in the cesarean rate. They also emphasized that a collaborative practice between midwives and doctors aided in everyone sharing a philosophy of protecting normal birth. Before the waterbirth program started the cesarean rate was close to 25 percent. At the end of the first five years of the program, the rate had fallen to 14 percent and has stayed at or just below that level.[21]

After converting all of their rooms to accommodate waterbirth, it was obvious that they didn't even need an anesthesiologist for the administration of epidurals, as the majority of women used the bath to manage their pain and didn't ask for an epidural. In early 2004, the hospital celebrated the one thousandth waterbirth, sending out press releases to local newspapers. Today more than 90 percent of laboring women utilize the water, with an average of 50 percent of all vaginal births occurring in one of their three birth pools.

The certified professional midwives who register their birth statistics with MANA report a great increase in the number of out-of-hospital births taking place in water.[22] It is rare to find a midwife who still refuses to attend a waterbirth. The educational component of Waterbirth International has provided workshops and lectures in all parts of the United States over the past ten years, ensuring a standard of care that midwives have put into practice.

American women reported high rates of satisfaction with the use of water in the 2002 Listening To Mothers survey sponsored by the Maternity Center Association. In that report mothers who used water during labor rated it as the most helpful of all pain management choices. Even though water was only used by 6 percent of the women, the approval response was surprising, especially given all the other methods of pain management available.[23]

My personal experience of assisting more than five thousand couples to rent birth pool equipment for use in homes and hospitals has been a challenge as well as a pleasure. To hear the reports of successful uses of water and listen to women glowingly describe their experiences makes every struggle worthwhile. Fathers, who often set up the birth pool and maintain the equipment, take a particular pride in being present at waterbirths. Many fathers will get into the pool with their partners and assist with the birth, receiving in love the baby they both created.

The intimacy that is present in a waterbirth is one of the most attractive benefits for couples. There is no better way to embrace the power of birth than to get into a pool of body-temperature water and let go of tension, anxiety, and expectations.

## THE UNITED KINGDOM TAKES THE PLUNGE

It is often the birth of our children that take us into the path of midwifery, childbirth education, or doula work. This was the case in England with Jayn Lee-Miller and her son, Nathan, born in 1989. She experienced a wonderful home waterbirth and soon created Splashdown Waterbirth Services, designing and renting birth pools for women all over the United Kingdom.

Jayn kept lists of independent midwives and physicians who were recognized specialists in home waterbirth, referring couples and educating them on their options. One such provider was Roger Lichy, an independent general practitioner whose specialty was obstetric homeopathy and home waterbirth. Now retired from his practice in Cornwall, Lichy published the first British book on waterbirth, *The Waterbirth Handbook,* in which he showed photographs of a portable tub on top of his van. Dr. Lichy kept track of the outcomes from his many years of facilitating waterbirth in the English countryside. His statistics match those of all the other practitioners of waterbirth: No one has seen any serious infections in mother or baby, there are fewer and less severe perineal tears, there is less demand for analgesia, and the length of labor is reduced.[24]

The women of England who heard about waterbirth and wanted to have it available to them often rented portable birth pools from companies like Splashdown or the Active Birth Centre in London. The women informed their doctors or midwives that they were going to labor in water. They asked the practitioners to help them work out the details with the hospital staff. The pioneering efforts of Janet Balaskas—founder of the Active Birth Centre and what she has termed "the active birth movement," and author of several books on natural childbirth including *The Water Birth Book*—has empowered thousands of women to speak up and demand change in British hospitals.[25]

Waterbirths have been taking place in several major hospitals in London since the early 1980s. One out-of-the-way place where waterbirth has been happening since 1986 is Maidstone Hospital in Kent, England. From the demands of one couple came the redesign of an entire delivery room, now affectionately called "the Lagoon Room" by the patients and staff. Senior Midwife Dianne Garland is an internationally recognized pioneer in waterbirth and has become a spokesperson for the very successful birthing unit. She says, "It took some convincing and a great deal of paperwork to push this through. Sometimes I feel like this has been my own little baby." There were just over three hundred waterbirths reported in the first five years. To date Garland and her team of National Childbirth Trust researchers have documented thousands of waterbirths and their outcomes.[26] Her book, *Waterbirth: An Attitude to Care,* is required reading in all midwifery courses in the United Kingdom.[27]

As early as 1992 the House of Commons Health Committee stated in the Winterton Report that, "We recommend that all hospitals make it their policy to make full provision whenever possible for women to choose the position which they prefer for labour and birth with the option of a birthing pool where this is practicable."[28]

England played host to the First International Waterbirth Conference in London in 1995, where providers from twenty-two countries filled Wimbeldon Hall and listened as case studies of 19,000 waterbirths were presented.[29] It was the first time that midwives and obstetricians listened to one another and agreed that indeed waterbirth was a different kind of birth experience for all concerned—mothers, fathers, babies, and practitioners.

In 2000 the Royal College of Midwives created a position paper on waterbirth, stating that more than 50 percent of all hospitals in the National Health System were equipped to offer waterbirths to women. This paper also recommends that all midwives should develop the knowledge and skills to assist women during a waterbirth.[30] The Royal College of Obstetricians published a similar report in 2001.[31]

Dianne Garland and her research team chose ten hospitals in 2002 to investigate variances in practice and outcomes. They wanted to see why one hospital would report a 60 percent birth pool usage and another hospital in the same system only reported a 17 percent use. As one would imagine the variability in practice is attributed to personal preference among care providers and in some cases the lack of proper training. The research team hopes to expand this collaborative audit to include more hospitals.

Garland was not surprised by the reaction of some midwives and nurse managers when they refused to offer waterbirths. She stated, "Change never comes easily and I believe that part of the problems that have been experienced may be due to the political and social arena within which we are working."[32] Despite this type of resistance waterbirth is still much more common today, easily obtained in home, hospital, or birth centers. The British Parliament mentioned waterbirth in a June 2003 publication by the Select Committee on Health Evidence, citing Garland's observations on negative attitudes about waterbirth.[33] The support and acceptance of current evidence by the British government is making the United Kingdom the leader worldwide in this new area of gentle birth options.

## WATERBIRTH AROUND THE WORLD

It is difficult to estimate the number of waterbirths that have taken place worldwide because of the exponential increase. Current estimates are that between 1970 and 2004 more than one hundred fifty thousand waterbirths occurred in hospitals, homes, birth centers, and even in the oceans worldwide, with the largest number occurring in the last decade. Waterbirths have been documented in at least sixty-nine countries. As information on the viability of waterbirth spreads, the number of waterbirths increases. What is evident from talking to numerous childbirth practitioners in different countries is that waterbirth is an appealing choice for women who want to birth their babies naturally, without medical intervention.

The birth practitioners who support waterbirth, whether physicians or midwives, have an underlying respect and reverence for the birth process. They respect the baby as a fully conscious being who deserves exquisite treatment at the time of his or her birth. Dr. Bruce Sutherland, an obstetrician from Australia, states, "Waterbirth is the most spiritual kind of birth experience." Often midwives and physicians become emotional while describing particular waterbirths they have attended. Without the distractions of a typical hospital birth, physicians and midwives experience birth as an important passage in which they feel privileged to participate.

### Australia

Waterbirth has gained more popularity in Australia in the past decade, in part because of the pioneering work of Dr. Bruce Sutherland, founder of the Hawthorn Birth and Development Centre. Home-birth midwives have been using water for

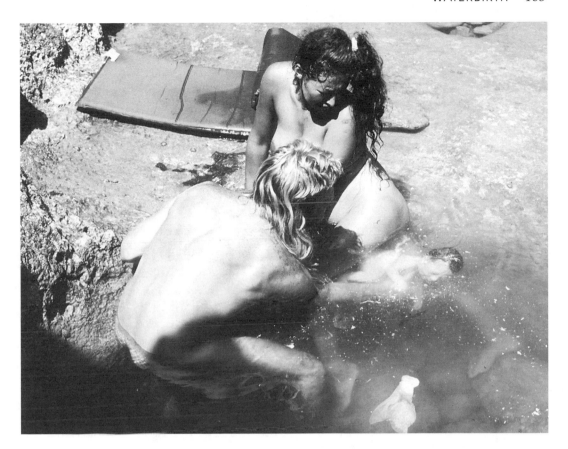

*Baby Sonoma floats in the clear ocean water for a moment before his father gently picks him up. (The white object in the foreground is a piece of the amniotic sac.)*

a number of years, and now several large teaching hospitals have installed new birth pools in their maternity units. The creative person behind the establishment of the Hawthorn Birth and Development Centre was actually June Sutherland, who is a traditionally trained midwife and mother of four. Several years before the 1983 opening of the center, June had taken over as office manager for her husband Bruce's busy obstetric practice. She immediately saw the need for change in the treatment of women in labor and during birth.

June and Bruce discussed the needs of his hospital patients and the fact that many women were dissatisfied with their experiences. The women all expressed regret over giving up the control of the birth to someone else. The Sutherlands were aware that there was a need for alternatives to hospital birth, even though Bruce had practiced gentle birth in the hospital for years. He was the first doctor in Australia to use Frederick Leboyer's approach to birth. June suggested that since Bruce could not possibly attend home births because of Australian governmental regulations, they should build a "home away from home" for pregnant women and their families. They encountered resistance from the traditional medical community, but June's determination never faltered. Even the health commission stood in their way by not approving the necessary building plans for the center. June went ahead and built the Hawthorn Birth and Development Centre without approved plans, paying very close attention to all the building codes. An essential part of this plan was the installation of a spa large enough to accommodate the birthing woman and all of her family if she should so desire.

Once the bath was operational, it was used for labor and birth by 80 percent of the women who came to their new freestanding birthing center. Women enjoyed the water so much that some were heard to remark, "This is better than making love." Bruce has been present at almost all of the water births at the center. Visibly moved when he speaks about water birth, he says, "It makes so much sense to me and it restores all the control to the woman. We encourage the dads to get in to 'catch' the baby if they want to. I just sit in a chair, sometimes rocking, and witness this magnificent process. It is quite a privilege to be included in such a sacred act. My fellow obstetricians accuse me of taking birth back to the dark ages. I feel sorry for them. They don't have any idea what they are missing."

All the staff of the Hawthorn Birth and Development Centre live by its motto, "Love creates and heals."[34] Today the birth center is also the home of the International College of Spiritual Midwifery, run by midwife Shivam Rachana. The school and birth center provide training for both midwives and doulas, with a specialty in waterbirth and lotus birth. Lotus birth is the process of leaving the umbilical cord attached to the placenta after the baby is born until it separates naturally—usually in three to seven days.[35]

## Japan

The Japanese have always incorporated the bath into their daily rituals for the relaxation and health of the family. The bath has been used as a social gathering for centuries. Prior to World War II, most births in Japan were home births attended by midwives. Formal midwifery education in Japan began in the late nineteenth century. The midwife in Japanese culture has always been respected and embraced as a member of the extended family.

During the American occupation following World War II, the medicalization of childbirth in Japan began. The scene for birth quickly shifted to the hospital and the comforts of home were left behind, including the use of warm water for labor.

In recent years there has been a resurgence of home birth in Japan. Another option for Japanese women is the use of a birth home, usually the midwife's personal residence. Despite the medicalization of childbirth in Japan, midwives continue to be respected, whether attending home births or hospital births. Today there are more than twenty-three thousand medically educated midwives in Japan, compared to the United States where there are fewer than ten thousand midwives.

One Japanese midwife, Fuseiko Sei, who runs her own birth home, offers women the choice to labor and birth in water. Sei has written extensively about her experiences, and has been one of the first Japanese midwives to present papers on her waterbirth practices, both in Japan and internationally.[36] Waterbirth has grown in popularity in Japan. Television specials, magazine articles, and acceptance among midwives have helped increase the numbers of Japanese women requesting water for labor and birth. One enthusiastic waterbirth midwife reports birthing her own child in water attended by her mother, who is also a midwife. Now she and her mother practice together, running their own birth house where waterbirth is an available alternative.

## China

A group of physicians in Shanghai obtained books and videos about waterbirth from Waterbirth International and other sources in 2002. The new Shanghai Changning Maternity and Infant Hospital installed a deep bath and began a randomized controlled trial of waterbirth from May to October 2003. Their objective was to investigate its safety and satisfaction among women, especially in pain relief. By early 2005 the hospital reported success on over 350 waterbirths. The group's published abstract of their initial work points out that the water group of women requested far less analgesia (8/51) as opposed to the control (24/51). Dr. Guixia Bao, M.D., chair of the department of Obstetrics and Gynecology at Changning Hospital, is hoping to expand the project and has invited midwives and doctors from different parts of the world to come to Shanghai to lecture and share information about waterbirth.[37]

## Malta

The island of Malta seems more like the backdrop for a great spy thriller than an environment that would support a natural birth clinic. There, Dr. Josie Muscat, along with several midwives, runs the St. James Natural Childbirth Clinic. Laboring women at the clinic experience such innovations as still-life videos showing scenes of waterfalls, oceans, birds, and flowers, accompanied by relaxing music. In an effort to achieve relaxation for women, Muscat has installed a large tub that was specifically designed to incorporate a birthing chair.

On November 11, 1987, less than one year after opening the clinic, Muscat "caught" his first baby in the water. Since that first birth more than three thousand babies have been greeted by the warmth and security of this "expanded womb," which contains the baby's mother and father as well. Muscat firmly believes that once a mother's fear threshold is reduced, her ability to give birth naturally returns without the need for intervention. The 2 percent cesarean section rate at his clinic speaks for itself.[38]

## Russia

Waterbirth in Russia has been the subject of discussion all over the world. Erik Sidenbladh's book *Water Babies,* which chronicles the life of waterbirth pioneer Igor Charcovsky, sparked much speculation about how popular waterbirth was in the former Soviet Union. Many mistakenly thought that it was a common practice in the maternity hospitals there.

On five trips to Russia, the Ukraine, and Georgia between 1987 and 1999, I visited Russian birth homes, called *roddoms* (from the Russian words for birth and home). They displayed the most terrifying conditions for childbirth that I had ever witnessed. Almost all women were drugged or unconscious, and physical brutality was common, with women being beaten or struck while in labor. Immediate separation of the mother and baby was standard and continued for two to three days, sometimes longer. Fathers were not only not allowed in the delivery room, they were not even allowed in the hospital!

There is a saying in Russia that a woman who gives birth to her first baby is a hero but a woman who gives birth the second time is a fool. This judgment says more about the tortures that a woman must endure to give birth than about the merits of limiting family size. No wonder waterbirth and home birth became popular options among people who were willing to take the chance to be different, risking arrest and a fine.

Dr. Zina Bakhareva endured her first birth in a Soviet hospital in Vladivostok, in the Russian Far East. Her story evokes horror and tears as she recounts giving birth to a baby boy and then not being able to see that child, by a series of circumstances and lots of bureaucracy, for over one month! Zina is a pediatrician who worked in the hospital system. The only way to "rescue" her baby from the medical system was to use her limited influence as a doctor and volunteer in the same hospital where her baby was kept under "observation." She literally kidnapped her own child from the hospital and took him home, thinking that he was dreadfully ill. In truth there was nothing wrong with him—he had been kept so long by mistake. She vowed to change things in whatever way she could.

She shared her unique story with others so they could be prepared for the worst-case scenario. More important was her use of exercise, both gymnastics and swimming, to increase her child's vitality. She shared these techniques with other parents as well, and soon experienced a small following of well-educated and concerned parents.

After a second, less traumatic hospital birth Zina finally gave birth in 1990 to a healthy baby girl at home in water. She has subsequently been midwife for hundreds of Vladivostok couples, preparing them for waterbirth and home birth with physical exercise, swimming, reading, and spiritual development. The majority of the babies are born in water, even though sometimes there is no running water in

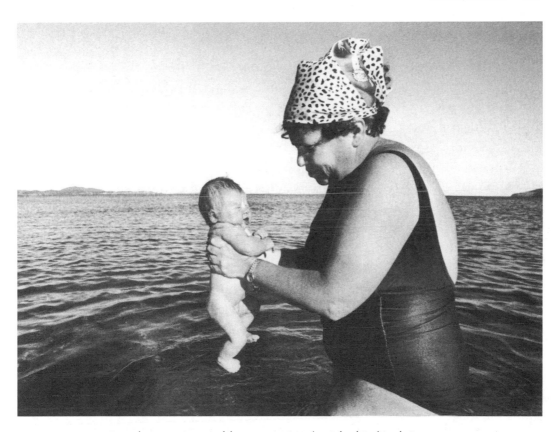

*Russian doctor Zina Bakhareva assisted with this birth in sea water on an island near Vladivostok.*

the apartment buildings, let alone hot water. Fathers have been known to carry enough water to fill an inflatable birth pool in buckets up five flights of stairs, and then heat it on a stove.[39]

Every year the family club which Dr. Bakhareva started, called Krepysh, which in Russian means "sturdy child," takes an excursion to an island in the Sea of Japan. They camp, hike, read, sing, cook, and eat together, and sometimes babies are born at the camp either on the shore or in the ocean. German photographer Michael Appelt documented one such camp in 2002, publishing a beautiful photo essay showing a waterbirth.[40]

The ocean water is sometimes too cold in this location for the mother to remain comfortable, so the men take the ocean water and heat it over open fires and pour it into an inflatable pool. These parents are more than dedicated—they are resolute in their desire for a gentle waterbirth. Their inspiration comes from Dr. Bakhareva's passion and dedication to her families. The camping trip in August 2004 welcomed over 200 community members ranging in ages from newborn to eighty years old.

Another midwife known the world over is Tatyana Sargunas in Moscow. Two of her own births are shown on the beautiful birth film, "Birth Into Being: The Russian Waterbirth Experience," along with two ocean births. She too had a horrendous first hospital birth, then three home waterbirths. Her midwifery training has been completely empirical, but she is respected by many. She and her former husband Alexi founded an organization that has taken many families to a camping site at the shore of the Black Sea.

When they hear "Russia" and "ocean birth" in the same sentence, not many people would think of palm trees, avocado groves, and citrus orchards. But every summer dozens of babies are born on the Crimean Peninsula in the Ukraine, in the waters at the edge of the Black Sea which are warmed by tropical breezes in the summer months.

One couple described their birth in the Black Sea as an incredibly unifying experience—unifying in the sense that they felt connected with all life on the planet by birthing into the abundant sea, out in the fresh salt air, with the trees above them and dolphins cavorting nearby. They felt that their baby's perceptions of the world would be very different from those babies who were born in a hospital and immediately separated from everything and everyone known and familiar. They called their birth an ecological birth and stressed that more couples should look at the impact of birth on our planet.

Although this type of birth experience sounds ideal for some women, certain factors must be considered. Currently the Black Sea is one of the most polluted bodies of water in the world. It suffers from the industrial waste of Eastern Europe and the dumping of radioactive material from nuclear power plants along its shores. For some parents the motivation for an ocean birth outweighs any risks of complications or environmental deterrents.

There are a few midwives around the world who will assist with an ocean birth experience but one must evaluate the reasons for wanting this type of birth and pursue it with care and caution. It can be a very difficult and costly task to arrange and sometimes involves tricky politics. A British group of pregnant women and their physician were asked to leave Israel while attempting ocean births in the Red Sea. My suggestion is to swim in the ocean during your pregnancy, but stay home with a trusted midwife and your family for the birth.

Besides the sensational ocean births, waterbirth has gradually found its way into many of the former Soviet republics and is now available in some hospitals in Moscow and St. Petersburg, as well as other cities. Dr. Bakhareva reports that one of the maternity hospitals in Vladivostok has installed a bathtub, but it is a very rare occasion when it gets used. It is true that if any country needed a complete overhaul of their maternity system, it would be Russia.

## Mexico

The introduction of waterbirth into Mexican hospitals has been a long and hard-fought battle. With cesarean birth rates in private hospitals sometimes soaring as high as 80 percent, the prevailing medical attitude toward waterbirth is that it is something out of the Dark Ages. The overuse of technology and the acceptance of interventions by physicians is not too difficult to understand given the fact that there are some area of Mexico that still suffer from extremely high infant and maternal mortality rates. There are very few remaining empirically trained midwives or Traditional Birth Attendants to balance the technologically dependent medical establishment.

Childbirth education societies like ANIPP (a Mexican Lamaze organization), private teachers, and a few enlightened doctors and midwives provide a beacon of light in this dark period in Mexican childbirth history. The power of women who want this experience has prevailed as some doctors begin to understand the value of allowing women to birth in peace and privacy.

One such physican in Guadalajara is Jose Luis Grefnes Sanchez, the director of Plenitud, a private obstetric and midwifery practice that facilitates both home and hospital birth. Sanchez is the quintessential country doctor, as kind as he is wise and always sporting a smile. After attending the 2000 International Waterbirth Conference in Portland, Oregon, he promised himself and his team from Guadalajara—pediatrician Rosa Gonzalez and childbirth educator and doula Joni Nichols—that he would create a waterbirth hospital in that city to accommodate the growing demand from their clients. He did just that, creating a beautiful birth clinic with a built-in blue tiled bath.

He and Nichols presented their incredible journey at the 2004 International Waterbirth Congress in Chicago, outlining just what it took to get approvals, remodel a building, and begin offering waterbirths in that setting. A doctor who attends home birth is a rarity but Sanchez performs this duty with ease. He feels that when "families are properly prepared and treated with love and respect the babies know to come in their own time and their own way."

Waterbirth has been successfully integrated in hospital practices in Mexico City, Monterrey, and San Luis Pitosi, and is offered by a number of home-birth midwives throughout Mexico.

## Switzerland

A pioneering group of physicians and midwives attending women in the Cantonal Hospital Clinic in Frauenfeld, Switzerland, introduced waterbirth in 1991. From 1991 to 1997 the waterbirth rate in their hospital steadily rose and then stabilized around 50 percent. Their success in this approach was due to the fact that this group of forward-thinking providers put women in charge of their birth choices and then observed them, deliberately restricting use of invasive obstetric procedures. They found that their episiotomy rate dropped from a high of 80 percent to a low of less than 15 percent.

In an article published in 2000, they looked back not only at their statistics but at all birth methods in Switzerland in order to put their experiments in alternative birth methods in perspective. They wanted to rate themselves and analyze their data in a larger context. Where do they stand in comparison with the rest of Switzerland? Their cesarean birth rate is less than 10 percent, whereas the national Swiss average is 15 percent. Their conclusion regarding this successful experiment was that if they could successfully implement waterbirth in their hospital, it could be done anywhere. Doctor Verena Geissbuhler concludes in her research paper that ". . . [waterbirth] can be well integrated into the security-oriented way of thinking of classical medicine."[41]

## Other Countries

Waterbirth has been documented in seventy-one countries to date—everywhere from Iceland to Argentina. The reports are all the same—more satisfied mothers, happier babies who are alert and active right away, less perineal tearing, faster labors, and happier providers. One of the most rewarding reports of waterbirth for me personally came recently from Iran. At the 2002 International Confederation of Midwives conference in Vienna, Austria, I gave several waterbirth videos as a gift to midwifery professors from Teheran with the request that they show them in their classes. Knowing the Muslim restriction on nudity, this was a lot to ask. In just one year I received an email from a doctor there stating that he had not only seen the video, but had it translated into Persian so he could share it with more people. He had also attended his first waterbirth.

## QUESTIONS EVERYONE ASKS ABOUT WATERBIRTH

When people first hear about waterbirth, there are common questions and concerns. These questions come from pregnant women and their families as well as doctors, midwives, and nurses.

### How does the baby breathe during a waterbirth?

This is almost always the first question that people ask. Understanding how a newborn takes his first breath helps to dispel any fears concerning the safety of waterbirth.

While the child is in utero, it has no contact with the atmosphere and no need to breathe. The fetus's lungs do not yet work the way they will once it is born and begins to breathe air. A baby in the womb "breathes" by receiving oxygenated blood from its mother via the placenta and the umbilical cord. The baby's heart pumps the oxygenated blood throughout its body. Once the blood becomes

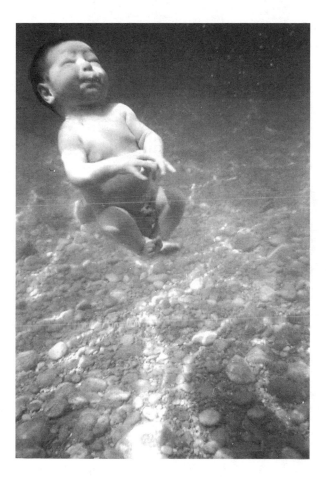

*Babies know how to hold their breath and instinctively swim.*

depleted of oxygen and full of waste materials, it is sent back to the mother via the umbilical cord and the placenta. The blood is purified and reoxygenated by the mother and returned to the fetus.

The baby in utero "practices" for future air breathing by moving his intercostal muscles and diaphragm in a regular and rhythmic pattern from about 10 weeks following gestation. This is why mothers feel their babies having hiccups late in pregnancy. It is part of their "practice" breathing. There is very little inspiration of amniotic fluid in utero. The fluids that are present in the lungs are produced there and are similar to gastric fluids. These fluids serve to protect the baby in a waterbirth, as we'll learn in a moment.

Twenty-four to forty-eight hours before the onset of spontaneous labor the fetus experiences a notable increase in the prostaglandin E2 levels from the placenta. This rise in hormone levels prepares the baby for birth by softening the cervix, making the uterus more irritable, and causing a slowing down or stopping of the fetal breathing movements (FBM).[42] With the work of the musculature of the diaphragm and intercostal muscles suspended, there is more blood flow to vital organs, including the brain. The baby in utero normally moves these muscles 40 percent of the time. By slowing this movement down, the baby saves a great deal of oxygen for the important task of being born. When the baby is born and the prostaglandin level is still high, the baby's muscles for breathing simply don't work, thus engaging the first of four inhibitory responses that prevent the baby from inhaling water.

A second inhibitory response is the fact that babies are born experiencing mild hypoxia or lack of oxygen. It is a built-in response to the birth process. Hypoxia causes apnea (the absence of breathing) and swallowing, not breathing or gasping. Another factor which is thought by many to inhibit the newborn from initiating the breathing response while in water is the temperature differential. The temperature of the water is so close to that of the maternal temperature that it prevents any detection of change within the newborn. This is an area for reconsideration after increasing reports of births taking place in the oceans, both now and in eras past. Ocean temperatures are certainly not as high as maternal body temperature and yet the babies that are born in these environments are reported to be just fine. The lower water temperatures do not stimulate the baby to breathe while immersed.

One more important inhibitory factor is the Dive Reflex, which involves the larynx. The larynx, a very small piece of flesh at the back of the throat, is covered all over with chemoreceptors, commonly known as taste buds. The larynx has five times as many taste buds as the whole surface of the tongue. So, when a solution hits the back of the throat, passing the larynx, the taste buds interpret what substance it is and the glottis automatically closes. The solution is then swallowed, not inhaled.[43] This autonomic reflex is built into all newborns to assist with breast-feeding and it is present until the age of about six to eight months when it mysteriously disappears. The newborn is very intelligent and can detect what substance is in its throat. It can differentiate between amniotic fluid, water, cow's milk, or human milk. The human infant will swallow and breathe differently when feeding on cow's milk or breast milk due to the Dive Reflex.

## What does cause the baby to take its first breath?

It is not until the newborn infant's skin, especially around the nose and mouth, makes contact with the air that the complex physiological process begins that results in the first breath. Water-born babies are slower to initiate this response due to the fact that their whole body is exposed to the air at the same time, not just the head as in a dry birth. Providers report that water babies take a few seconds longer to initiate the breathing process, thus remaining a darker color, but their tone and alertness are just fine.

There are several things that happen all at once for the baby upon contact with the air. The shunts in the fetus's heart, which bypass the lungs, close; fetal circulation turns to newborn circulation; the lungs experience oxygen for the first time; and the umbilical cord is stretched causing the umbilical arteries to close down. Nursing and medical schools taught their students for years that the first breath was dependent on the pressure of the passage through the birth canal and then a reflexive opening of the compressed chest creating a vacuum. Actually, there is no vacuum created, and that action has little or no bearing on newborn breathing.

All the fluids that are present in the lung alveoli are automatically pushed out into the vascular system from the pressure of pulmonary circulation, thus increasing blood volume for the newborn by 20 percent. The lymphatic system absorbs the rest of the fluids through the interstitial spaces in the lung tissue. The increase of blood volume is vital for the baby's health. It usually takes about six hours for all the lung fluids to disappear, but in some cases it can take as long as forty-eight hours.[44]

In the mid-1980s a baby in the United States was reported as dying from being born in the water. This particular newborn death was caused not by aspiration, but by asphyxiation due to leaving the baby under the water for more than fifteen minutes after the full body was born. At some point the placenta detached from the wall of the uterus and stopped the flow of oxygen to the baby. When the baby was taken out of the water, it did not begin breathing and could not be revived. On autopsy the baby was reported to have no water in the lungs and its death was attributed to asphyxia.[45]

Reacting out of fear and bringing a baby out of the water too quickly can be just as traumatic, and it can also lead to either torn or broken cords. This has been reported by a few midwives and doctors.[46] Problems with the baby's cord can be avoided by bringing her out of the water slowly and gently. Mothers and fathers who desire to pick up their own babies need to be reminded to do it slowly and with care.

The most striking example of the gentle-birth concept of allowing a baby to emerge in his own time is the baby who is born in water with the amniotic sac intact. Many providers report that the water cushions the sac and the baby is born completely inside this protective bubble. The baby floats in the water of the amniotic sac, cradled and buoyant, supported by the water it has just been born into, until it moves and possibly pokes a finger through the sac. The provider or mother gently pulls the sac open and lifts the baby out and into his mother's arms. The child's first breath is initiated in exactly the same manner as babies born directly into warm water.

## Will the mother get an infection from the water?
In the 1950s women were told that it was unsafe to take a bath in the latter stages of pregnancy because the cervix was opening and the uterus could be infected by germs in the water. This edict against bathing is still printed in some childbirth books read by women today. If a woman's bag of water (common term for amniotic sac)

has ruptured before labor begins, most providers will advise her to stay out of the bath until labor is initiated and progressing. Otherwise bathing, especially in labor, is encouraged without worry of possible infection. The only precaution is to make sure that the water for bathing is clean. Some couples go to the extreme of using purified water for the bath in which they intend to give birth. Regular tap water is usually sufficient.

During labor everything is moving down and out. The baby is descending into the birth canal. It does not make sense that bacteria from the water would go up into the uterus. In fact, the concentration of bacteria in and around the vagina is actually diluted by the water, lessening the possibility of infection. Perhaps the old adage "the solution to pollution is dilution" is applicable here. A study of 1,385 healthy women in 1996 reported that 538 of these women, all of whom had premature rupture of membranes, bathed during labor, while 847 did not desire a bath. When the infection rates of the two groups were compared, no significant difference was found between the two groups for infections either in the mothers or their babies, even when the membranes had been ruptured for up to seventy-two hours.[47]

Infection control, especially in a hospital setting, requires diligence and following a strict protocol for cleaning the birth pool between uses. This will be an effective way of preventing any postpartum infections in mothers or babies.

All the way back in 1960, the question of bathing in pregnancy and labor was addressed in an article published in the *American Journal of Obstetrics and Gynecology,* titled, "Does Bath Water Enter the Vagina?" Comments at the end of the article by Doctor Seigel, whose study proved that it was an impossibility, stated his hope that this study would forever put the question to rest. Unfortunately it is still alive today in some discussions about water labor and birth.[48]

## Can the water become contaminated?

Related to the discussion of infection, one of a mother's major concerns is what happens if she accidentally looses stool while laboring in the water. A simple reassurance from her nurse or provider that this situation is normal and not to be worried about is usually enough to set a mother's mind at ease. When a woman is pushing out her baby it is impossible for her to control the anal sphincter at the same time. Everything comes out with the baby.

A long handled fish net, affectionately known as the "pooper scooper," is used to remove any particulate matter. If the water becomes too dirty or cloudy, the mother may be asked to leave the water.

It is commonly believed that the mother's own bacteria and blood pose no risk for the baby. On the contrary, it is important for the baby to become colonized with the mother's bacteria, which offers some protection to the baby, helping develop its immune system.

Infection control nurses and risk managers in hospitals worry about what to do with a large supply of water filled with blood and by-products of conception (membranes, vernix, etc.) The protocol is to empty the birth pool into the sewage system of the hospital via the toilet. A sanitized or new submersible drain pump with hose attached is used to remove the water. Proper universal precautions are taken when handling waste water.

At home, the couple make the decision on where to dispose of the birth pool water. Some run a hose out to the garden and give the lawn a nitrogen-rich watering. Others send the two hundred gallons of water down the toilet, which will not overflow, but flush with the pressure of the water.

The fact that there is an extremely low infant infection rate with babies born in water indicates that waterbirth is safe even in situations where there may be possible contaminants. As mentioned before, it is necessary to start out with clean water. Everyone who is going to join the mother in the birth pool either during the birth or directly afterward should be certain to be free of communicable disease and to shower completely before entering the water.

## When should a laboring woman get into the water?

Before beginning the discussion about when to enter the water, we must have a clear understanding about the types of baths or pools into which a woman is entering.

The ordinary home bathtub is definitely not deep enough to provide a woman with enough room to move comfortably and stretch out in the water. Typical baths in the United States are a mere twelve to thirteen inches from the floor to the overflow drain. That provides enough water to make her bottom feel good, but for a woman about to give birth, it is a difficult place to be.

A pool or bathtub must be deep enough to create buoyancy. The phenomenon of buoyancy was explained by the Greek mathematician Archimedes. (Interestingly, he discovered how buoyancy works while he was bathing and thinking about a difficult math problem involving the weight of gold.) Archimedes' principle states: Any object [the mother] wholly or partly immersed in a fluid [the birth pool] is buoyed up by a force equal to the weight of the fluid displaced by the object.

The deeper the water, the more weight is displaced; the more buoyant the woman becomes, the lighter she feels. The pregnant mother who enters the immersion pool immediately feels her body weight disappear and she becomes buoyant. She will experience a loss of 75 percent of her body weight, making her feel like a slippery dolphin in the water now capable of swaying, dancing, and quickly changing positions.

Let's put this into perspective with the dimensions of a proper birth pool—at least twenty inches of water, preferably twenty-two inches, yet small enough to be able to grip the sides to provide adequate support for kneeling or squatting. The water needs to almost cover her breasts while sitting and should cover her belly while squatting, leaning over the side of the pool, or kneeling upright in the pool sitting back on her heels.

In this type of birth pool or bathtub she is now able to move into any position that is comfortable. There is also a physiologic response to her now buoyant body. After about twenty minutes of immersion there is notable redistribution of blood volume, which stimulates the release of atrial natriuretic peptide (ANP) by specialized heart cells.[49] There is a close and complex relationship between the natriuretic peptide system and the activity of the posterior pituitary gland, producing more oxytocin.[50] More oxytocin is a good thing in labor, especially to help the mother's labor become more active. In a recent study in England water immersion was found to be better and more productive than augmentation by Pitocin for a slow or stalled labor.[51]

The higher levels of oxytocin seem to peak after about an hour and then reach a plateau. If the mother gets out, walks, showers and then gets back into the pool the whole process starts all over again.[52]

The immediate pain reduction upon entering the bath is quite noticeable. It is what I refer to as "the ahh effect." The smile, the sound, and the inner peace that mothers display are unmistakable. This response can happen at any point in the labor, but most notably when contractions are long and strong and close together and the water suddenly provides a sense of relief. Some midwives and nurses who assume that there is little or no progress in dilation because the mother is not displaying any outward signs of discomfort are often surprised to find rapid dilation in the first hour of immersion.

Having experienced a waterbirth myself, I can verify the incredible difference in perception of pain from the room to the water. I conducted a small study in a local Portland hospital that confirmed my experience was not unique. For women in active labor, the fetal monitor strip is usually calibrated at a starting point of twenty. As soon as a contraction begins the numbers on the machine start to rise and the woman, tethered to the bed and uncomfortable to begin with, starts to react. A strong contraction might peak around seventy-five and then drop and the mother, who was breathing hard, gripping a hand or making noise, finally relaxes. With the advent of waterproof monitoring I was able to compare a woman's out of water response to her contractions with her response to the same contraction pattern, when she was immersed in water. She did not even react when the monitor began to register a contraction. Twenty—no response; twenty-five—no response; thirty, forty, forty-five—she finally began to moan or change positions and focus. To the untrained eye it would appear that her contractions had become shorter in duration and less frequent when in the water. In actuality she was simply not responding to the sensation in the same way. Her coping skills were better in the birth pool.

The mother experiences more than the sum of her physiological responses to warm-water immersion. Most women feel inherently safe in the water. The water creates a wonderful barrier to the outside world. It becomes her nest, her cave, her own "womb with a view." If the pool is large enough to include her partner or husband, it then becomes an intimate place for the two of them to labor together and experience the love dance of birth. If the midwife or physician wants to do a vaginal examination while the mother is in the water, it is much easier for the mother to refuse.

The control that women gain by being able to move freely in the water often aids them in assessing their own progress either through feeling the movements of the baby more intensively or actually being able to examine themselves internally. Women report that the water intensifies the connection with the baby at the same time that it reduces the pain. They can feel the baby move, descend, and push through the birth canal. The prospect of the attendant becoming an active observer increases as mothers assume more and more responsibility for the birth and have the ease of mobility in the water.

So, the decision to enter the birth pool should be up to the mother, with the understanding that the earlier in labor the more likely her relaxation may slow labor progress.

## Why do women seek the comfort of water?

Most will head for the pool to avoid pain. Pain is such an individual perception. In speaking with thousands of mothers who have used our birth pools, the majority want to use the water in order to avoid drugs or epidural, thinking that it will help them cope without those interventions.

If a woman is planning on birthing her baby in a hospital, she should plan on staying home until her labor is well established with contractions that are long and strong and close together. Before going to the hospital she may want to enjoy a relaxing bath. This is perfectly fine as long as she is willing to keep her early labor active by frequently moving from one place to another—the bed to the bath, the bath to the toilet, indoors to outdoors. Most providers recommend using the water in early labor for no more than an hour to an hour and a half, then getting out, walking, squatting, moving, and being as normal as possible.

The most benefit is usually derived when a consistent labor pattern has been established. A consistent labor pattern does not always mean "active labor," which according to traditional definitions means four to five centimeters of dilation. For some women the relaxation effect may cause her to let go of inhibitions, producing a more rapid labor. Many home-birth midwives report watching women progress from one centimeter dilation to complete in less than two hours.

Delta County Memorial Hospital in Delta, Colorado, built a brand-new hospital from the ground up in 2004. The director of nursing, Krista Lewis, was adamant about including deep labor pools in all the birth rooms and building them as part of the room, not sealed off in a bathroom. Several months after the opening of the new unit, she reported an amazing result. Mothers started using the baths and the nurses were often taken by surprise with how fast the labors progressed. They made a rule that if a woman gets into the bath after five centimeters' dilation, the delivery cart should be set up in the room.[53]

It seems that if a woman waits until her labor is progressing well before getting into the water, then the contractions are more effective and complete dilation is often accomplished faster. There are a number of studies that compare early and late entry in the bath, concluding that labors are shorter if a labor pattern is well established before entering the birth pool.[54]

Women planning on using a portable birth pool in a hospital often report that just the thought that they can use a birth pool will keep their labor strong and help them progress. The setting up and filling of the equipment can sometimes take an hour so it is best to plan ahead and not be disappointed when the baby comes before the water is in the pool.

The smaller the pool, the less physiologic the response. When using a blow-up kiddy pool, the baby derives the most benefit, as opposed to the mother. A baby born in any amount of water still constitutes a waterbirth. Mothers who have used both a small bath and a larger birth pool report the incredible difference the freedom of movement and buoyancy made in their labors. Archimedes was on to something!

Some women who have had waterbirths comment that, in retrospect, they would prefer that their midwives not tell them when to get into the birth pool. After a certain point in labor many mothers don't want to move, be touched, or make any extra effort and the thought of getting into the birth pool may be distressing to them. On the other hand, my own midwife, due to her inexperience with waterbirth, advised me not to get into the birth pool until I was already eight centimeters dilated. My thought upon getting in and experiencing that buoyant feeling was "Why did I wait so long?"

My next birth in water was spent almost entirely in my outdoor hot tub. The labor was only four hours from start to finish and even though I tried to get out of the water, when I stood up and felt the difference that gravity made on my belly, I sat right back down and refused to get out.

Waterbirth, although a desirable choice for many women, is simply an option, not an end to be achieved in every birth. When women have the birth pool available, many gravitate to it without hesitation and feel safe staying in and birthing their babies.

### Do you deliver the placenta in the water?

Childbirth practitioners are somewhat divided on this issue. Some allow the woman to stay in the birth pool for the expulsion of the placenta, and some ask the woman to stand up or leave the birth pool to birth the placenta. Although opinion and practice is divided on this issue, physicians and midwives who allow women to deliver the placenta in the water report that it is safe and without side effects. Using this method, the umbilical cord is not cut or clamped until the placenta is out of the woman's body. Doctors and midwives have observed that there is less bleeding this way and that the babies almost always start nursing immediately after birth, which helps with the expulsion of the placenta.

There are some restrictions to staying in the birth pool after the baby has been born. These would include excessive bleeding, problems with the baby's cord, severe tearing in the perineal area, or if the mother was feeling exhausted or faint.

In a physiologic birth where no artificial hormones have been used the placenta usually only take a few minutes to expel. One can almost set a watch by the reaction of the mother. She is relaxed, extremely happy, and holding her baby in the water. After about twelve minutes she gets a puzzled look or a grimace on her face. You know that contractions have started and at that time you can ask her to push and the placenta generally plops out into the water.

Some midwives state that the time allowed for the passage of the placenta increases slightly with birth in water. It is their general feeling that the water relaxes the uterus and that the contractions for birthing the placenta are less effective when a woman stays in the water after the baby's birth. When some women stand up to get out of the tub, however, the placenta virtually falls out.

Some women who have "planned" to have a waterbirth and then birth outside the birth pool get back into the water to birth the placenta. Other women who have had a waterbirth and get out to birth the placenta often get back into a clean bath to relax and float the baby. Once again, this seems to be a matter of choice and judgment. There are no set guidelines to follow.

## How are emergencies handled in the water?

The physicians and midwives who include waterbirth in their practices carefully monitor the progress of the birth and the baby's status throughout labor, just as in any birth. If an emergency is encountered, the situation is assessed and the proper course of action taken. The mother may be required to get out of the birth pool or simply change positions. Practitioners use their own judgment and level of experience during labor and birth to guide them.

A decrease in the baby's heart rate, detected through the use of a waterproof Doppler or fetal monitor, is often seen as a cause for concern, especially in the hospital. Sometimes this situation can be easily remedied by simply asking the mother to change positions. Almost all birthing positions can be assumed in the water with minimal effort because of the water's buoyancy. A woman can squat, sit, kneel, be on her hands and knees, or sit on someone's lap. She can even lie down on her side if the birth pool is large enough. In some instances changing positions will not resolve the problem and the mother is asked to leave the pool for more careful monitoring.

There are absolute reasons to discontinue a birth in water or not plan one in the first place. The most important reason not to do a waterbirth is a fearful attendant. The midwife or doctor who has no experience and has not yet learned how to relax and allow the mother to be in control of her own body and birth has a higher risk of causing the complications they wish to avoid.

Waterbirth is a very hands-off experience. A doctor in Illinois, after attending one of my waterbirth workshops, innocently and rather sarcastically asked how he could justify his fees if he was not required to "do" anything at the birth. I prayed for a quick response and was happy when I used a creative analogy to illustrate the importance of his job. I replied, "Does the lifeguard on the beach get paid if no one drowns?"

The best way to handle an emergency situation in the water is to avoid having one. Careful screening and watchful monitoring of labor progress and fetal well-being will help avoid potential problems. Any problems associated with the actual

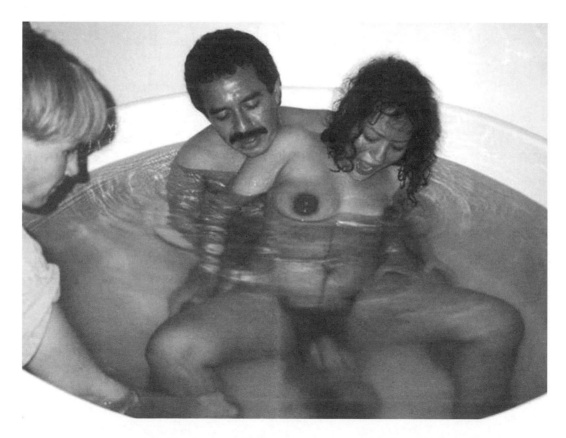

*Most waterbirths occur without anyone ever touching the baby.*

birth can also be assessed and handled quickly when a woman is in the water. Some problems are actually resolved more easily because of the water. Midwives report that a cord around the baby's neck is much easier to remove while the baby is still in the water. When the baby's head emerges under the water and a cord is felt, it is either lifted over the baby's head or a hand is slipped under the cord so that it can be passed down over the body when the baby comes out.

Another concern is that the baby may inhale meconium, the baby's first stool, during the birth. Although a rare occurrence, this is a situation that must be monitored closely. Inhaling this thick, tarry substance can be life-threatening to a baby. Midwives have stated that their ability to deal with meconium is so much better in the water. If the meconium staining is what they classify as light or medium, they allow the birth to proceed in the water and watch as the water "washes" any meconium off the baby's face. Some midwives gently massage the baby's face during the time between the emergence of the baby's head and the birth of the body. This may help to expel any plugs of meconium from the baby's nostrils and sinus cavities. If the meconium staining is classified as heavy, most practitioners ask the mother to stand as the baby's head is crowning. As soon as the head is born, the baby can be suctioned with a DeLee mucus trap to remove the meconium.

Breech position has traditionally been a reason for a more controlled birth or even an automatic cesarean section. But there are practitioners throughout the world who recognize that even for breech births there is increased safety for the baby if it is born in water. A doctor experienced in breech birth in water is Hermann Ponette, an obstetrician who practices at H. Surreys Hospital in Ostend, Belgium. He has attended well over two thousand waterbirths including dozens of breeches and twins. He uses a frank breech position as an *indication* for a waterbirth.[55] There are other reports of a few hospitals in the US attending breech waterbirths and hundreds of reported breech births in water at home.

Shoulder dystocia is considered an obstetric or midwifery emergency by most practitioners. Protocols require mothers who are anticipating large babies to leave the bath. Now there is a growing body of experience that suggests that shoulder dystocia can be managed more easily in the pool. Canadian home-birth attendant Gloria Lemay has written a protocol for management of shoulder dystocia in the water. It appears that tight shoulders happen more often because of practitioners or mothers trying to push before the baby fully rotates. Position changes in the water are so much easier to effect and the mother doesn't panic but remains calm. A quick switch to hands and knees or even to standing up with one foot up on the edge of the pool if shoulders are really tight can help maneuver the baby out.

The use of water often transforms what could be considered an emergency and possibly require a cesarean into an experience that is handled efficiently because of the water.

### How can I have a waterbirth in my hospital, and will my insurance company pay for it?

Hospitals in the United States have made incredible advances in the waterbirth movement. In almost all of the more than 250 hospitals where there are successful waterbirth programs, they have been started by Certified Nurse-Midwives. Midwives are more open to exploring the issue with their clients and doing the research necessary to get protocols accepted in hospitals. Some midwives have even purchased portable birth pool equipment with their own funds in hopes that it would pay for itself by generating more business. In most instances that investment has paid off. The use of birth pools in U.S. hospitals is at least five years behind the European movement, but home-birth midwives in the United States have been offering waterbirth longer than most of their European counterparts.[56] The United Kingdom has had the benefit of government-sponsored research and data reporting. One of the barriers to acceptance of waterbirth in the United States is the lack of published studies. I wrote to the practice committee of the American College of Obstetricians and Gynecologists (ACOG) in 1995, sending them all the printed studies available at that time. I wanted to know their opinion of waterbirth. Dr. Stanley Zinberg wrote back and cited that due to the lack of evidence ACOG could not have an official opinion and would wait until there were randomized controlled trials with large numbers, whose outcomes were published in U.S. peer review journals, before issuing an opinion.

Some of the states that have made the most progress for hospital waterbirth are Maine, New Hampshire, Vermont, Illinois, Ohio, North Carolina, and Massachusetts. Obviously, the East Coast is changing faster than the West Coast. It is surprising to some people when they find out that the whole state of California only has a handful of hospitals that provide waterbirth services.

For mothers who want their hospital to provide this service it is good to know how to navigate the political and social culture of hospitals. I have worked with many women who call during their pregnancy and want a hospital waterbirth.

It takes three ingredients to make policy changes within a hospital setting:

1. a motivated mother;
2. an open and supportive practitioner;
3. a compassionate nurse manager or perinatal coordinator who is willing to take on the training of staff and the creation of new policy.

Waterbirth International will supply the necessary research studies, the sample protocols, the pool kits, the videos, and the experience to help couples get policy changed, but without these first three components some hospitals will continue to deny the request. Time is the other factor. The more advance notice a hospital is given, the better chances there are for change.

Hospitals in England that have installed birth pools or allow women to bring their own rented pools are not hampered by the restrictions of the insurance companies that govern policy in American hospitals. The most successful way of negotiating change in hospitals is consumer advocacy. One couple's request may be easily overlooked, but ten couples asking for the same service are more difficult to ignore.

Lisa and David Blake were preparing for their second baby when they felt motivated to investigate using water for labor. Their first calls to the hospital in Yuma, Arizona, were not returned. Their provider, a certified nurse-midwife, was open to exploring the option of water labor and possibly waterbirth. Lisa downloaded articles from the Waterbirth International Web site and shared this information with her midwife and doula. The stumbling block was the nurse manager at the local community hospital. I called the nurse manager, and we had a frank discussion about clients bringing in their own birth pool equipment. I faxed her engineering details and mailed her a packet of materials with protocols and names of other hospitals in Arizona that have already adopted water labor and birth protocols. Everything seemed to look favorable for the Blakes.

After about three weeks, Lisa called the nurse manager who told her that it was not possible for her to bring in the pool. She stated that the engineering department did not approve its use. Lisa called me, quite discouraged, and I assured her that we still had plenty of time to reverse this decision. I laid out a plan to call the engineering department directly and then the CEO of the hospital, if that did not work. We joked that she should rent the pool kit anyway and set it up on the sidewalk outside of the hospital. Her husband thought that was a good idea.

When I reached the hospital engineer, he informed me that he had no objections but the nurse manager had refused to allow the birth pool onto her unit. I am very familiar with this game of approval ping-pong. Getting bounced between departments is sometimes a deliberate stall tactic. If a delay is long enough, the mother goes into labor, has her baby, and everyone can go back to practicing standard obstetrics.

I called the nurse manager and confronted her with the engineer's words. At that point we started getting somewhere because she then admitted that it was beyond her ability to decide and in the hands of the hospital management. A letter seemed in order. Advising Lisa and her husband on how to compose an effective letter, I also told them to call the local newspaper and television station to offer them a story about a proposed waterbirth. Both the TV and newspaper were interested and even arranged for a photographer to record the birth.

The letter that David and Lisa wrote mentioned that laboring in water was their chosen method of pain management and they fully intended to comply with the wishes of their midwife in case anything went wrong. All the approvals from the hospital came just two weeks prior to Lisa's due date and she was thrilled, but worried that the baby might arrive before the birth pool did. In the end, baby Annika arrived in the birth pool exactly on Lisa's due date, with a photographer and television reporter attending along with midwife and doula.

The nurse manager of any unit, large or small, has an enormous responsibility and has to answer to as many as nine department heads in order to make policy revisions or inclusions. This is why it may take as long as three to five months to seek approvals. Having the patience to work with the various departments usually pays off.

A few insurance companies have refused to cover providers who offer waterbirth to their clients. After educating most of the insurance executives about waterbirth, they continue to insure the doctors and midwives. The state health insurance agency in Washington in 1998 attempted to make waterbirth illegal by refusing to reimburse for services if the baby was born in water. Waterbirth is extremely popular among women giving birth at home or in birth centers in Washington. The Midwives Association of Washington State (MAWS) appointed a committee to investigate and form a rebuttal to this uneducated reaction. The midwives were successful in having this state ruling overturned.

When waterbirth is offered in a hospital or birth center as part of the program, it is usually not even mentioned to the insurance company that the birth took place in the water. A vaginal birth is a vaginal birth, no matter where it takes place. If a woman needs to rent or purchase equipment for her water labor or birth she can submit a claim to her insurance company for reimbursement. There are only a few pool rental companies in the United States and none of them bill for third-party reimbursement. There is currently no unified insurance billing code for the use of a waterbirth pool for labor. There should be a code, just as there is for an epidural or a shot of pain medication. The water is the best non-pharmacological method of pain management and insurance companies will eventually pay for it. Some already reimburse their subscribers for renting birth pool equipment.

If you would like waterbirth available at your hospital, consult your provider first, do your homework, and make your wishes known in the form of a letter to the hospital nurse manager of the maternity unit (see Appendix D for a sample letter). If you don't get any response the first time, send a follow-up letter within two weeks. Get other couples to do the same thing. Don't be afraid to send a copy to the newspaper, either.

## JUST FOR PROVIDERS

Even though a waterbirth is a very hands-off procedure there is a great deal of very useful information that doesn't come from the literature, but from attending births and seeing what does and does not work. The International Waterbirth Conferences yield a great deal of information every three years. Here are some "helpful hints" from providers around the world.

1. Add a few extras pieces of equipment to birth bags or equipment carts.

   *A waterproof mirror.* Very useful in placing underneath a woman if she is squatting and you want to visualize the perineum. A regular mirror will get water trapped behind the glass and distort the image.

   *A waterproof flashlight.* If the room is dark, you can hold the flashlight above the water and shine it down toward the perineum, or place it on the floor of the pool so that it reflects in the mirror.

   *Floating bowl.* Bring your own placenta container and know how much it holds.

   *A roll of duct tape.* A small piece of duct tape on the top of your shoulder-length glove will keep it in place. A bigger piece will keep towels used as head rolls in place on the edge of birth pools.

   *Pool noodle.* Mothers can lean over it and experience more flotation.

   *Aromatherapy drops for water.* Discuss this before labor and know what the mother's preferences are.

   *Extra clamp ready for cord.* If you do intend to cut the cord while the mother is still in the water, have a second clamp handy. Polly Malby, CNM, reports that the cord is not as sticky in the water and she has seen a clamp come off and float away.

   *Small plastic footstool.* Can be easily placed under the mother after birth while she is still in the water to raise her up slightly higher. Babies sometimes have difficulty reaching the breast when the water is deep.

2. *Bend, don't lean.* Good body mechanics will prevent a backache. Reaching over a birth pool is too difficult, so keep your knees bent and use a birth ball to sit on.

3. *Keep your hands out of the water.* Practice leaving your hands off the perineum. It is better for mother to reach down and guide her baby out and your back will appreciate the rest.

4. *Practice assessing blood loss.* Some midwives practice visualizing blood in the water by placing a few tablespoons of cow blood (obtained from a butcher) at a time into a birth pool. The practice makes some feel more comfortable and better able to judge how much blood is too much.

5. *Keep extra towels on hand.* Cleaning up water spillage quickly will prevent any slips. A non-slip bath mat beside the birth pool is useful.

6. *Waterproof watch.* Make sure you either remove your wrist watch or have a waterproof one.

7. *Basin of water.* Keep a basin of water beside the birth pool for bathing the feet of mothers who walk around the house or yard and then get back in the pool.
8. *Spray bottle.* A spritz of cool water on the face and neck helps keep the mother cooled and prevents her from overheating. It feels good too!
9. *Extra tee shirt.* Just in case you get wet, it is a good idea to have something to change into.

## THE FUTURE OF WATERBIRTH

A midwife's or physician's hesitancy about allowing labor or birth in water can be felt by the mother and she often acquiesces just to make her practitioner feel more comfortable, instead of following her own instincts and staying in the water. Many women in hospitals get out of the pool because they don't want to get their midwives "in trouble" by insisting on giving birth in water. Conversely, midwives often must insist that a mother get out of the pool because protocols have not been set up for birth or the practitioner is just not comfortable with the process.

The decision to birth in the water should be left up to the mother, but based on sound advice and assessment of fetal well-being by the practitioner. The mother who presents prenatally and is insistent that she is going to have a water birth no matter what is usually destined to birth anywhere but the birth pool. Flexibility is always required in birth, but especially for those women who add the element of water.

Waterbirth has taught us a great deal about normal labor and birth. Watching a woman labor and give birth without interference of any kind renews our faith and trust in the birth process. Many other practices are changed in hospital environments due to the amazing success of the waterbirths. How can a provider justify cutting an episiotomy on women birthing on a bed, when they have been totally eliminated for women birthing is water? Why are women told not to eat or drink in labor when a woman who is laboring in water must drink a glass of fluid every hour to prevent dehydration? When a water pool is placed on a busy maternity unit, unnecessary obstetric practices have a better chance of dying out. I call it the "K-Mart" theory. You go to K-Mart to buy a sale item and you come out with a whole lot of things you didn't even know you wanted.

A woman who has experienced one waterbirth will *almost always* seek to repeat her experience. Here is what some women have to say about their waterbirths.

## Women's Voices

*"I experienced relaxation, total peace. I felt very loose, my body just melted, my face dropped, it was wonderful."*

*"I felt more in control of the situation instead of at the mercy of doctors and nurses."*

*"Simon's waterbirth was the most euphoric experience of my life. It was calm, relaxed, powerful, natural and blessed. We all have the capability to transcend the stereotype that birth has become in our society."*

*"Our birthpool was invaluable during an intense four-hour labor!"*

*"I couldn't imagine giving birth any other way than in the comfort of our home and in water. I loved it so much I did it a second time!"*

*"It was so great to be able to move and change positions without help or hindrance as I needed to during labor. I had absolutely no tearing even though he was actually 'born' really quickly. I only pushed twice. My husband caught him, rocked him underwater for a minute, then brought him up to me. He was pink and perfect from moment one. He is almost 6 months old now and this whole time—really from his first days—people have been commenting on his alertness and strength. I think it stems from having an unmedicated, gentle birth. We had only candlelight to see by and the only people in attendance were people I loved and who loved me."*

*"2.5 hours of labor from the first contraction. She never cried, and ever since then has been the most peaceful baby (compared to my first daughter!). The hot water was instrumental in relieving my pain as I did it naturally, without meds."*

*"The water helped me to relax and prepare for the next contractions. . . . Even my doctor was impressed with how well everything went, from 6cm to delivered in 11 minutes, without an episiotomy."*

*"Addison's birth in water was mind-blowing, mystical, life changing, invigorating, powerful, validating and much more. I would encourage everyone to try water as a soothing and healing way to give birth. Absolutely incredible."*

*"The birth of my son was beautiful, every contraction, every moment of labor, every ounce of pain. Declan was born in the water. He was calm and relaxed. His eyes were wide open and his limbs extended. I can not think of a more peaceful way for a child to enter the world. If it were possible I would give birth 1,000 times."*

# CHAPTER SEVEN

# The Mind-Body Connection

The cooperation between mind and body is most evident during pregnancy and birth, and an integrated approach to health can be very effective during these times. As the option of gentle birth becomes more available, we have the opportunity to observe the birth process in its natural form. We can talk to women about why they did not need intervention or medication and what helped them to be able to give birth gently. In this chapter we will explore the connectedness between mind and body, thoughts and actions, mother and baby.

Many childbirth educators have recognized the importance of the mind-body response. In *Childbirth Without Fear,* Grantly Dick-Read noted that when a woman experiences fear (an emotion), her body tightens (a physical response), which causes pain. When she experiences the pain, her level of fear increases, causing more tension and thus more pain. A cycle of fear, tension, and pain becomes established and often leads to a prolonged birth process.[1] Without explaining this cycle on a cellular or chemical level, Dick-Read correctly identified the cause-and-effect relationship of emotions and the mind-body response. He emphasized the importance of using awareness of the biological functions of the body as a method of dispelling learned fear and also stressed how valuable the presence of a calm and reassuring person can be throughout a woman's labor and birth.

Ferdinand Lamaze also worked within the area of mind-body response using the conditioning techniques that he perfected for labor and birth. By replacing their current anxious thoughts with more positive ones, women were able to learn a new response to stimuli that would have otherwise produced pain. They conditioned their bodies not to respond to the pain in the way that they had previously learned.

It is impossible to ignore the dramatic and dynamic changes that take place in the body during pregnancy. It is important for a woman to have an understanding of the physical changes that occur during her pregnancy. Focusing attention on the growing fetus and its development helps a mother shift into thinking about herself. She now has a reason for paying attention to the inner workings of her body; she may now be motivated to evaluate her diet and her lifestyle in general.

## WOMB ECOLOGY

Your womb is the sacred space for the baby's growth. There are many factors that influence the growth and development of the baby—physical, emotional, and spiritual. Your baby's body and all the biological systems within it—including the skeleton, brain, kidneys, liver, lungs, and heart—are formed in the first six weeks. This is one of the most vital times of the baby's life and yet some women don't even realize they are pregnant at this early stage.

Diet plays a vital part in fostering a good mind/body connection and a safe and secure womb environment for your baby. An inadequate diet will not only contribute to problems during the birth but it will also lead to permanent and life-long difficulties for your child. It might be burdensome to consider that your choice today may affect your great-grandchild, but everything you eat, drink, and think becomes the inner ecology of generations yet to be born.

Forty years of research in prenatal nutrition yields scientific evidence that good nutrition is directly related to preventing problems that include:

- Birth defects, such as spina bifida
- Stillbirth
- Premature or low-birth-weight babies
- Lower intelligence
- Diabetes
- Irritability and behavior disorders
- Autism
- Allergy and skin conditions, such as eczema

You are "eating for two," but you need to do this in a healthful and conscious way. The best recommendation that I can make is to follow closely the "Blue Ribbon Baby Diet" that Dr. Tom Brewer and Gail Brewer created and promote in her book, *What Every Pregnant Woman Should Know: The Truth About Diet and Drugs in Pregnancy*.[2]

It goes without saying that tobacco smoke and alcohol consumption puts the growing baby at risk. So do many other substances that most pregnant women aren't even aware of. We can't always be conscious of what is in our water or food supply, but scientists, ecologists, and researchers have clearly identified some devastating connections between fetal brain development and certain metal compounds. The baby is extremely susceptible to even the minutest amounts of chemicals and toxins. My rule of thumb about consuming things that may be harmful, even when not pregnant, has been "when in doubt, don't."

## Fish and Mercury

During the second half of pregnancy, when the fetal brain undergoes a big growth spurt, omega-3 fatty acids (DHA and EPA) are required for the sudden growth of fetal neurons and blood vessels. You have probably seen the eggs in the supermarket that boast of containing omega-3. It is now clear that omega-3 fatty acids are of major importance for proper nutrition during pregnancy.

DHA (docosahexaenoic acid) is a vital component of the brain and is needed to create specific nerve pathways including the light-sensitive parts of the eye. DHA is like the connector piece in a Lego set. If there aren't enough of them, then certain areas of the pathways in the brain just don't form. After the baby is born, breast-feeding is essential because the DHA content of the infant's brain triples during the first three months of life. DHA is the most abundant omega-3 long chain fatty acid in breast milk and formula makers can't replicate it. Studies show that breast-fed babies have IQ advantages over babies who are fed formula.[3]

Fish is well known to have the highest content of omega-3 fatty acids, so it would seem that we should just eat more fish. Well, it is not quite as easy as that due to air and water pollution. The Environmental Protection Agency maintains a national database on U.S. rivers and lakes. Their concern for pregnant women is that one out of three lakes and 25 percent of rivers have toxic levels of pollutants, especially methyl mercury, that have been linked to birth defects and illnesses in infants and children. Women who eat fish more than twice a week have blood mercury levels that are seven times higher than women who eat no fish. Mercury, like lead, wreaks havoc on fetal brain growth and must be avoided.[4] Prenatal exposure to mercury has been linked to deficits in memory, learning, and attention span that persist into adolescence and appear to be irreversible.

Mercury gets into fish due to air pollution by way of toxins from coal-burning power plants, incinerators, and from the manufacture of soap and of wood pulp for paper products. Paper towels, napkins, tissues, and even disposable diapers all contribute to the mercury content of fish, which could potentially damage your baby's brain. To date, no federal laws require existing power plants to control mercury emissions.

Once in the atmosphere the mercury floats around for up to a year, coming back down in rain and snow. When it reaches our water supply the mercury attaches to plant life and becomes the highly toxic methyl mercury. This toxin magnifies itself through the aquatic food chain, becoming more and more concentrated. Each time a bigger fish eats a smaller fish, the toxin levels get higher and higher. Top-feeding fishes like tuna carry levels that are a million times higher than the water they swim in.

The good news is that not all fish is bad, and if strict guidelines are followed you should be reasonably safe. The Food and Drug Administration (FDA) now advises pregnant mothers to eat no more than two six-ounce cans of light-colored tuna per week (or no more than one can of albacore tuna). Swordfish, shark, tile-fish, and king mackerel should be avoided completely. The July 2004 issue of "Consumer Reports" advises women to eat no more than three ounces of albacore tuna each week. This is half the FDA's recommended weekly limit. Because mercury is stored in our body fat, just as it is in fish, women planning to have children should also avoid high-mercury fish well before they become pregnant. Shrimp, pollock, salmon, and catfish are low-mercury fish and are good choices.[5]

The presence of mercury in fish is an environmental issue and now a political one. It is interesting to note that the largest disposable diaper manufacturer in the country, Procter & Gamble, which also makes soap and other paper products, is opposed to any regulations on mercury emissions. One would hate to think that the seemingly simple choice of whether to use disposable diapers or cloth diapers might contribute to mental retardation and attention deficit disorders in children. This is an example of how interconnected all of the choices we make as consumers, and especially as parents, really are.

Creating a nourishing womb environment may mean cleansing the body of toxins prior to conception and avoiding all persistent organic pollutants (POPs) and all heavy metals throughout pregnancy and nursing. There are very gentle homeo-pathic formulas that can assist with detoxifying the body.[6] Before starting any pro-gram to rid your body of heavy metals it is best to check with a naturopathic or holistic physician for testing and guidance.

Here are some suggestions for both preconception and prenatal diet regimens that create a nontoxic womb environment.

- Eat organic foods whenever possible.
- Drink filtered water—8 glasses a day.
- Eat a natural, seasonal cuisine.
- Cook in iron, stainless steel, glass, or porcelain cookware.
- Salt your food only after tasting it.
- Alternate foods, especially common allergens, trying not to eat the same things every day, such as milk products, eggs, wheat, and yeast foods.
- Include fruits, vegetables, whole grains, legumes, nuts and seeds.
- Avoid or minimize red meats, cured meats, organ meats, refined foods, canned foods, sugar, salt, saturated fats, coffee, alcohol, and nicotine.
- Avoid seafood known to contain mercury.

- Supplement diet with 400 mcg of folic acid daily. This is the B vitamin needed for healthy development of the spinal cord.
- Supplement with some form of omega-3 fatty acid (cod liver oil being the best) by mid-pregnancy.

## MIND-BODY RESPONSE

Amazingly enough, our bodies know how to heal themselves, filter waste products, fertilize an egg, grow a baby, and give birth. These processes that we take for granted are not things we can consciously control. They all require an uninterrupted flow of energy. The body actually experiences an energy current that flows through and around it much like the electricity that flows through the wires in the walls of your house. You don't think about electricity flowing through your house until the light doesn't turn on.

The concept of a vital energy force is shared by cultures throughout the world. Unconscious functions of the body, such as healing cancer or birthing a baby, can be strongly affected by thoughts and emotions that block the flow of this energy, or chi, through the body.

Labor is extremely physical, but it is also emotional and spiritual in nature. Medical science is now discovering that the body is made up of thoughts and emotions in addition to its physical components. Creating a harmonious womb environment requires the baby to be bathed in positive thoughts and healthy emotions. Many respected physicians and scientists believe that the mind can no longer be considered separate from the body. Intelligence, once believed to be contained only in the brain and nerve cells, is now known to be an integral part of each of our cells. In his book *Quantum Healing,* endocrinologist Dr. Deepak Chopra explains that everything we experience in our lives—memories, emotions, thoughts, and stimulation—is stored in each of our cells, thus expanding our understanding of what really forms the intelligence of our minds.[7]

Every emotion we experience is accompanied by a thought; every thought we think is accompanied by an emotion. All of the thoughts and emotions we think and feel emanate from our bodies on a cellular level. This is one reason that we have such intense physical responses to what we "feel. " Modern research shows that anything that influences our minds also influences our bodies. All forms of stress put strain on the bodily systems and our behavior becomes affected, especially during pregnancy. The body expresses the results of stress often with subtle or chronic symptoms, such as hypertension, rashes, headaches, irritable bowel, or simply making other conditions worsen. In pregnancy and labor we can predict complications sometimes based on how much anxiety and stress the woman is exhibiting. Too much stress can cause uterine blood vessels to constrict, reducing oxygen to the baby. Anything that decreases the amount of oxygen that a baby is able to receive from the placenta will cause problems, such as fetal distress or premature birth.

The interesting phenomenon of the mind-body connection is that the same mechanism that can make you sick can also be used to heal you. That is, your thoughts, emotions, responses to the environment, lifestyle, and inner conflicts can be experienced as stressful, or they may be used in a positive manner to create healing responses. Understanding our responses to stress and examining all the influences in our lives—environmental, emotional, physical, spiritual—both present and in our past, will help in coping with the stress of pregnancy and in preparing for a gentle birth. One must be willing to do the necessary work in examining all the issues, and create a plan to overcome any obstacles.

Besides "eating for two," research shows that "sleeping for two" helps reduce stress levels. A report suggested that the length and quality of sleep in the last month of pregnancy even effected the length of labor and the outcome. Women who slept fewer than seven hours a night had a much greater incidence of cesarean births.[8]

Some external influences can be changed but the majority of what we experience as stressful is often out of our control. By choosing responses which reflect compassion, forgiveness, and faith, we can often mitigate the detrimental effects of stress and experience a healthy gentle birth. Pregnancy is a perfect time to take new approaches in learning about yourself. Pregnancy is, after all, the time in your life when you express the most creative potential.

## LISTENING TO YOUR BODY

Women usually want to know if what they are experiencing during pregnancy is normal. They look to others for the answers to these questions, especially in a first pregnancy, which can be a new and possibly frightening experience. The medical model, described in chapter 4, encourages an outward focus by insisting that pregnant women go to experts who will tell them what they are feeling. Pregnancy has to be officially diagnosed by a doctor before some women will trust what they are feeling in their bodies. The midwives model empowers a woman to become mindful of her body, explore her inner feelings, and question *herself* about their meaning instead of asking an expert for an outward interpretation.

In order to be in touch with yourself it is important to be aware of the ongoing dialogue between the physical body and the mind, including emotions and thoughts. By taking time each day for an inner dialogue, you can begin a process of self-discovery. It is not necessary for this process to be mystical or complicated. It can be as simple as lying quietly and asking yourself, "What is going on in my body and how do I feel about it?" It may mean taking a walk by the ocean or in the woods. The object is to reduce the amount of outward stimulation and focus inward. Some people achieve this through prayer or meditation; others simply become "mindful." With all the distractions of our busy lives, it is sometimes difficult to set aside the time to focus inward, but when practiced daily, mindfulness becomes a valuable tool for the rest of your life, not just during pregnancy.

Pregnancy is a time of increased awareness. Most women are amazed at the process that takes place within them. For some women, being pregnant is the deepest connection that they have ever felt within themselves. Some women may be afraid to become a mother because of unpleasant experiences in their own childhood. It is important to ask yourself questions like, "How do I really feel about becoming a mother?" or "What did I like about the way in which I was mothered?" These questions will allow you to explore your feelings.

Emotions at a birth can be extremely intense. Having a baby is a major transition in a woman's life. It can be fulfilling and empowering, or it can be a struggle with unresolved emotions that can produce long-lasting effects. Many pregnancies are accompanied by feelings of ambivalence. The sooner those feelings are resolved, the less chance there will be for complications during labor and birth.

Many women, including grandmothers, describe their births as if they had just taken place. Their stories have the emotional intensity of the original experience. The remembrance of a woman's birth experience, if it was a negative one, needs to be cleared or processed in order to integrate it into her consciousness. If this is not done, this remembrance may influence other births and how she feels about herself and her children. When Nancy Wainer Cohen founded Cesarean/Support, Education, and Concern (C/SEC), a cesarean counseling group, she was flooded with over forty thousand letters from women who still could not deal with the emotional issues surrounding their cesarean births.[9]

The object of being aware is not so much to be in control of your body or its emotions but to recognize and work with them. This allows you to take charge of your life. A woman who keeps herself from expressing or releasing emotions is storing them on a cellular level somewhere in the body. The hormonal shifts in a woman's body during pregnancy make her emotionally vulnerable. Many people view emotions as being either positive or negative, but expressing all emotions is healthy. The key to dealing with emotions during pregnancy and birth is to first recognize them and then to release the negative ones. Most women need a support person who can encourage them to express their feelings without judgment. This person could be a friend, partner, professional counselor, doctor, or midwife.

When Eleanor became pregnant with her second baby it was a shock and a disappointment. She had been using birth control. She was divorced with one child already and not sure she wanted to be in a permanent relationship with this baby's father. She also distinctly remembered the pain and suffering of her first birth experience and vowed never to repeat it, even abstaining from sex for five years. Part of her wanted to lovingly accept the pregnancy, but the other part was terrified. The ambivalence was tearing her apart; she was experiencing intense nausea and sleep difficulties and she noticed that her three-year-old was acting out. Her life was in turmoil.

Accepting her pregnancy, she consciously decided to seek counseling and support so that she could prepare for this birth differently. She went first to a traditional psychotherapist, but felt that it might take too long to dredge up all the horrors of her past. In choosing her maternity care provider, a midwife, she was introduced to a woman who used a combination of hypnosis and breathwork to address emotional issues. Her sessions with Linda were comfortable and focused on her power of choice.

Eleanor felt a breakthrough when she understood the impact that her behavioral choices were having on her mental state as well as her physical feelings. She began to understand that she might not be able to choose how she was feeling about a situation or event, but she had the power to choose what to think and speak about it.

She remembered feeling powerless in her first birth and very frightened about becoming a mother. Her labor had lasted almost two full days. The turning point in her labor came when she admitted she was afraid. She recalled that she suddenly dilated from 1 to 7 centimeters in about fifteen minutes after finally saying that no matter what, she wanted this baby. It was her first conscious admission of wanting to become a mother. Her body responded when she unblocked this energy.

So, for this new pregnancy she practiced witnessing her feelings and choosing how to think and speak about them. In essence she harnessed them and used positive affirmations to counteract her fear. Although she still sometimes felt afraid and reluctant, she spoke to herself in positive terms. This time her labor only lasted two hours, with the midwife barely making it to her home.

## LISTENING TO THE BABY

For many years professionals have thought that a baby's biology and behavior was determined only by the quality and number of genes that he or she received in utero. Today, there is a growing awareness that what goes on in the womb from a hormonal and emotional perspective profoundly affects not only the life of this child, but actually influences future generations. In his ground-breaking work on nature versus nurture, Dr. Bruce Lipton states that "maternal behaviors and emotions profoundly impact the child's physical development, behavioral characteristics, and even its level of intelligence."[10]

One striking example of the generational legacy of the womb experience can be found in children born to Dutch women who were on starvation diets during the famine of World War II. The women produced smaller than normal babies.

Interestingly, this pattern of stunted growth continued into the next generation even though there was an abundance of food and not one single mother was starving.[11] This phenomenon has been called "the grandmother effect." It demonstrates that we have the power to alter brain chemistry and genetic encoding.

Babies demonstrate most dramatically the mind-body response. When a baby is born, she has been in close physical contact with her mother and has lived within her womb environment of thoughts and emotions. If we perceive these emotions to be stimulated and released on a cellular level, as Dr. Deepak Chopra illustrates in *Quantum Healing,* then it is likely that the baby also perceives them in utero. Mother and baby share the same bioenergy system. Chopra describes this shared system as *entrainment,* a rhythmic relationship between the physical bodies, including all cellular activity.[12]

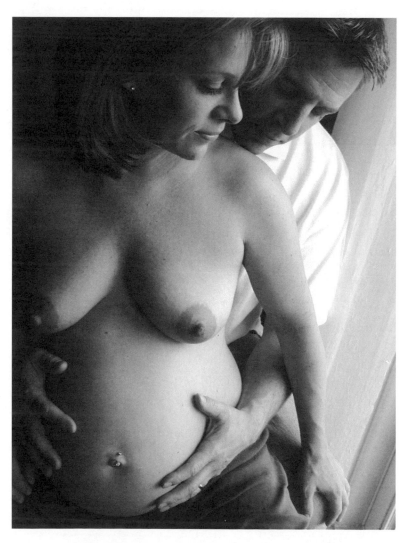

*Communication with the baby starts during pregnancy.*

Dr. David Cheek was a noted San Francisco obstetrician who, after a long and successful career, turned his attention to prenatal life. He published extensively on prenatal communication. In a study in which he used hypnotic techniques that he had developed, over one thousand subjects related incidences of prenatal communication. The doctor noted that "fetal channels for information are psychic (telepathic and or/clairvoyant) and possibly hormonal."[13]

This connection does not end at birth; in fact, it becomes stronger because the infant now has the basis for his own emotional life. While perceiving his mother's mind-body state, an infant cannot communicate with words but uses his cries and body postures as cues to indicate what is going on inside of him and what he perceives in his environment.

Dr. Wendy Anne McCarty was a therapist and former obstetric nurse attending a pre- and perinatal psychology conference when she heard Dr. William Emerson introduce his work—diagnosing birth trauma and defining a course of treatment for a three-month-old baby.[14] "Can someone actually do psychotherapy with an infant?" was the question that McCarty kept asking herself. But what she witnessed during a videotape presentation of the therapy was not only a communication between therapist and baby, but a deep and quiet stillness in the baby, who emanated an expression of gratitude. Gratitude for being seen and heard.

Dr. Emerson works exclusively with birth trauma. This particular infant was portraying movement patterns and emotional expressions associated with a difficult portion of his birth. By quietly speaking to the baby and acknowledging how similar the baby's present experience felt to that particularly difficult time during his birth, the doctor empathized with the baby's experience and the baby responded.

Dr. McCarty was fascinated by this demonstration. She went on to cofound with Dr. Ray Castellino one of the first training programs in birth trauma awareness and resolution. BEBA (Building and Enhancing Bonding and Attachment), based in Santa Barbara, California, is a school for future therapists, but more importantly it serves families with immediate needs for healing. Brain and nervous system development, immune system strength, learning capacity, stress coping strategies, emotional stability, and physical coordination are all dependent on experiences in the womb, at birth, or in early childhood.

As Dr. Lipton revealed in his work on the importance of a loving womb environment, nature or genetics is only part of what creates a normal, healthy child. The sequence of development is laid out genetically but the early environment is the major contributor to how well the systems work. Optimal development occurs with the timely resolution of early trauma and the resulting secure attachment between parents and children. Secure attachment provides the base for a healthy life with healthy relationships. This is the good news. Even if the birth experience was less than optimal, parents can still work with their children to make up for the loss and adults can resolve trauma at any age.

Birth memories reflecting early perceptions have been activated in adult clients in response to hypnosis, psychoanalysis, LSD, psychodrama, sensory deprivation tanks, and certain breathing techniques.[15] In each experience the spontaneous "remembering" of the birth experience reveals just how great its influence was on the entire psychological patterning of the individual. Psychiatrist Stanislav Grof states, "Reliving biological birth and integrating the experience into one's way of being seems to offer possibilities of psychosomatic healing, personality transformation and consciousness evolution that by far exceed therapy limited to work with biographical material from childhood and later life."[16]

Dr. David Chamberlain, psychotherapist and past president of the Association of Prenatal and Perinatal Psychology and Health (APPPAH), came to similar conclusions, stating that "when we believed that no mind could be working at birth, we never had to consider the consequences of needless pain and suffering on our personal lives or on our social order."[17]

Out of the many therapies that help people remember and resolve birth trauma, hypnosis gives us the most detailed accounts, often moment-by-moment birth reports. These amazing stories give us the advantage of a mature adult with the full use of language, but they reveal the clear thought processes and deep feelings of the infant at the time of birth. From these accounts we can now learn what birth and newborn care are like from the baby's point of view. Dr. Chamberlain did a cross-matching of mothers' accounts of birth compared to their adult children "remembering" and found an amazingly consistent correlation between perceived memories and actual events. Children even reported what their mothers were thinking during labor and birth! A short example of a taped hypnosis session will give you a much better understanding of the thoughts of a newborn.

[Dr. Chamberlain explains that Deborah, when only halfway out of her mother's body, begins to make a series of sharp observations.] The doctor is looking around for something. I'm coming out, but just my eyes, I think. The doctor has black hair and a white coat and he's looking at a tray of instruments. He's turned away from me. I don't think he knows I'm coming out. Somebody better tell him I'm going to come out! I think I'm just going to do it by myself. . . .

I feel awful cold all over, especially my hands and feet. I think I'm not supposed to be this cold. My mom's trying to look around and see what's going on. They keep pushing her back down on the table. She's starting to cry because she doesn't know what's happening, and she thinks something is the matter with me. I'm all right. They're pulling on my hands and feet, kind of rubbing on them real hard. Why don't they just leave me alone? I'm all right, really I am. Just leave me alone. Everybody's all around, pulling on my fingers and rubbing them. I guess they think I'm the wrong color. That's what it is—my fingers are blue. That's why they are so cold. They put me by somebody now, on a blanket, lots of blankets.

Somebody's holding me. It's the nurse with the yellow hair. I'm all wrapped up real tight now. I can't wiggle around anymore but at least they quit mashing me. They let her [Deborah's mom] hold me for a little while. My hands are still cold, wrapped up. Mom's still crying a little bit but not like she was before. Everything's okay now, so I can go to sleep. I knew I was okay. I tried to tell everybody, but they wouldn't listen. I was trying to talk but they didn't understand me. And I was trying to push them away with my hands, but there were too many of them. I was crying, trying to talk, but I guess it was just crying to them.

One of the things that really made me mad about the whole situation is this: All the time I was in there by myself, everything was just how I wanted it. And I figured that was it. I sort of had a feeling there were other things around but not people like me. But they didn't really matter because they were outside. Then when I came out, it made me mad because I didn't have anything to say about it. When I tried to, nobody paid any attention to me. That made me mad, too, because I always thought I knew what was going on. I felt I knew a lot—I really did. I thought I was pretty intelligent. I never thought about being a person, just a mind. I thought I was an intelligent mind. And so when the situation was forced on me, I didn't like it too much. I saw all these people acting real crazy. That's when I thought I really had a more intelligent mind, because I knew what the situation was with me, and they didn't seem to. They seemed to ignore me. They were doing things to me—to the outside of me. But they acted like that's all there was. When I tried to tell them things, they just wouldn't listen, like that noise wasn't really anything. It didn't sound too impressive, but it was all I had. I just really felt like I was more intelligent than they were."[18]

Many mothers experience what they call a psychic or spiritual communication with their unborn children. They hear their babies' voices and sense their presence. Dr. McCarty, after a decade of working with mothers and their babies, verifies this phenomenon, stating that even in the womb babies communicate with a sense of self. All humans need contact and recognition. This contact begins while we are still in the womb.

Part of the process of listening to your baby is listening to yourself. If the baby is particularly active or seems restless, ask yourself, "How am I feeling? Is there anything that is bothering me?" Remember, the baby responds to your mind-body state with a mind–body state of its own. Babies are wonderfully accurate mirrors for us, even in utero. We have the opportunity to bathe in the spirit of our baby's love and wisdom, to accept their unconditional love and their need to be seen, heard, touched, valued, and included. By listening to our babies, we have a rare opportunity to nurture ourselves.

Dr. Fred Wirth, a neonatologist and founder of the Institute for Prenatal Parenting, recommends that mothers take "prenatal love breaks" several times a day. He advises that your baby's personality will be predisposed to love and peace if you can simply slow down, listen quietly to peaceful music, and breathe deeply, achieving a sense of inner peace.[19] Just make sure the baby can hear the music, too. You can converse with your baby and massage your belly at the same time. This has been a tradition in many cultures for centuries. There are posters on the walls of prenatal clinics in China which remind women to look upon lovely things, think good thoughts, listen to gentle sounds, and speak only positive words. In the fast-paced Western culture it is a good reminder that a rest time for pregnant mothers and a focus on happy thoughts will actually contribute to a happier, healthier baby. "Don't worry—be happy" takes on a new meaning for both mother and baby in this context.

The right kind of music helps create a happy and welcoming womb environment. The calming and language-building qualities of listening to music in the womb have been widely discussed and promoted in the past decade.[20] Current research tells us that prenates would prefer to hear lullabies sung by their mothers. Michel Odent has written extensively on the value of the indigenous lullaby. Every mother has an innate song, which is evidenced in more primitive cultures.[21]

I created and sang different songs for all three of my children. I listened to Pachelbel's Canon in D so much during my second pregnancy it was not surprising at all when my son, Sam, at age nine, played it on his violin after only a few lessons. He even asked me where he had heard this song before. Baroque music by composers such as Pachelbel, Vivaldi, Telemann, and Handel have a tempo resembling our own heart beat at rest. Research has shown that four-month-old infants demonstrate an innate preference for music that is consonant rather than dissonant. The objective in listening to music is to help create not a musical genius but a person well integrated in mind, body, and spirit. Prenatal music is a wonderful way for parents to bond with their babies in utero and set the stage for early and successful attachment.

Babies do have thoughts of their own, but they are also sponges that absorb everything around them. This becomes even more evident after birth. Babies know when we are tense or upset. Their mind-body state will not allow negative emotions to be stored long, and they will cry to send the energy through. It is their natural way of moving energy to cry or fuss for us. Many mothers complain about their babies being fussy at the end of the day, commonly between 5 and 7 p.m. Nothing can calm them. Mothers who take time to sit and relax in order to release what they are storing up inside before they try to comfort their crying babies report that their babies calm down in half the time.

Many different mind-body activities will help you get in close contact with your baby in utero. Of all the things a mother can do to bond with her baby, my favorite was definitely singing to my babies. It was something that came from the heart and continued throughout their childhoods. And it doesn't matter how you sound to yourself—your baby will love it.

## MIND-BODY PREPARATIONS FOR GENTLE BIRTH

### Prenatal Yoga

Yoga is truly an ideal activity for pregnant women. It reflects the essence of the mind-body connection. When practiced mindfully, yoga increases flexibility, strength, circulation, and balance. Yoga allows mothers to adapt more gracefully to the rapid physical changes in the body and fosters a sense of integration and appreciation for the miracle taking place. One of the primary benefits of regular yoga practice is breath awareness. In the process of becoming more aware of your breath and gaining control over it, you suddenly awaken to your intuition and, often, to repressed feelings. Yoga assists in going deep within yourself.

It is best to work with a reputable teacher who has been trained to specialize in pregnancy. There are many prenatal yoga videos and DVD programs now available, which are almost as good as attending a regular class. Just remember to pace yourself and never force your body into a pose or breathing pattern, especially if you are experiencing pain or discomfort. It is best to work at your own pace, even staying with one or two postures, than to rush though a routine.

Some women are afraid of practicing yoga, mistakenly thinking that it is part of a religious practice. While it has been an integral part of some Eastern philosophies and religions, as practiced today by housewives, business executives, students, and health-care professionals yoga has taken on an entirely new meaning. At the core of all yoga practice is a desire to focus the mind, to concentrate on an object and sustain the focus without distraction. What could be a better goal for a woman in labor? By focusing inward and surrendering to the body, a woman can experience the force and intensity of labor and at the same time remain still and open. Practicing yoga and meditation can help her achieve this state of relaxation.

### Prenatal Pilates

Pilates is a system of exercises developed by Joseph Pilates, a German national, while he was interned in England during World War II. Using a simple resistance machine that he built out of bed springs and wood, he devised an exercise regimen to help injured soldiers regain their strength and vitality. Adopted by ballet dancers to retain their flexibility and strengthen their abdominal muscles ("the power-house"), Pilates is now a worldwide exercise phenomenon which has been adapted for pregnant and postpartum women.

The same long-term benefits that yoga offers can be obtained by practicing the exercises of a Pilates routine. Each movement in the routine is tied to a specific manner of breathing. The overall goal is to become calm and relaxed. Using the breath helps accomplish this. Concentration is increased even though the movements do not require a great deal of exertion. They are specific and intentional movements, which yield a fluid and graceful body.

Prenatal Pilates teachers focus on pelvic floor strengthening, deep abdominal conditioning, breathing and relaxation, posture strengthening, and overall body conditioning and toning, which results in a healthier pregnancy, easier labor and birth, and a speedy recovery.[22]

## Prenatal Aquatic Exercise

When Françoise Barbira Freedman founded Birthlight, a nonprofit organization in Cambridge, England, she was already an accomplished instructor of yoga, an ocean swimmer, and a medical anthropologist. Even though she is a distinguished professor of anthropology at the University of Cambridge, she considers her finest accomplishment the birth and rearing of her four children.

The basis for her holistic approach to maternity care came from her interaction with the lighthearted and gentle mothering she witnessed in her anthropological fieldwork with a Peruvian Amazonian culture. She developed an original approach to prenatal and postpartum holistic care that combines yoga and swimming into a distinct form of "aquatic yoga."

Aquatic yoga workouts are the ideal form of prenatal exercise. In water, fitness can be achieved and maintained without stress or strain on the body. Even the most difficult or advanced yoga poses, hard to do even when you are not pregnant, become easy in the weightlessness and buoyancy of the water. All the benefits of controlled breathing, focus, and meditation can also be experienced in the aquatic environment. Mothers who investigate aquatic prenatal yoga classes need not be either swimmers or experienced in yoga. The exercises are usually done in the shallow part of warm pools. Many aquatic classes encourage women to come back after the baby is born and join other mothers in aquatic swim and yoga exercises for babies.

While visiting the United States on a lecture and cultural exchange trip, Russian pediatrician Zina Bakhareva shared her expertise in baby swimming instruction by teaching classes for several weeks at a local indoor pool in Portland,

Oregon. Seventy-five babies, with their mothers and a few dads, participated in the program, out of which grew a local postnatal swim club.

Reactions to the baby class were all the same. Mothers reported healthier, more alert babies who slept and nursed better and spent less time being fussy. Dr. Bakhareva and other professionals like Dr. Freedman attribute this to the close attention that is paid to the babies in the water. The child experiences the constant and undivided attention of the person holding them. This contact allows the child, even very small babies, to communicate in ways that are extremely rewarding and satisfying. As a result babies display more confidence.

## Visualization

Visualization is intentionally imagining a situation or desired goal as if it is actually happening. Behind every action there is first a thought. If a pregnant woman is afraid of giving birth, her fear will affect the birth process in a negative way. However, if she can visualize herself relaxing, letting go, and birthing her baby with ease, it may help her to actually have an easier birth.

It is very important for a woman to have an image of the way in which she would like to give birth. A group of twenty women who had had cesarean sections were asked if they had visualized themselves giving birth before they went into labor. Amazingly, only one woman had seen herself actually giving birth.[23]

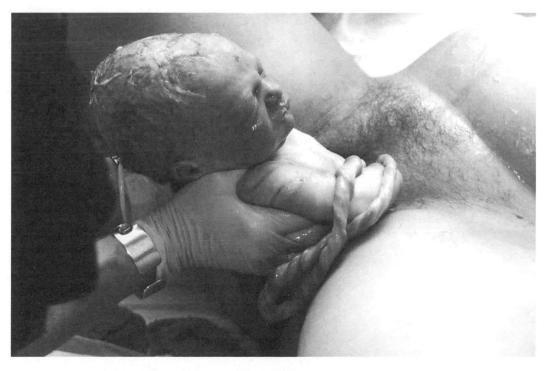

*The more a mother can visualize the baby being born, the easier her birth will be.*

To be most effective, a visualization should be built with imagery that supports a full range of feelings. In visualizing how you would like your birth to be, you make it a conscious part of your mind-body state. A creative visualization is a consciously chosen reality—one that is not subject to past thoughts and emotions.

The use of positive imagery has been proven to be beneficial in many areas of health and healing. Oncologists have used visions of healthy T-cells battling cancer cells, often with the result that "terminally ill" cancer patients experience remissions. Dr. Deepak Chopra uses imagery and suggestion with patients who come to the Ayurvedic Clinic in Massachusetts. Gayle Peterson and Lewis Mehl elevated guided visualization to a science in their clinic in Berkeley, California. Their work is described later in this chapter.

There are distinct methods to help a mother relax in order for her visualizations to be most effective. Women need to be receptive in order to really take in the positive messages and store them for later use. Gayle Peterson usually uses visualization imagery with women following a massage. How does visualization work to dissolve a woman's fear and help her achieve a normal birth? Peterson explains, "Suggestion can only serve that part of the person that desires a particular outcome. When personal motivation is not present, hypnosis does not work. For example, a woman may feel that she is too "nervous" to relax effectively for natural childbirth. She does, however, wish that she could relax. She just does not believe in her ability to do so."[24]

The relaxed woman is in an altered state in which she is able to suspend her own ingrained belief system long enough to receive a suggestion that matches her desire for a particular outcome. During labor, women experience an altered state of consciousness as well. We discussed earlier that in a gentle birth the environment that a woman has created supports her in shifting between this inner-focused state to a lighter state where she can communicate her desires. During labor the mother is suggestible to words and visualizations used by her support persons to help her create the birth experience she desires. If she has heard these words during her pregnancy while in a state of deep relaxation, they will be even more powerful in helping her overcome her resistance. The use of imagery and visualization can support the mother by allowing her to trust in her ability to surrender to the power that moves through her.

Following are a few examples of gentle visualizations for relaxation. These visualizations can be practiced throughout pregnancy and used during labor and birth.

### The Wave

This particular visualization can be done on the floor or on a bed. It is most effective when done in a pool or hot tub. When the practitioner holds the woman as she relaxes and breathes in the water, the woman feels total support and comfort. Women who have used this process say they felt like a baby in the womb.

*See yourself lying on a warm, sandy beach with the waves softly moving up and back just beyond where you are lying.*

*I hear the waves and note their rhythmic consistency.*

*I listen intensely to all the sounds around me.*

*I breathe lightly and effortlessly.*

*I feel all the feelings in my body.*

*As I listen to the quiet between the waves, I anticipate the movement of the water.*

*I hear the waves coming in closer and closer until they break just beyond my feet.*

*As I become more aware, I feel the water touch my feet.*

*I do not draw away from the water.*

*The water is warm and soothing, comforting and relaxing.*

*As the next wave moves over my feet, I breathe in.*

*As the wave recedes, I breathe out, opening every part of my body, flowing.*

*I release all tension from my body as I breathe out.*

*The warm, nurturing, comforting waves continue to move over my body. With each wave I breathe and I become more relaxed and open.*

*Before long the waves have carried me into the water.*

*I now relax in the warm weightlessness of the ocean.*

*The more I relax and breathe, the more I am carried and supported by the wave.*

*My body opens and releases as the wave carries me.*

*The movement of the waves comforts me.*

*The waves are pleasurable.*

*I relax and breathe with each wave.*

*The wave intensifies. I breathe.*

*The wave is powerful. I breathe.*

*The wave is flowing. I breathe.*

*The wave eventually comes to the shore. I breathe.*

*The wave is calm. I breathe.*

*The wave is quiet. I breathe.*

*I now see myself lying on the warm sand.*

*The waves are receding.*

## The Rose

This short visualization can be used at any time during pregnancy or labor. I have brought a single rose to many mothers in labor and reminded them to watch as the rose opens, telling them that their cervix is just like the beautiful pink blossom. Every time I have brought a rose to a laboring woman, it has fully opened by the time the baby was born.

*My cervix is like a rosebud.*
*Ready to open.*
*I am nurtured by those around me as the rose is nurtured by the soil.*
*The rosebud gradually, ever so softly, opens and blossoms.*
*I open and blossom.*
*My cervix is soft and ripe like the rosebud.*
*I see the outer petals of the rose falling away.*
*I see my cervix yielding like the outer petals of the rose.*
*Every contraction opens another petal of my rosebud cervix.*
*I welcome each contraction, which helps me open my rosebud cervix.*
*I welcome and receive all the nurturing around me, which helps me open.*
*Just like the warm sun opens the rose, the warmth I receive opens my cervix.*
*I yield and open.*
*The rose does not resist.*
*I open and blossom.*

## The Candle

Women who want to use this visualization during labor often buy a special large candle just for labor, one that is likely to burn for at least twelve hours. They can use the sight of the candle to remind them to melt with the contractions.

*Imagine that your pelvis is a candle with a flame in the middle.*
*As my contractions come, the flame burns brighter.*
*My body is the wax of the candle, warming and yielding to the flame.*
*The more I breathe, the brighter the candle burns.*
*The wax melts and drips with each contraction.*
*My body becomes looser and opens to the flame.*
*I see my pelvis becoming soft and warm and pliable.*
*I breathe. With each contraction the candle becomes softer.*
*I melt with the candle.*
*My breath helps the candle burn brighter, melting quicker.*
*I remain soft, warm, and yielding.*

## *Hypnotherapy*

HypnoBirthing has gained much popularity in the past few years with appearances by instructors and mothers on TV talk shows and in Hollywood magazines extolling the great benefits that hypnosis and deep relaxation provide. Mickey Mongan, the founder of HypnoBirthing, proclaims that this approach to prenatal preparation is "taking the world by calm."

It is a firmly held belief by HypnoBirthing practitioners that there is no physiological reason for experiencing pain during birth. Mongan explains, "We teach the
pregnant family to understand that when mom is relaxed, and free of the fight-
flight-or-freeze response, her own autonomic nervous system steps in to release
endorphins and enables her to bring herself into a state of well being that negates
the secretion of catecholamines—those constrictor hormones that are believed to
be heavily present during birthing."[25]

Caity McCardell used HypnoBirthing to prepare for her labor and birth. She
describes how she drew on this experience for comfort during her labor:

> I imagined with each surge of energy that I was a mermaid in the ocean. I
> would swim down to the sea floor, pick up a seashell and bring it to the sur-
> face where my baby was sitting on a float. Each time, the baby would be
> delighted at mummy bringing a gift, and I felt a strong sense of loving con-
> nection with the baby. Sometimes, when a surge was particularly strong, I'd
> imagine a sea creature stuck to my abdomen as I was swimming down for
> shells, but it would smile at me and I'd acknowledge that it was just taking a
> little ride and that it would soon be gone.

Caity describes her labor and birth as more than manageable.

> It was truly amazing relaxing through the surges. Somewhere along the line I
> realized I had a choice. I could either respond to the pain by freezing up,
> screaming, tensing my body—which all made it unbearable—or I could go
> into a deep state of relaxation. The relaxation and visualization actually made
> me much more aware of the experience. I never felt distant from my body. I
> looked like I was asleep, but I was really quite present and focused inwardly on
> everything that was happening in my body. I could actually feel the baby twist-
> ing and turning. Stefan and I attended a prenatal HypnoBirthing class where
> we had watched many birth videos of other couples who had used hypnosis.
> They all looked relaxed and peaceful. We thought the combination of hypno-
> sis and waterbirth would be a good choice. And it was.
>
> At one point our midwife, Maria, asked Stefan, "Is she even having any
> contractions?" Stefan knew that I had three in the last ten minutes. He was sit-
> ting right next to me and could see how my breathing changed when an
> energy rush took over. Other than that indication no one could tell how strong
> or powerful my surges were. Maria was amazed and later called me "Amazon
> Woman of the Month."
>
> I took everyone by surprise when, between pushing surges, I sponta-
> neously exclaimed, "I feel great!" Maria said that statement is the stuff of

midwifery legend—the kind of experience midwives talk about to inspire other clients.

My bag of waters released only ten minutes before Gianna was born. The water was clear and it was wonderful to know it had kept baby safe and sound for so long!

I pushed for a total of only twenty-five minutes. When Gianna's head was halfway out, I heard Marcelle say, "I can see the ears!" I think that made it real to me and inspired me to push harder. So at the peak of the next surge I pushed really hard and the entire baby came out! Suddenly, this beautiful, pink angel was on my chest! I was overwhelmed. It was the most amazing, profound experience of my life. A little person had come out of me and was there on me in the warm water. Not bad for a first baby. Ten hours of labor, twenty-five minutes of pushing and a beautiful waterbirth. I can do this again!

HypnoBirthing teaches dissociation, but it is dissociation from the myths and the scenarios of complicated and pain-filled births that healthy women are subjected to in this society. Detailed explanations of birth complications are deliberately missing from all HypnoBirthing training courses. Other birth hypnosis training courses for pregnant couples use similar techniques.

In a study conducted at a Gainesville, Florida hospital in 2000, a group of forty-two teenage mothers was divided into two groups during their pregnancies, one of which received only standard counseling, while the other group was trained, utilizing hypnosis, to relax, breathe, and use imagery techniques during labor. The hypnosis group were all encouraged to talk to their babies with birth affirmations during pregnancy and labor.

According to the report, none of the girls in the hypnosis group needed surgical intervention, compared with 60 percent of those in the non-hypnosis group. Dr. Paul G. Schauble, who participated in the study, evaluated the results and concluded, "The use of hypnosis in preparing pregnant women for labor and delivery reduces the risk of complications, decreases the need for medical intervention . . . and results in a more comfortable delivery for mother and child."[26]

## Vocalization

Encouraging the use of the voice is a technique first popularized by Dr. Michel Odent in Pithiviers and subsequently adapted by many midwives. Midwife Hideko Suzuki runs a birth center in Kagawa, Japan, where all the women are encouraged to sing during pregnancy and labor. A rousing piece of opera is practiced during prenatal visits, with the midwife coaching her clients with great enthusiasm.

Singing through pregnancy and birth is a way of opening the body and mind. The vibration that moves through the body when we sing also moves blocked energy

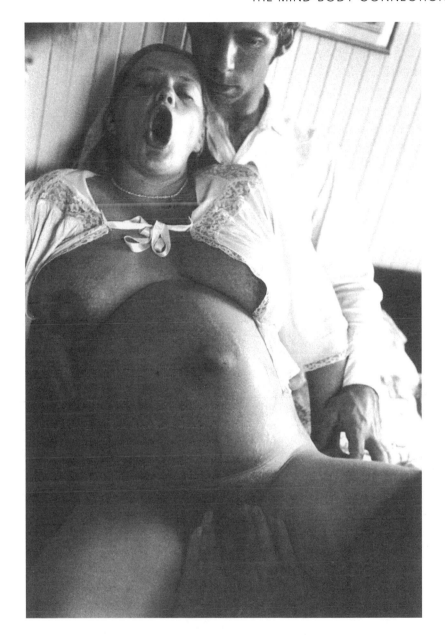

*Vocalizing during labor opens the throat and relaxes the jaw,*
*which helps relax the whole body.*

and makes us breathe. Women who sing during pregnancy and feel the energy surge that singing can bring are often more open to vocalizing during birth.

Women who are encouraged to open their throats and make natural sounds during labor relax their jaws. As the body relaxes, the cervix opens. *As above, so below.* When Trudy, a singer, was laboring with her second baby, everyone in the room matched her original intonations. There were two men and two women attending the birth. Trudy experienced her labor as being powerful and amazing. "The sounds that everyone made went into me and helped me open even faster. It showed me that we were all working together. The energy of each contraction was matched with a very positive vibration that I could feel in every fiber of my being. It really helped me surrender to the power that God was moving through me. I could actually sense my cervix opening."

## Acupuncture or Acupressure

Acupuncture is the oldest known treatment modality, and has been practiced with continuity from ancient times until now. More and more hospitals and clinics are integrating the use of acupuncture in maternity care.

The classical Chinese explanation for how acupuncture works is that channels of energy run in regular patterns through the body and over its surface. These energy channels, called meridians, are like rivers flowing through the body to irrigate and nourish the tissues with chi (energy). An obstruction in the movement of these energy rivers is like a dam that backs up, causing organs to react by producing symptoms.

The meridians can be influenced by placing needles at the acupuncture points, using degrees of pressure and sometimes heat. The acupuncture needles unblock the obstructions at the dams, and reestablish the regular flow of energy through the meridians. Acupuncture treatments can therefore help the body's internal organs to correct imbalances in digestion, absorption of nutrients, and energy production, and in the circulation of energy through the meridians. Treatments usually last about an hour and are extremely relaxing.

The traditional explanation of how acupuncture works is sometimes difficult for the medical mind to grasp. Let's examine this in more scientific terms.

Needling the acupuncture points stimulates the nervous system to release chemicals in the muscles, spinal cord, and brain. These chemicals either change the experience of pain, or trigger the release of other chemicals and hormones which influence the body's own internal regulating system.

The improved energy and biochemical balance produced by acupuncture results in stimulating the body's natural healing abilities, and in promoting physical and emotional well-being. The lack of side effects, if proper rules are followed, makes acupuncture extremely safe for mother and baby during pregnancy and labor.

Regular acupuncture sessions have been reported to help women cure the nausea of pregnancy and even cure a condition called hyperemesis gravidarum (a long name for frequent and severe vomiting). Using needling techniques has been documented to turn a baby from a breech position to a head-down position, thus avoiding a cesarean.

Catherine Lowe is a certified nurse-midwife and licensed acupuncturist working in Portland, Oregon. She often attends the hospital births of women who have chosen to use acupuncture as a pain management technique. She is frequently called by other midwives to assist with inducing labor using this natural form of stimulation, especially when a woman is past her due date and facing a drug-facilitated induction.

Acupuncture treatment during pregnancy can be used not just for specific conditions or problems, but for overall health benefits for both mother and baby. I used acupuncture during my last two pregnancies. My acupuncturist explained that traditional Chinese doctors understand fetal development and have a whole system of needling the mother so that organ systems and brain development in the baby are stimulated. When I consented to this approach, I was advised that I had to know my conception date precisely* so that the right points could be stimulated at the right times during pregnancy. My children have certainly been healthy throughout their childhoods, not needing a single pediatric visit other than normal checkups. I believe the regular balancing acupuncture treatments I received throughout my pregnancy may indeed have influenced the healthy development of my children.

## Affirmations

Affirmations, or positive statements, are positive visualizations in miniature. They counteract negative thoughts that may be hidden on a subconscious level. Your life is a manifestation of what you are thinking, so even a tiny positive thought will bring more positive actions into your life. Ending a counseling session or rebirthing with several positive affirmations that can be written down and repeated can help carry the momentum of that session forward into your daily experience.

Susan Fekety is a certified nurse-midwife and graduate of Yale who practices midwifery in Maine. She developed a series of affirmations to be used during pregnancy and birth. She describes how her work with affirmations began:

> We would frequently encounter fears and worries in the women in our prenatal clinic. Women would come to my office troubled about this or that: something someone said, something they'd seen on TV, something they remembered happening in the past, something that happened to a friend, or some bad dream they'd had. One of the first things we would do is develop an affirmation to serve as a touchstone for moving past the tough spot. Over the years, I observed that the same issues showed up again and again. I started keeping track of them and out of that list developed a handy little book that we now have available for all our clients.[27]

*The practice of "conscious conception," explained by the Bakers in their book of that title (see Bibliography), makes us aware of the spiritual energy of conception, and makes it possible to know exactly when you become pregnant.

You don't necessarily have to believe an affirmation to use it and have it produce results for you. All affirmations act on the mind-body connection. You also don't have to say it out loud. If your mind only hears the affirmation while you are reading it or listening to it, it still has profound effects. Some women like to tape affirmations on their bathroom mirrors so they can see them when they get up and when they go to bed. Affirmations can be used to help you feel safe, strong, relaxed, and at ease or at peace. Some of my favorite ones are:

*I am a wonderful mother.*
*My body is safe, even though I may feel afraid.*
*I am loved and appreciated.*
*My strength is abundant.*
*God takes care of me.*
*The more I breathe and feel, the more I relax.*
*I welcome every rush of energy through my body.*
*I open to receive life.*
*I receive all the love and support I need; I deserve it.*
*My baby is perfect.*
*There is no limit to how good I can feel.*
*I love and trust my body.*
*God's love and power flows through me.*

A good way to practice affirmations is to record them on a CD, in your own voice and with your favorite music. You can even use the recording during labor. There are numerous affirmation CDs and cards now available for those who don't want to create their own.

## The Power of Prayer

Human beings often turn to faith and prayer when a situation looks bad or is difficult. But regular devotion and prayer is a powerful tool to help women through pregnancy and birth. Just as visualization brings desired results, the outcome of prayer can be nothing less than amazing.

The physical drama of birth makes it very clear that we are not in control. When women surrender and literally give up trying to control the pain of labor, their bodies take over and do the work that they were designed to do. Life is very much like birth. When we surrender and commit ourselves to letting a higher power do the work, we accomplish far more. The phrase "let go and let God" has greater implications than we know.

For many women with strong religious convictions, having a baby any other way than the way God intended us to birth is letting man assume too much control. For many couples, a life without prayer would be like a life without food. It is not always easy to pray, but it can give us a time to be mindful and thankful. Prayer gives us a time to quietly assess what our needs are and to ask for help in working out the solutions.

I have seen many women suddenly turn devotional in labor. They will light candles, say prayers, and ask for protection. Some women will put on a necklace symbolizing their particular religious beliefs. They are reminded through powerful and awesome emotions and physical responses that there really is a creative and powerful force outside of themselves. I often give women a prayer to be said just before they go into labor or when they are in the early stages of labor:

*As I quietly sit with you, my child, nestled here inside of me,*
*I ask God to hold your hand and guide you in your journey.*
*I accept the gift that you are and I am thankful for it.*
*I ask that I be made strong and loving so that I will be a good parent.*
*I ask that I be blessed so that I may be a blessing to you, my child.*
*I ask that I be uplifted so that I may have words of encouragement for you.*
*You come to me with all the innocence and love of God.*
*It's time to say good-bye to my pregnant body and open to receive the fullness of your love.*
*I pray that our home together will be filled with peace, love and joy.*
*May your life always be filled with light.*
*Amen*

Midwives honor women and meet them where they are in their spiritual lives. Many Christian midwives pray devotedly during a birth and have a support team of other midwives around the country praying for the mother through her pregnancy and birth. Christian Midwives International has organized prayer chains via the Internet. When someone calls with a particular need or request, the chain is activated. The end result is sometimes over one thousand women praying together for a particular person or situation. This network is growing and proving to be very effective.

The work of Japanese doctor Masaru Imoto has given us remarkable, tangible images of the power of prayer and intention. Dr. Imoto photographs the crystal structure of droplets of water before and after a group of people intentionally prays over the water. His photographs visually demonstrate the transformation that the water undergoes as a result of the prayer. Even the use of a single word, such as "love," can change the structure and appearance of the water crystal.

Many cultures around the world emphasize the opportunity for a woman's spiritual awakening during the process of birth. This tradition has developed many rituals to guide and protect the mother on her spiritual journey. Archetypal symbols such as Artemis, the protector of both mother and midwife, provide women with images both of power and of surrender. Artemis, the goddess of the seasons, celebrates the rhythmic changes of the earth. As a woman's body changes during labor she mirrors this ebb and flow, this constant rhythm of creation. When a woman realizes that she cannot control the powerful rhythms of her laboring body, just as she cannot control the rain or the wind, she surrenders to the process of bringing new life into the world.

Native Americans traditionally prepare women for birth through a ceremony known as a Blessing Way. During the ceremony the pregnant woman is pampered, cared for, sung to, and made to feel totally at peace. She receives special gifts to help her through her journey. Her feet are rubbed with cornmeal, symbolizing her connection to the earth. Birth is seen as both of the earth and of the spiritual world. Native Americans recognize that we are all spiritual beings living an earthly existence, and that childbirth opens a woman to her spiritual self like no other practice.

Adaptations of this sacred Native American tradition are becoming as common as baby showers. In her book, *Blessingways,* author Sheri Maser shows how easy it is to create a sacred circle of support for a mother, which will ultimately ease her fears and empower her as she approaches the birth of her baby.[28] A mother-centered shower can be tailored to each woman's need and cultural heritage. I have attended and given many blessing ways for women. Some were Christian-based and others more traditionally focused.

Native Hawaiians encourage the mother to search deep within herself and resolve any past traumas before baby arrives. Members of the community gather together and pass a talking stick—an object used to give each person a chance to speak and hold the undivided attention of everyone in the group. In this gathering, as each person receives the talking stick the mother either shares her appreciation of the person or expresses a buried or forgotten hurt. Forgiveness abounds and by the end of the gathering the mother is clear and clean from all possible negative emotions.

Many East Indian cultures purify and pray over the pregnant woman, knowing that she will be closer to the spiritual world when she is in labor. Dr. Geetanjali Shah, a pediatrician in Mumbai, India, describes the spiritual aspects of pregnancy from pre-conception to birth:

> Women pray for blessings and communicate with the spirit of their baby so that it may recognize where it is to go. The mother is purified and instructed to eat certain foods to ensure conception and to be in an excellent state of health. She practices yoga postures and breathing. Once she conceives, she again prays and is blessed many times throughout her pregnancy. She must prepare her body and her spirit for this important task.[29]

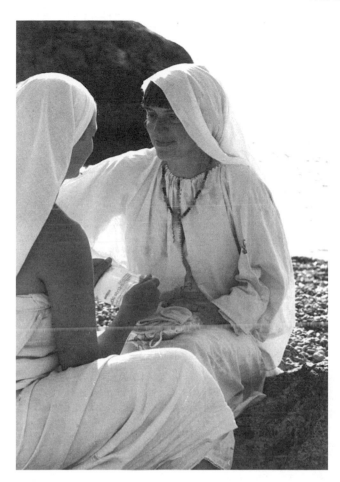

*Lithuanian women create a Blessingway on the beach before a birth in the Black Sea.*

Many gurus claim that giving birth and raising a child provides far greater spiritual growth in a much shorter time than years of living a contemplative life.

The Lithuanians have an ancient tradition of consecrating a pregnant woman much in the same manner as Native Americans. A white dress is handmade and embroidered with red thread, symbolizing protection from fear and misfortune. A group of women gather with the pregnant woman very close to her time of labor and present her with gifts, sing her songs, and say special blessings. She is then washed, dressed in her new white dress, and given a necklace of amber, wood, and clay—symbolizing her connectedness to the earth, which can give her strength during labor.

No matter what a woman's religious beliefs, there is an undeniable connectedness with all of life while a woman is giving birth. Resistance and fear, or trying in any way to control the birth process, denies her the opportunity to experience the divine nature of the creative power within.

## THE SEXUALITY OF CHILDBIRTH

Surrendering to the energy that flows through her during labor and birth requires that a woman be aware of the mind–body relationship, including her feelings about her sexuality. Sexuality is our way of expressing who we are as men and women in all aspects of life. Western culture has tried to limit our sensual natures to the sexual organs and the bedroom. The guilt associated with sex is often extended to birth as well.

A woman giving birth experiences many of the same sensations as a woman making love. In both processes, she relaxes, opens, and surrenders. The hormones that flow through her body during lovemaking are the same ones coursing through her during labor. Because the baby is moving through the vagina, a sexual organ, some women see birth in a sexual context. Women sometimes block the energy in their pelvis in an effort to shut off the sexual feelings or sensations they are experiencing. When these women shut down, the cervix may stop opening. In many cases this energy blockage is the reason epidurals are given or cesarean sections are performed.

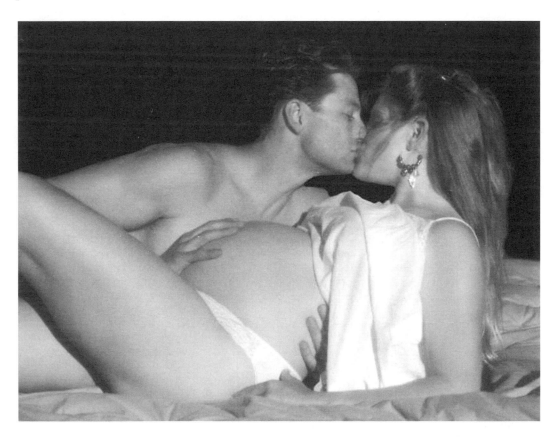

*Feelings of intimacy and expressions of love help women open
to the sensual and orgasmic nature of birth.*

Women who have been sexually abused as children or young adults are very susceptible to shutting down during birth. Childbirth expert Penny Simkin teaches a workshop for providers on how to recognize the signs of prior sexual abuse and how to assist those who are survivors prepare for a gentle and empowering birth experience. Approximately 20 to 45 percent of American women are survivors of sexual abuse. Behavior patterns in these women range from complete denial to destructive behavior such as self-mutilation.[30] Abuse survivors most often seek alternative care, due to their need to control the birth situation. As a result, midwives see a disproportionate number of women with an abuse history.[31] It is very important for providers, doulas, and nurses to help women sort out and separate the act of giving birth from the prior abuse. Sensitive, caring practitioners can help women work through emotions that might be devastatingly painful, thereby avoiding the additional trauma of cesarean section.

Many midwives encourage couples to express physical affection during labor. Kissing, holding, and fondling will often help a woman open up and give in to the power and intensity of her labor. I have even known midwives to recommend orgasm as a way of bringing on hard labor or helping with a stalled labor. A woman in California was giving birth at home in a portable birth pool and feeling very sexy and loving with her partner. Each time she had a contraction she would cry out, "Oh, baby, I love it. More . . . more!" Her windows were open because it was July, and soon a crowd gathered outside her home. When the baby was born amidst shouts of, "Yes!! Yes!! Oh, my God, yes!!!" her neighbors gave her a great round of applause. They only realized that it was a birth after they heard the cries of the baby.

It is not too often that women associate the act of giving birth with the possibility of sexual pleasure, but when a woman is completely in charge and left undisturbed, she can easily move from experiencing pain to intense pleasure. If a woman feels safe, the instinctual nature of birth allows her to forget her inhibitions. Preparation, positive visualization, and mindfulness can all help a woman open and release during birth. There is a tremendous energy release when the baby emerges. Diane describes the birth of her daughter as "splitting open, having an orgasm, and seeing God all at the same time."

Many women cite similar experiences and recount having powerful and life-changing orgasms. When a woman experiences joy with her body and feelings of love, acceptance, and support during her pregnancy, she often experiences the release of the baby in the same powerful way.

## HOLISTIC PRENATAL PREPARATION

An integrated approach to prenatal preparation, one that involves the whole family and examines not just the physical but the emotional dynamics of the couple, will produce healthier, safer births. Many midwives support and honor the use of a balanced approach to prenatal preparation that focuses on ensuring the emotional readiness of the family for their newest member.

Parenting starts with pregnancy or before. In his book *Parenting from the Inside Out,* Dr. Daniel Siegel helps couples understand that it is never too late to look within and sort out the trauma of their own lives so that they aren't forced to repeat the same mistakes their parents did. Ideally, all high school students would be given the education and tools not only to learn about the reproductive system, but to understand the incredible forces at work in producing the next generation of society. But most people don't even think of birth and parenting preparation until they are actually pregnant.

Dr. Siegel's work is ground-breaking because it uses a combination of psychology, neurobiology, physiology, and a healthy dose of common sense to foster loving relationships with our children. It blends subjective and personal reflections with objective scientific knowledge.[32] At no other time have we had as much knowledge and understanding about how the developing mind creates intelligence and lays down patterns for health and disease not just in infancy and childhood, but prenatally. It is becoming imperative that we understand and appreciate the critical impact that the family's emotional health and stability has on each of our lives.

By preparing a woman for a gentle birth experience, supporting her with loving relationships, and allowing her to birth undisturbed, we lay the groundwork for the most important part of this equation—secure attachment of the infant. It is not so much the attachment of the baby to the parent, but amazingly the other way around. The mother must have a clear and accessible psyche so that the baby can base its responses to the environment, like an anchor in a harbor, on her responses to him. The baby must receive signals from its parents from the earliest stage possible (even conception) that it is being acknowledged, listened to, and cared for. Childbirth education and preparation that encourages parents to examine their issues and focuses on self-healing will set the stage for vibrant healthy children. There are a great many providers today offering this type of guidance.

As early as 1978 physician Lewis Mehl and social worker Gayle Peterson clearly demonstrated the relationship among emotional factors, body image, attitudes, and cultural patterning in their research with pregnant women in Berkeley, California. Each woman who used the clinic for prenatal care was evaluated by completing a comprehensive and detailed assessment of health and probable health risks. This health-risk assessment as outlined in their book, *Pregnancy as Healing,* guides the practitioner into evaluating many different aspects of a woman's life.[33] It is important to incorporate her self-image, her past and present emotional states, and the amount of stress in her life into the evaluation. Mehl and Peterson believe that physical health reflects a combination of these factors as well as many others. Many techniques are made available to women so that they can become more aware of their thoughts and behavior patterns. Taking advantage of these techniques puts women in charge of their emotions, allowing them to be fully available for their babies.

Peterson used her extensive experience in working with pregnant women to create an extremely useful book, *An Easier Childbirth*. Peterson used the earlier risk assessment as a guide to help women keep an "emotional" journal during pregnancy. She says, "When women use the assessment to uncover their emotional states, their labors are easier. Women need to be listened to. If a woman is allowed to talk about her feelings, she can usually find her own answers." Peterson uses a combination of active visualization and body-centered hypnosis in working with specific issues about birth. She relates that first-time mothers who have processed emotional issues in this way often will have easier labors.[34]

It is Peterson's hope that providers of maternity care and birth centers will provide a person in their offices who is trained to deal with emotional issues, thus giving women a new integrated approach to labor and birth. She says, "The tremendous change in identity that women go through with each pregnancy, but especially the first, is not often addressed in our culture. Medical practitioners can be very sensitive, but they will unconsciously divert a woman from actually addressing her emotional concerns."

There are many techniques that can help people access buried emotions, and many practitioners who know how to use them. Sandra Bardsley is a registered nurse, a Lamaze-certified childbirth educator, and author who founded and ran a counseling center for childbearing families in Ashland, Oregon. The community focus was on providing women with all the tools to assist in preparing them for ecstatic birth experiences, which included resolving previous birth trauma. Bardsley used unique art therapy sessions, drawing exercises, and writing with the non-dominant hand and to aid women in revealing emotions.[35] She also developed birth journaling techniques and asked the moms and dads to record their thoughts, draw pictures, and discuss their relationship, and to begin early to develop a partnership with their babies. By working prenatally women drew on their strong bond with the baby to accompany them into the labor.

Other options offered through the center were chiropractic adjustments during pregnancy, acupuncture, aromatherapy, and homeopathy. Assuring that the spine is in alignment enhances health by improving the quality of messages from the brain and spinal cord to all major organs. The pelvic bones can often move out of place during pregnancy, and a quick manipulation by a chiropractor will realign them. Pregnant women who receive regular chiropractic or osteopathic adjustments state that their backs don't hurt and their labors are faster and less painful.

Other therapists and writers have used innovative techniques to help women prepare for the experience of labor. Certified nurse-midwife Pam England has created a unique way for women to focus inwardly. Her workshops and her book *Birthing From Within* (BFW) use metaphor, spirituality, and art to help couples look deep inside themselves in order to access both rational and irrational fears and worries. Women participate in art and writing projects and work in small groups with a "mentor."

One of the symbols commonly used in BFW classes is that of the labyrinth. Instead of envisioning labor as an almost insurmountable mountain top, women are encouraged to see labor in the pattern of a labyrinth of dimly lit corridors lined with hedges or walls that conceal the entire pattern.[36] You never quite know where you are in relation to the end goal (the birth) and you have no control over the direction the labyrinth (labor) takes you. While traversing the hairpin turns and switchbacks, ever spiraling inward, the movements evoke patterns of response to the unknown, such as impatience, or perhaps anger, or deep despair. Each turn may bring on a new emotion ranging from elation and confidence to disorientation and exhaustion. During these exercises the mentor helps the mother visualize the journey and the response to the journey, not the end goal. Women get to experience the "hidden agendas" that come into play during the birth process *before* labor begins.

Although the partner of a pregnant woman does not experience the birth on the physical level, he (or she) experiences it on his own emotional or mind–body

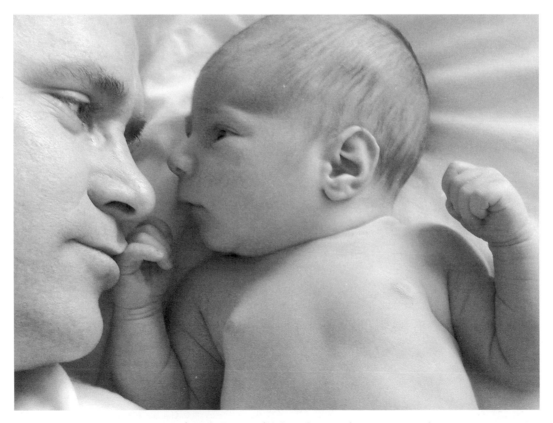

*Were you met by someone who loved you when you were born?*

level. The partner gains the ability to be more relaxed if he too has experienced himself as being supported and loved, through regression or rebirthing sessions. Some practitioners have taken the process one step further and recommend that all the people chosen to attend the birth of a child prepare themselves by examining their thoughts and beliefs about birth. Many providers feel strongly that other people's emotions and thoughts can influence the outcome of a birth. Dr. Robert Doughton has observed that "[I]t just takes one fearful person, one who has not dealt with their own feelings about love and acceptance, to stop a labor."[37]

## MIND, BODY, SPIRIT IN UNITY

The more we can associate childbirth with life, the more we can see the influences of energy and the mind–body relationship. Childbirth is a time for exploring, examining, and realizing the creative power of life. Each and every one of us has a responsibility to live life according to our highest potential. For a baby to begin life being recognized, loved, and accepted creates a new paradigm, a new understanding of just how incredible and creative our lives can be. When life is lived in cooperation with the power of the universe—in balance—it will be lived in cooperation with everyone and everything around us. Creating this internal balance from the very beginning is one enormously important way to create balance in the world. Gentle, conscious birth can lead the way to a better understanding of the true nature of our being. Through this understanding we can birth ourselves into the beings that we were brought here to be.

> From the most ancient of days,
> women have worn a wreath upon their heads.
> With this wreath they are said to have pronounced
> the most sacred incantations.
> Is it not the wreath of unity?
> And this blessed unity,
> is it not the highest responsibility and beautiful mission of womanhood?
> From women one may hear that we must seek disarmament
> not in warships and guns
> but in our spirits.
> And from where can the young generation hear its first caress of unification?
> Only from mother.
> To both East and West, the image of the Great Mother—
> womanhood, is the bridge of ultimate unification.
>
> NICHOLAS ROERICH (1874–1947) FROM SHAMBHALA

# CHAPTER EIGHT

# Creating Gentle Birth Choices

## PLANNING YOUR BIRTH

### Choosing a Maternity Care Provider

The first and most important decision that couples need to make, ideally before they become pregnant, is who they will hire to provide prenatal care and to attend their birth. It is a decision that needs careful attention. Many factors determine the type of care a woman will choose, and choosing where you want to give birth often goes hand in hand with whom you choose as a provider. Some doctors only have privileges at specific hospitals, and you may like the doctor but not the hospital. Not all midwives have hospital privileges, just as not all midwives will attend home births. Let's first look at choosing a practitioner.

The very first factor to investigate is who the care providers are in your area. There are many places to look for all the different kinds of care offered. Physicians will be listed in the Yellow Pages or may be found by contacting the local medical society. Often certified nurse-midwives will also be listed as providing hospital or home-birth services. Within the last few years, direct-entry midwives have taken ads in newspapers and telephone directories. The availability of midwifery services (other than CNMs) is usually determined by the legal status of midwives in each state (see chapter 5). If a state regulates midwifery, as Oregon does, direct-entry midwives practice and advertise openly. But in states like Illinois and Indiana, where selective prosecution for practicing medicine without a license has still threatened midwives, they tend to keep a low profile.

How does one find a good midwife? The Internet can assist women in finding midwives both locally and nationally. There are numerous Web sites which assist in locating midwives, doulas, childbirth educators, and alternative health practitioners. Some of them are listed in the Resources section of this book (Appendix E). Individual state midwifery organizations, all online, keep records of midwives who are members. The Midwives Alliance of North America (MANA) and the American College of Nurse Midwives (ACNM) both have databases of member midwives who are listed and can be found through their Web sites. Both organizations also will help you find midwives in your area over the phone. Waterbirth International provides a computer referral network of all providers in the United States and in many foreign countries who have registered as supporting gentle birth and providing water labor and birth. Check local alternative and parenting newspapers, resource centers, and bulletin boards in children's stores and health-food stores.

Talk with friends and family members and other women with whom you share common values concerning birth. Ask them about their birth experiences. If you know women who have had one cesarean and then a successful vaginal birth, find out who their care provider was. As soon as you have a few referrals, make interview appointments. Remember that you are the prospective client conducting the interview and doing the hiring. You will find convenient lists of questions to ask potential care providers, both midwives and doctors, in Appendices A and B.

Finding a caregiver who will truly support you in having the best birth experience possible will, in most cases, automatically determine where you will give birth. If you are unable to find a referral in your local area, look a little farther afield. Think about driving to the next city or even across state lines. Most first labors progress slowly enough to allow time for travel, although riding in a car while in labor is not one of the most thrilling experiences of a woman's life.

Many couples do choose to travel in order to find the care they want. Women have even reported giving birth in plush hotel rooms in the city where their home-birth midwife resides. This is sometimes a decision forced by winter weather, but some choose this option because no midwives are close enough to their homes. The good thing about hotels is the constant supply of hot water for water labor and the supply of fresh towels. Instead of the honeymoon suite, you can turn it into the maternity suite! (Actually, many birth centers around the country feel like luxury hotels.) Some couples have stayed in a hotel or apartment close to the birth center for the last few weeks of pregnancy and then given birth at the birth center.

Expectant parents have traveled halfway around the world seeking extraordinary birth experiences, especially those wanting water births. I most often recommend that keeping the birth simple and close to home usually works the best. But if you have no other choices, traveling can be worth the added inconvenience.

## *What Does It Cost To Have a Baby Today?*

The cost of maternity care and insurance coverage is the next major determining factor in seeking the care you want. Doctors' and midwives' fees vary among individual practitioners and in different geographic areas. Most providers charge pregnant women a set fee that includes prenatal visits, labor and delivery management, and postpartum follow-up. Not included in this fee are required blood tests, diagnostic testing such as ultrasound or amniocentesis, all hospital or birth center costs, anesthesia and anesthesiologist fees, newborn care, and pediatrician charges.

In determining where you want to give birth and with whom, cost is all too often the most influential factor. The cost of a normal uncomplicated vaginal birth in most hospitals is between $5,000 and $8,500. The average physician fee is $1,800. The cost of a cesarean birth ranges between $12,000 and $26,000 depending on cost of anesthesia and assistant surgeons. The cost of neonatal intensive care for one low-birth-weight infant with no other complications is approximately $18,698.[1] The charge for full maternity care in birth centers varies between densely urban areas like Los Angeles and Houston and more rural areas, such as Columbia, Missouri, or northeastern Ohio. In Los Angeles, couples may pay as much as $8,500 for midwifery care and birth center services, but in Ohio the charge may only be $2,500.

Midwife fees also vary drastically because of differences in education, qualifications, and geographic location. The average cost of a midwife-attended birth in the United States is $2800 and includes far more quality hours of prenatal care, labor and birth support, and postpartum visits than a physician-attended birth.

Before making any decisions about maternity care, take out your insurance policy and read it. Write a letter to the company if you are in doubt as to whether the type of birth experience you want is covered completely, partially, or not at all. Group insurance plans, such as Health Net and some others, may restrict choices. With this type of coverage you are usually restricted to choosing from a pool of physicians who provide services for that insurance company.

A young couple in Brooklyn, New York, was determined to have their second baby at home even though their insurance company would not pay for the services of a CNM. They wrote letters to the insurance company and found out that the midwife expenses would be covered if a doctor in their medical group would refer them to a qualified CNM for care. Of course, none of the doctors was willing to do that. But after their daughter was born at home, they went back to one of the doctors in the medical group and asked him to retroactively refer them to the CNM who had attended their birth. The insurance company not only reimbursed all their midwifery expenses, they also paid for her birth pool purchase and doula services. The combined fees of all her choices were far less than an uncomplicated vaginal birth in the hospital, and some clear-thinking insurance adjuster saw the efficacy of paying this expense.

As mentioned previously, over eleven million women have no health care coverage for pregnancy and birth. When a woman is forced to seek public assistance through Medicaid or another state health insurance plan, her choices are automatically limited. Health care costs may be covered, but she becomes part of a heavily burdened system that usually does not allow for individuality. Her voice can be heard if she herself knows what she wants.

Julie, who had no insurance coverage when she became pregnant, applied for Medical (California Medicaid). There was only one doctor, in the town of over ninety thousand people, who would provide care for Medical patients. Even though Julie was forced to go to this particular physician, she supplemented her regular prenatal visits with a birth class at a local resource center. There she was encouraged to ask for what she wanted. The course included writing a birth plan, which plainly stated that she would like freedom of movement and nothing to initiate or augment labor unless it was medically advisable.

When she awoke one morning having mild contractions about a week before her due date, Julie called her doctor and he told her to meet him at the hospital within the next hour. She was placed on a fetal monitor as soon as she checked in; a vaginal examination by hospital staff revealed that she was only two centimeters dilated. When the doctor arrived, he also examined her, taking an unusual amount of time. When Julie asked him what he was doing, he didn't answer her but the nurse told her that he was preparing to break her bag of water. She was shocked and asked him if he had forgotten the birth plan they had discussed. He told her that he was the one in charge and that he viewed it as necessary to speed up the labor. When she refused, he became defensive, trying to make her feel guilty for her choice. " You might be in labor for a long time. Do you want to be responsible for what may happen to your baby? " She assured him that she was quite willing to take on all the responsibility for her decision. She checked out of the hospital against his advice. Her mild labor stopped, probably from the emotional stress of the confrontation.

Julie gave birth easily a week later to a healthy boy. She knew what she wanted and she had acted on it. Not having the financial power to purchase the health care that you ideally want does not preclude the option of taking control of your birth as Julie did.

After reviewing financial concerns, some couples decide to forego insurance coverage and opt for a home- or birth-center birth that may not be reimbursable. Jim reluctantly went along with Maggie's desire to have a home waterbirth, even though his insurance policy could afford them the "best" doctor and hospital. Their location restricted them to the choice of a reputable but nonreimbursable direct-entry midwife. Jim talked about the experience after his son's birth: "At this point I don't care what it would have cost me. To know that Maggie was in control and that she wouldn't have to have another cesarean was worth every penny. I've decided to start a fund for our next baby's birth. It's the best investment you can make for your child's future—a gentle birth."

## Writing a Birth Plan

A written birth plan is a tool that can be used for negotiation in any birth setting. It helps define what you want and how you may possibly give birth. A birth plan needs to be well thought out and clearly written, depicting your desires for your birth and for postnatal care. The details may vary according to where you choose to give birth, but there are many similar elements. A careful consideration of all your needs is important. Many childbirth instructors will assist women in creating a plan. Some hospital personnel look disdainfully at birth plans and become defensive if a woman presents what they perceive as a demand list. Others welcome the plan and understand that it represents a woman's desire for having the birth she wants.

One objection to birth plans is that they may create false expectations and result in disappointment if the plan is not followed. Flexibility is necessary in birth, but a birth plan keeps everyone aware of the mother's desires and allows the woman to be more in charge of her care. It is at times difficult for some care providers to simply turn over the decision-making process to someone else, but a well-thought-out plan shows that the woman is not only willing but able to accept that responsibility.

Preparing a birth plan is an educational process that can help you focus on what you want your birth to be like. A key point to keep in mind is to always keep the request or desires in a birth plan in the positive. The brain does not do well with interpreting negatives, such as, "I don't want an IV." The brain only sees the "I want" part of the statement. It is best to reframe the directive into a positive statement, such as "I want to drink fluids freely instead of having an IV."

Creating a comprehensive birth plan takes cooperation between you and your care provider. It is also a beneficial process for a woman who is planning a home birth. It can be fun deciding simple things like the kind of food to have available or the kind of music to play during labor. For a sample birth plan for a hospital birth, see Appendix C.

## Where to Birth Your Baby

Choosing a caregiver and deciding how you'll pay for maternity care sometimes automatically determines where you will give birth. Yet often the decision process is reversed. You may already know that you want to have the baby at home or in a hospital. You must then find the practitioner who will work with you. Where you give birth will greatly affect just how many options you have in achieving a gentle birth. Let's take a look at some of the considerations in creating choices in all birth settings and environments.

## Home Birth

The demand for home birth is increasing, but the number of qualified midwives is lagging behind the demand. There are seven thousand American CNMs, the majority of whom work in hospitals, and two thousand members of Midwives Alliance of North America—compare that with England's *thirty-four thousand* midwives. In a landmark 1992 report, the British House of Commons Health Committee stated that "the needs of mothers and babies [should be] placed at the centre, from which it follows that the maternity services must be fashioned around them and not the other way round."[2] Now any woman in England can request a home birth; it is up to the local health service to work out the details. The out-of-hospital rate in the United Kingdom remains at about 4 percent, with a shortage of home-birth trained midwives reported.[3]

Women who want to be in charge of every element in their environment usually elect to have their babies at home. Many couples find that their desire for privacy and intimacy takes precedence over any financial or legal obstacles they may encounter. Many must finance the birth out of their own pockets because of lack of insurance coverage or refusal of third-party reimbursement for midwives. Couples who choose a home birth often accept more responsibility than those who choose to birth at a hospital or birth center.

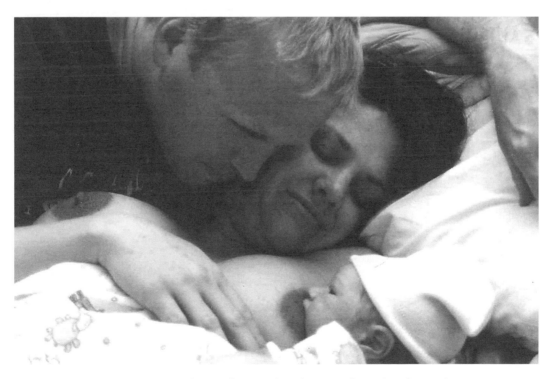

*Babies need to know they are loved, wanted, and welcomed.*

Many prospective parents who are considering a home birth wonder if it is legal. Home birth is absolutely legal. As witnessed in England, it has now become a legislative mandate. Here in the United States, the legal gray area still depends on the status of midwives in each state. The midwife who provides prenatal care and attends the home birth assumes the legal responsibility for the life of the mother and baby. If there is no midwife involved, the parents then become legally responsible if anything happens to the baby during the birth. There are child abuse and neglect laws in force now in every state. If a child dies during an unattended home birth any third party can conceivably charge the parents with child abuse and manslaughter. These instances are very rare and are seldom carried through the court system.

Parents who decide they want a home birth are often faced with the lack of doctor support or backup. Some couples who are committed to home birth hire a midwife but also see an obstetrician throughout their pregnancy, just so they have help available in case of an emergency. When midwives work independently, without doctor backup, they must rely on the doctors in the local emergency room to take over if there is a complication that requires transport to a hospital. In states where midwifery is not licensed or regulated, midwives often cannot even accompany their clients into the hospital for fear of prosecution. A midwife who is lucky enough to develop a working relationship with a doctor and hospital is considered a respected member of the health care team. Her presence and expertise are not only acknowledged but called upon.

Couples often wonder about the materials and supplies necessary in a home birth. Not much is really needed. Home birth kits are readily available from birthing supply companies (see Appendix E, Resources). The kits contain sterile gloves, gauze pads, straws, a cotton hat for the baby, drop cloths, waterproof covers for the bed, a thermometer, and a pan for sitz baths after birth. Midwives bring everything else needed, including the technology of birth, to the home. Fetal heart tones are monitored with fetoscopes or Dopplers. Oxygen tanks stand ready in case either mother or baby needs oxygen. Midwives carry drugs that can be administered to slow or stop a hemorrhage. Most midwives also bring with them special herbal preparations, homeopathic remedies, massage techniques, and even acupuncture needles. IV lines can be started at home; tears or episiotomies can be stitched.

Choosing to have a home birth demands commitment, cooperation, and trust. For many couples, however, it is the most satisfactory choice. Trudy and Ned recall feelings of absolute awe overwhelming them after the birth of their second son at home. Their first son was born in the hospital and it was a good experience, but Trudy said of her second birth, "I just didn't realize there could be so much difference between home and hospital. Here [at home] everyone was focused on me and my needs; there [the hospital] everyone just wanted the baby to come out. I almost felt like I wasn't a part of it. Having everyone here and feeling the baby come out and having his dad be the first one in this world to touch him. . . . That's the way God intended birth to be."

There are literally thousands of home birth stories—Web sites are full of first-hand accounts just like Ned and Trudy's. Many couples who have one or two births in the hospital and then try a home birth come away with a confidence that is unparalleled.

### Unassisted Home Birth

Hundreds of couples each year make a conscious decision to birth at home without the assistance of any medically trained professional. The level of experience and expertise varies from couple to couple, but the one thing that all of these parents have in common is extreme confidence in their ability to birth with ease, following their instincts. Jeannine Parvati Baker refers to couples who choose this option as experiencing "free birth"—free from all the trappings of the medicalization of the birth event.

One such couple in southern California who knew they were having twins chose to stay at home, by themselves, and film their birth when it happened. Mindy and Alex Goorchenko have produced a DVD of their birth experience, showing both twins, birthed almost an hour apart, being born in the bathroom of their small apartment.[4] The first twin was born in a head down position. The second twin was born feet first (footling breech).

Despite the ease with which Goorchenko gives birth to both her babies, calmly talking to her husband and her two-year-old son, some people who have seen the filmed birth are very perplexed by her choice. Questions immediately emerge, ranging from, "What if something had gone wrong?" and "Why would anyone take such an enormous risk?" to "Who is going to clean everything up?" All reasonable questions, considering this society and its cultural norm of technology-based hospital births. Couples who choose to stay at home or on the beach or in the forest are simply returning to their instinctual roots. Gentle birth is exemplified through the undisturbed nature of an unassisted birth.

There are those who question whether a birth that is attended by a midwife or physician who merely sits quietly, sometimes in another room, and does nothing qualifies as unattended. What is important to remember is that women have amazing, empowering birth experiences every day with the midwife either on the way to the birth or in the other room. Birth must first happen in your head. The confidence and utter determination that unassisted birth couples demonstrate can give other women the courage to take control over their birth process no matter where it is taking place.

## Birth Center Birth

When Mary Breckenridge founded the Kentucky Frontier Nursing Service in 1925, she understood that health care starts in the home with the women who take the responsibility for raising children. Breckenridge had a deep love and concern for children; she also knew that if you take care of a mother, she is better able to care for her baby. Freestanding birth centers, offering care based on the midwives model, are designed to take care of mothers for almost a year or beyond. The total focus of care is on the development of health through creating a balance in women's lives. Women are nurtured, and their self-confidence in their inherent abilities to give birth and nurture their children is increased. Kitty Ernst describes birth centers as "family places where there is no generation gap and where children and grandparents alike are invited to share in one of life's most special events. They are places where health care for all can begin now and grow."

There is a vast difference between birth centers that are attached to hospitals and birth centers that are freestanding and owned and operated independently by midwives or physicians. Besides the absence of expensive medical equipment, there is an obvious difference in attitude about birth. You already have a good idea of birth center philosophy and of the family-centered care they offer. Freestanding birth centers focus on serving the needs of the women and families who use them.

Because women who have access to care from a birth center are more involved in their care, birth centers can offer a viable alternative to the dilemma of high infant mortality. They have more prenatal visits, fewer instances of prematurity, and babies with higher birth weights. The National Association of Childbearing Centers (NACC) has been working since 1983 to help establish a network of community-based birth centers throughout the United States.

One of the first jobs that CNM Kitty Ernst tackled as founder of NACC was the licensing and regulation of freestanding birth centers. A task force was set up to create the guidelines that individual states would eventually adopt as their licensing procedures. Licensing legitimized birth centers and allowed insurance companies to reimburse fees.

The majority of birth centers serve primarily the educated middle class, who either have the money to pay out of pocket for their births or have an insurance provider who will cover it. Access to birth centers for poor or working women has been limited, which is why Sister Angela Murdough founded a birth center in Raymondville, Texas in 1972. Now located in Weslaco, Texas, only eleven miles from the Mexican border, Holy Family Services, a Catholic charity, offers prenatal care, well-baby visits, natural labor and birth, and other health services to mostly Spanish-speaking families who often have nowhere else to go. In return, many families work at the center, doing laundry, yard work, and cooking. Their children play on the grounds. At midday, they sit down to a nutritious meal, sometimes the only one they'll have.

Sister Angela, a Franciscan nun, also happens to be a certified nurse-midwife and an advocate for the advancement of the midwifery profession. Her untiring efforts resulted in Medicaid reimbursement for the services of nurse-midwives in Texas, with Holy Family receiving the first provider number. The tradition, which started over thirty years ago, continues in the Rio Grande Valley where Holy Family is also known as a training center for midwives and nurses who want to improve their clinical skills. Sister Angela also helped write the National Association of Childbearing Center's "Standards for Birth Centers" and serves as a site visitor to birth centers seeking accreditation based on those standards.

It's difficult to say which of Sister Angela's accomplishments has made a more profound difference: advancing the profession of midwifery through years of advocacy, or improving the health and well-being of thousands of the nation's poorest women and their children. The infant mortality in her area has been cut in half, mostly due to the tireless efforts of the birth center staff. The state of Texas decided all of her efforts made her worthy of the honor of being inducted into the Texas Women's Hall of Fame in 2002.

Sister Angela's latest achievement at the birth center is the creation of a new waterbirth room. Starting out with one small portable birth pool, the center now boasts a beautiful garden cottage equipped with a deep bath for labor and birth. Very soon after offering this new room to the clients at Holy Family their rate of waterbirth climbed to over 60 percent.

Kate Bauer, NACC's executive director states, "NACC refers thousands of parents a year to birthing centers in their areas. . . . Birth centers offer quality nurse-midwifery care for half the cost. When mothers realize just what they could be getting for half the price of a two-day stay in a hospital, they will begin to demand these services. As taxpayers we should be looking at this because of all the dollars that go into medically subsidized maternity care."[5]

Whole Health Family Birth Center in Columbia, Missouri, focuses on women's needs by giving families complete freedom of choice. Founder and medical director Dr. Laurel Walter had a vision of what equates to the old-fashioned country doctor, who provided services for the whole community. She opened this holistic health center in 1999, offering her clients the option of home, hospital, or birth center births as well as complete family health care. Doctor Walter has been so successful with her birth and wellness center that she and her staff have helped over one hundred families in this rural Missouri area achieve gentle noninterventionist births. Two-thirds of these births have been in warm water.

The success of this center and Walter's desire to help a broader section of rural Missouri led to the building of a second birth center—this one intended just to serve the nearby Amish community. Horses and buggies park outside the new birth facility which also offers waterbirth. Starkly and serenely decorated, with handmade quilts on the wall, this center provides a valuable community service—one that Walter admits is time-intensive. "We put women in charge of their birth experience," she states, "and keep the costs reasonable."

The mother of four children, three born at home in water, Walter values the concept of centrally located birth and wellness centers. "When our family experienced midwifery care, we greatly valued the support, education, encouragement, and continuity." She champions the right of families to make their own best choices concerning their maternity experience. And in doing so she proves that even physicians can practice and fully integrate the midwives model of care into any setting. The overall cesarean birth rate for her practice is 5 percent, as compared to the national rate of close to 30 percent! She can't remember when she last did an episiotomy, and 96 percent of the mothers who use her services are still breast-feeding at their six-week postpartum visit.

There is great client satisfaction at birth centers. The homelike atmosphere and relaxed attitudes help make women feel safe. Women bring their personal items, their chosen music, and most important, any and all of their family members. The birth center is the heart and the home of midwifery care.

## Hospital Birth

Negotiating for what you want in a hospital birth can be a challenging but rewarding experience. In the last decade many couples throughout the United States have succeeded in having satisfying birth experiences within an institutional setting.

Not every hospital is resistant to change. Hospitals in Europe, especially in the United Kingdom, are adjusting to requests for waterbirth by installing birth pools. Slowly, more and more American hospitals are remodeling their birthing units to also include water for labor and birth. Some are even using double beds, so families can cuddle together during and after the birth. They are providing rooms in which the mother may labor, give birth, and stay with her baby after birth.

Some of these birthing units, however, have become masterful reproductions of homelike environments that merely conceal the standard hospital technology. Everything needed for a medically controlled birth either pops out of the wall or conveniently rolls into the room. The consumer must be aware of whether a hospital just advertises the availability of gentle birth or truly provides it. Make sure you talk with both the hospital and your provider so that you feel confident you will be allowed to create the experience you want within the hospital. Some doctors will sit with women in labor and let the process unfold in an undisturbed way. The majority of CNMs work in hospital settings and we have them to thank for many of the changes that have taken place in the past ten years.

Don't be dependent on your provider to tell you everything about the hospital. Call the nursing administration yourself and ask about their policies and whether they offer tours of the maternity area. Even if you have a great relationship with your provider and you write a detailed birth plan, you may be faced with the limits of hospital policy the minute you are admitted. You might set aside some time to visit the maternity unit and talk to some of the nurses who work there. If they are too busy to answer your questions, ask for their phone numbers and set a time to call them at home. Talk to other women who have given birth at that hospital. Write down your questions so you know what to ask. By asking questions, sometimes simple ones, you make hospital staffs more aware of the growing concerns for gentle birth choices. You will find a very complete list of questions for doctors and midwives, any of which may be addressed to hospitals, in Appendices A and B.

When Peggy toured the maternity unit three weeks before her second baby was due, she suddenly changed her mind about giving birth in that hospital. Fortunately she was able to hire a CNM at that late date, and she had a beautiful and quick home birth. She said, "It's not that I didn't have a good experience with my first baby in the hospital, but I just knew it wasn't for me after I saw it again." Find out what you really want before you are in labor, and don't make the mistake of assuming anything.

Many hospitals today call their maternity units "Birth Centers." Yes, they are places where women give birth, but do not confuse a free-standing birth center accredited by NACC with a hospital birth center. There are a handful of hospitals

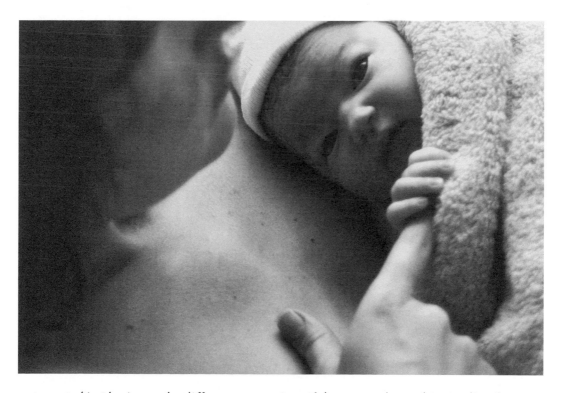

*Babies' brains make different connections if they are welcomed immediately and allowed to bond with their family undisturbed.*

that actually have a birth center within the walls of the hospital, like the BirthPlace at St. Mary's Hospital in Waterbury, Connecticut.

Family Beginnings Birth Center at Miami Valley Hospital in Dayton, Ohio, is an example of one that actually has adopted the midwives model of care for the birth center, leaving the fetal monitor upstairs on the OB unit and offering women the ability to give birth in a large jetted bath. But when Margaret Hayes, a successful attorney in a small city near Dayton, wanted to have her fourth baby at Family Beginnings, the hospital stated that it would not be possible. Hayes was intending to give birth to her fourth baby after having had two previous waterbirths at the birth center, but her first baby was born by cesarean due to a breech position. With the new hospital restrictions on VBAC birth, mothers with previous cesareans were no longer allowed to use the birth center. They had to be on the OB unit for their birth. The disappointment that Hayes and her husband felt only lasted long enough for them to plan to rent a portable birth pool and bring it upstairs with them onto the OB floor. This was not as easy as it seemed, since the hospital, even though they had been assisting with hundreds of successful waterbirths in the same building at the birth center, had no policy covering a waterbirth or the use of a birth pool on the regular maternity floor. Hayes' determination, letter writing, and legal expertise resulted in a beautiful waterbirth for Emily, her fourth baby, in a rented pool on the OB unit.

Carefully examine the actual pattern of care that any birth setting offers and compare it to what you want to achieve in your birth experience. For decades now a safe birth just meant that everyone survived the experience. A gentle birth is so much more than survival; it is the basis for creating a loving, peaceful world.

## The Value of Continuous Labor Support

Sheila Kitzinger calls the people you choose to support you at your birth your "birth companions." Who they will be is a very important decision to consider. Many women say that one of the reasons they chose a home birth was that they were able to have friends and family around them. More hospitals are allowing mothers to have more than one person with them for birth. The baby's father is usually the one person most women want to be with them. They draw on the strength and love of their partner and seek his support through this most powerful and emotional transition. Most couples find that sharing the birth experience strengthens their relationship and bonds them as a family. Some women want only their partner and their doctor or midwife in order to maintain intimacy, but most women like to have at least one other woman as part of her support team.

Mothers, sisters, or close female friends are most often chosen by pregnant women as that added support person. Women need to feel mothered during the birth process. The emotional demands of labor can often be met by another woman who has given birth herself. Midwives sometimes fill this role for women, especially if they have formed a close bond with the mother during her pregnancy. A few progressive hospitals provide doula services for women or have volunteer doula programs.

There have been numerous studies that show that continuous support throughout labor affects the course of the labor. The first study published in the United States was actually carried out in Guatemala where it was seen that labor time was cut in half and the number of complications was reduced.[6] Studies also show that mothers receiving continuous labor support have a stronger response to their newborns, cuddling and bonding with them in the first hour after birth.

There are a growing number of professionally trained doulas present in hospitals and birth centers for the sole support and comfort of the mother. The creation of this additional support for mothers grew directly out of the medicalization of birth. One could say it was a pleasant side effect of the overuse of interventions. Mothers would not need protecting and comfort if the environment of birth were supportive and if we respected the intimate nature of birth, so that a mother could give birth undisturbed. But until we reach that place of respect and environmental redesign, the professional doula provides women with a protective and necessary ally.

A number of programs offer labor assistant or doula training, which can lead now to certification. Doulas range in age from young unmarried women to grandmothers. Although predominantly a female occupation, there are a few male doulas, who care deeply for the women whose births they attend. One grandfather in Maine stated that after raising six children and being present for all their births, he was delighted to assist families on this important journey. He is a retired civil engineer, turned professional doula. If you are interested in becoming a doula, contact one of the birthing organizations listed in Appendix E for more information.

Robin and Ted had decided to have their first baby in the hospital and to hire a doula to be with them for their birth. The doula came to their home when Robin was in early labor and stayed with her there for several hours. The three of them worked and bonded well together. When the doula suggested that they go to the hospital, they made a smooth transition. Her support continued in the hospital and their baby was born after thirty minutes, much to the surprise of the hospital staff and doctor.

When considering hiring a doula or labor support person, you need to interview a candidate just as you would a midwife or doctor. What is her education and birth experience? What does she charge? Is she available and on call any hour of the day or night? Does someone take over for her if she cannot come for some reason? Are you able to discuss your specific needs with her, and is she flexible?

In consciously deciding whom you want around you at your birth, it is beneficial to choose someone with whom you share a deep love. Think about those people who are willing to give to you physically and emotionally without putting demands on you. The last thing you need during your labor is to take care of someone else's needs. This is why some women don't want to be responsible for their small children during labor and birth. Women know that the children may demand their attention and may not understand why mommy is making funny noises and can't talk or play with them. Most children do very well at birth when they are adequately supported, especially when birth is viewed as normal and natural. Children who grow up actually experiencing birth have a much broader view of life than those who only see pictures or movies about birth.

A woman must choose the number of people who will be present at a birth with caution. Often if there are too many people, it will slow down or stop labor. Women who invite their entire family to their births often report afterward that they felt like they were performing. Diane and Allen had decided early in their pregnancy that they wanted their home birth to be very intimate, with only the midwife and Diane's mother present. When Diane's stepfather came during the night with her mother, Allen very quickly asked him to find a hotel room in town until the baby was born. It may have been difficult, but Allen truly supported Diane in respecting her plans of whom she wanted with her. It is very important to be able to clearly communicate your needs to the people you invite to attend your birth.

A postpartum doula can be extremely helpful after the birth as well. You might find a doula who provides both birth and postpartum services. If this is the case your doula may continue to come to the home to help for up to two weeks. A post-partum doula traditionally takes care of the mother and provides whatever service she may need, like watching the new baby while the mother bathes, eats, or takes a nap, or taking care of the other children so the mother can focus her attention on the baby. So much attention is focused on the birth that sometimes it is hard to conceive that there is actually going to be a baby to take care of and parent for the next twenty to twenty-five years. A postpartum doula adds a very meaningful component to creating gentle birth choices for women.

## WHAT WOMEN WANT

Choices in childbirth are governed today by several major factors. To be able to choose how you give birth or what quality of care you receive, you must first have access to available and affordable options. There are far too many women who have no options. Over seventy years ago President Herbert Hoover asked the U.S. Congress to recognize children's rights by enacting legislation to create programs providing adequate prenatal and infant health care for every woman and child in the United States.[7] Though Congress acknowledged that there was a need, very few programs came into being. The health care needs of poor urban women, blacks of the rural South, and uneducated young women has remained a low priority.

The present statistics on infant mortality in the United States, especially when divided into specific regional areas, are no less than shocking. In 2003, 6.63 out of every 1,000 American babies died during their first year of life.[8] A baby born in Cuba has a better chance of survival than a baby born in the United States, especially the American South. The Southern Regional Project on Infant Mortality, which encompassed twenty southern states, was created in 1984 to investigate and create solutions for this incredible dilemma. A major cause of neonatal and infant mortality is low birth weight, predominantly due to inadequate prenatal care. Babies who are born to women who receive no prenatal care are three times more likely to be born weighing less than five pounds. Babies who weigh less than 5.5 pounds at birth have a 40 percent higher mortality rate in the first month and a 20 percent higher death rate within the first year.[9]

In 1960, 25 percent of all pregnant women in the United States received no prenatal care during their first trimester; that figure has remained unchanged for the past thirty years. In many counties, a doctor or midwife is simply unavailable. But the more prevalent problem by far is the lack of affordable health insurance. Eleven and a half million women in this country have no medical insurance to pay for prenatal care and childbirth. Understanding the problem and having compassion for the women and babies who suffer accomplishes nothing. A radical change in the health care delivery system must be set in motion.

Nearly one out of five women of childbearing age (15-44) went without health insurance in 2003.[10] The figure is higher for Hispanic, African-American, and Asian women. Texas has consistently had the highest rates of uninsured women of childbearing age compared to the rest of the United States. Medicaid, a government-sponsored insurance program for families below the poverty level, has adjusted their income markers making it possible for more families to be served, but there is considerable room for improvement.

A bill was introduced in the Senate in 2001 which received significant attention and debate. The Mothers and Newborns Health Insurance Act of 2002 is still waiting for approval. This act would raise the income eligibility of families to 185 percent of the poverty level and give states more flexibility to cover the infants of women who receive Medicaid benefits. This is the same level of income that the Women Infants and Children (WIC) nutrition program uses to award assistance.

Uninsured women are less likely to seek medical care during pregnancy and experience more complications, such as low birth weight and prematurity, which result in extended hospitalization, expensive medical treatments, and ultimately increased costs to public assistance programs. Women want and need access to health coverage for themselves and their children. Testimony before the Senate Committee on Health, Education, Labor and Pensions in October of 2002 brought together notable heads of organizations including Dr. Nancy Green from the March of Dimes, several senators, and Dr. Laura Riley, professor of obstetrics from Harvard Medical School.

Every person testifying pointed out that creating safe and acceptable alternatives to our current system of maternity care access must be identified as a top priority. The health and safety of all children is at stake until there is unlimited coverage to ensure the health and safety of all pregnant and postpartum women and their children through age five.

We now know statistically what women experience in maternity care from a groundbreaking study by the Maternity Center Association, which released its findings in October of 2002. The "Listening to Mothers" report was the first national survey of women's childbearing experiences in the United States. The comprehensive survey, done by phone and Internet, looked at all aspects of maternity care, including prenatal access, continuity of care, labor and birth routines in hospitals, types of providers, pain management, place of birth, childbirth education, and postpartum depression. The findings were extremely revealing, although not surprising in the face of heavy reliance on technology and science in the birth place:[11]

- 97% of births took place in hospitals
- 80% of births were attended by obstetricians
- 93% of mothers were attached to fetal monitors
- 63% of mothers used epidural analgesia
- 85% were connected to intravenous lines
- 49% had their labors induced
- 55% had their membranes ruptured artificially
- 52% had bladder catheters
- 52% had the repair of an episiotomy or a tear
- 74% of women were on their backs while pushing their baby out
- 42% of women who had a previous cesarean were denied a VBAC
- 47% of babies were not with their parents in the first hour after birth
- 80% of mothers were given free formula samples

In addition to recounting what women experienced, the survey also gave us this picture of what women wanted from their birth experience:

- Mothers want continuity of care. An incredible 20 percent of women had never even met the provider who ended up attending their births.
- Mothers want to decide when they become pregnant. Many women had planned to become pregnant at a later date or not at all.
- Women want to be supported during labor. Mothers loved their doulas, rating them the highest in terms of their satisfaction with supportive care during labor.
- Women wanted water during labor—it was rated as the most useful of all drug-free pain relief techniques.
- Women want to eat and drink in labor, but were denied access 88 percent of the time.
- Women want to give birth vaginally after a previous cesarean.
- Women want their babies with them after birth.
- Women want more time for labor, stating they felt "rushed" by their providers.
- Women prefer vaginal birth over cesarean by five to one.
- Women feel that birth is a natural process that should not be interfered with unless absolutely necessary.

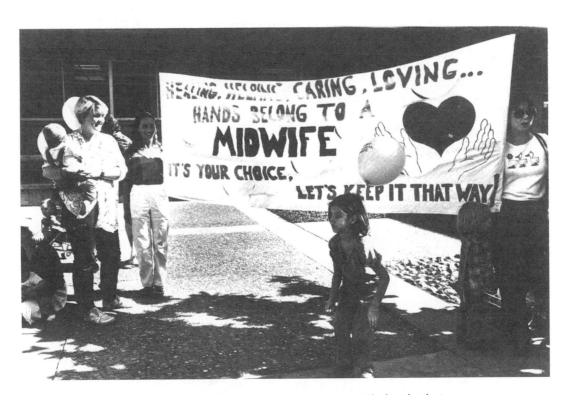

*Consumer advocacy is one way to create gentle birth choices.*

What resulted from "Listening to Mothers" was a stronger, more urgent advocacy for providers to use the principles of mother-friendly, baby-friendly, and gentle birth practices. The survey was a powerful stimulus for more discussions and a roadmap for the urgent changes that need to take place in our maternity care centers.

Women in England were surveyed in 2004 in a similar process, but with an even larger segment of birthing women responding. The editor of *Mother and Baby Magazine* stated in response to the survey, "I think women think giving birth is going to be much more of a holistic experience—the whale music, the soft lighting, the water birth. The reality is most women end up having a birth with intervention. This discrepancy between the dream and the reality can be quite disappointing."[12]

Prolific author and childbirth advocate Sheila Kitzinger feels that epidurals and caesareans are becoming the pervasive norm in British maternity care. Kitzinger runs a help line for women wanting to resolve issues around birth. She states, "I have so many women ringing up finding it hard to come to terms with having felt like meat being butchered—feeling they're tied down, trapped, that people are pooh-poohing their birthing plan. Women feel they have no control over what's happening. They've been smooth-talked into feeling they have control, that they have a say in what happens, and then they feel they don't."[13]

These feelings are universal. Women want control over their birth experiences. They want to be acknowledged and listened to. Helping women achieve a gentle birth will give them what they want. The time has come, for the sake of our children and future generations, to exchange our myths for facts and turn our visions into a reality that creates safe and gentle births for all women and children.

## CONSUMERS CREATE CHOICES

By demanding options and taking steps to create them, the consumer has made progress in taking back control of the birth process. Changes have taken place in hospitals where administrators have been willing to listen and in legislatures where lawmakers have been influenced by politically active individuals and groups. Consumer Advocates for the Legalization of Midwifery (CALM) organized a statewide campaign in California in 1991 to spread public awareness about midwifery.[14] That organization, along with the state organization and a barrage of consumer letters, helped enact midwifery legislation in California. Groups like CALM and Citizens for Midwifery are powerful tools for negotiating change. Some, like the Coalition for Improving Maternity Services, are helping to define what "good medical practice" is. Lamaze International and Maternity Center Association are at the forefront of providing consumers with the very best information possible on the standards for normal birth. Change will come when consumers and professionals combine forces, using gathered data to demonstrate that gentle birth choices, like home birth and waterbirth, are not only desired by the parents but safe and reasonable for the baby.

There is now a growing mothers' renaissance, a blossoming of communication and awareness that has never before taken place. The Internet is a powerful force that is bringing mothers from all walks of life together. They are beginning to see that how they give birth and how they raise their children are political statements. Small decisions sometimes have global repercussions. The recipient of the Nobel Peace Prize in 2004 was Wangari Maathai, a woman from Kenya. An educated woman, she had a simple yet powerful vision: Plant trees. Not for the global environmental impact, but to help women sustain and recover economic stability in Kenya by fulfilling their basic needs: firewood, clean drinking water (the trees prevent the mud from running into the river), balanced diets (with fruit and nuts from trees), shelter, and income (from the sale of wood and fruit). Women all over the country learned how to plant and nurture trees.

In her desire to help women, Maathai has helped an entire world. thirty million trees have been planted in thirty years. I believe women the world over should remember what Wangari stated in her acceptance speech in Oslo:

In the process, the participants discover that they must be part of the solutions. They realize their hidden potential and are empowered to overcome inertia and take action. They come to recognize that they are the primary custodians and beneficiaries of the environment that sustains them. Entire communities also come to understand that while it is necessary to hold their governments accountable, it is equally important that in their own relationships with each other, they exemplify the leadership values they wish to see in their own leaders, namely justice, integrity and trust.

There is a great lesson to be gained in looking at the impact of the Green Belt Movement in Africa. The environment there had been plundered, much like our birth environment here. It took women working together planting one tree at a time, in one village at a time, to produce a harvest of fruit and firewood. The movement to restore our trust in birth, to keep mothers and babies together, and to protect the lives of our children has many faces and millions of people involved. A Gentle Birth Movement requires putting aside personal and political agendas and striving to do what Maathai did—plant trees, one at a time. But instead of planting trees, we are creating healthy vibrant children one gentle birth at a time.

On a daily basis I counsel mothers throughout the world. I listen to their stories of birth disappointment and birth triumph. I advise them on how to change things in their communities or in their own lives. But most of all, I listen. And when I listen, I hear strength. I hear commitment. I hear resolve. I hear joy. I hear passion. Passion for the lives of children and passion for being mothers, no matter what their age, race, heritage, color, or socioeconomic status. And in that passion I hear hope.

## HEALTH CARE FOR ALL WOMEN AND CHILDREN BY 2015

We have looked at why the medicalization of childbirth took place, the effects that this has had on women and families, and why it is necessary to give birth to a cooperative and systematic restructuring of maternity care. Women need to know that they can create the alternatives they want, not just by demanding necessary change, but by living it—by making choices that reflect their understanding of the power they hold to create a world of loving, balanced people. The World Health Organization has created Millennium Development Goals to reduce maternal deaths by three quarters, and child mortality by two thirds, by the year 2015.

Motherhood is a privilege and a powerful force. In order to create a healthy society, we must give birth to healthy, whole children and we must take care of them in balanced, loving, joyful, and financially stable environments. The barriers to achieving this ideal are found not only in our resistance to leave technology out of the birth place. These barriers exist in all segments of our society—including business, economics, and politics. Here in the United States, we live in a society where just the act of becoming a mother puts a woman at risk of falling into poverty. With all of our wealth and technology, it is impossible to justify a society that has the highest rate of child poverty in the entire developed world.

Families deal with the reality that our society ranks fifty-fourth among nations in access to health care for all mothers and children. In a society that is only one of six countries in the world without paid maternity leave, women are forced back into the work place, abandoning their babies to underfunded childcare programs, creating the highest percentage of infants in day care among all developed nations. The early cessation and interruption of breast-feeding helps contribute to a society that ranks thirty-second in mortality rates for children under the age of five. These terribly frightening and real problems would not exist if children were seen as our most valuable economic resource and mothers were treasured as the greatest wealth producers in the nation. Our society will change dramatically when we realize the impact of keeping the mother-child continuum intact, but this will not be easy.

Creating gentle birth choices has become absolutely necessary. We must change the way birth is managed and the way babies are brought into their new lives. These changes will not happen overnight, but the sheer numbers of mothers who are banding together in small groups, national coalitions, and world organizations have the potential to create a revolution. Author and environmentalist Paul

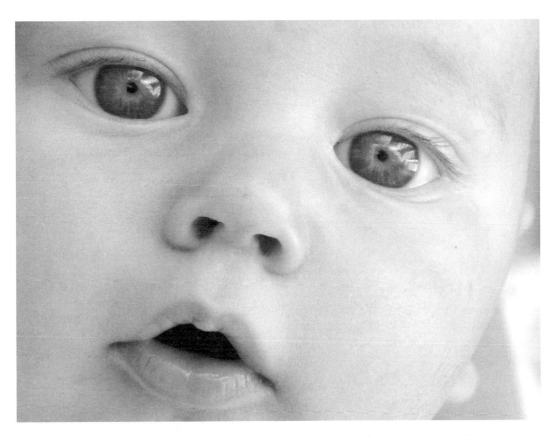

*What do babies want and need? Respect, reverence, and breast milk.*

Hawken reports that nearly 200,000 groups—more groups than at any other time in history—are working worldwide for social justice. He predicts that "we the people" are the next superpower.[15]

We have an opportunity, if not an obligation, to take our new understanding and create a maternal-child health care system that works: a system that acknowledges that birth is a normal physiological process and not a medical event; a system that embraces the midwives model as the best possible care for healthy birthing women; a system that recognizes and keeps the mother-baby continuum intact at birth and for the first year of life; and a system that allows women to choose how, where, and with whom they give birth. When we develop and utilize a health care system based on these precepts, we will begin to see healing take place in all levels of our society. Our families will be stronger, babies will be healthier, women will glow with self-confidence and power.

Birth changes women's and children's lives forever. Let us make sure that women's and children's lives are changed in positive, healthy, and empowering ways and that all parents have plenty of gentle birth choices.

# APPENDIX A

# *Questions to Ask a Doctor*

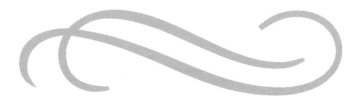

### What is your general philosophy concerning pregnancy and birth?

When you interview obstetricians, it is important to assess right away how liberal or traditional they are in their own practice. Are they open to new ideas or do they practice by the book?

### How long have you been practicing?

Some women may want a doctor who has attended a few thousand births, others may want to work with someone who is just starting out in practice and has fresh energy and openness about all birth situations.

### Are you board-certified? If not, why?

Each specialty of medicine has its own examining board that certifies doctors by written and oral examination. Being board-certified states that this doctor holds to a very high set of standards within the obstetric profession; however, this is no assurance of a particular physician's ability. Some physicians voluntarily choose not to be certified; others have been denied certification.

### Do you have any children and how were they born?

Having a female obstetrician will not automatically guarantee a lower intervention rate. Sometimes you will find a compassionate male doctor who actually gave birth at home or in a birth center or who has caught his own children. They are more likely to understand your requests for freedom of choice.

### Do you use midwives in your practice?

Not all obstetricians will advertise the existence of midwives on their staffs. If they do work with a midwife, request her services.

### What are your guidelines for "normal" and "high-risk" pregnancies?

Screening requirements vary from doctor to doctor. Some view all women over thirty-five as high risk; others do not see age as a significant factor. Standard obstetrics today views a woman who has had three children as high risk as well as the woman who is having her first baby. The set of guidelines that each doctor uses provides him or her with a picture of possible complications. By concentrating on the person and not the picture, better maternity care can be provided.

*What is your regular fee? What does this fee include?*

Normal prenatal care usually includes all tests performed within the doctor's office (blood tests for hemoglobin, urinalysis, and blood glucose levels) and delivery at the hospital. What fees do not cover are extra lab tests or the initial diagnostic work-up. These fees are paid directly to the laboratory.

*What routine tests do you require?*

*Under what circumstances would you require ultrasound during pregnancy, alpha-fetoprotein (AFP), chorionic villi sampling (CVS), amniocentesis, glucose tolerance test (GTT)?*

*How often do you do cesarean sections and for what reasons?*

Definitely assess this doctor's cesarean-section rate and ask for the reasons for them.

*If my baby is breech, can I give birth vaginally?*

By 1990 most medical schools were no longer teaching the procedures for vaginal breech birth. A breech baby, no matter what position, was classified as an automatic reason for a cesarean. There have been a number of studies that show that breech births are safer for mother and baby and there are some doctors who will agree to at least a trial of labor and possibly a vaginal birth.

*Do you encourage women who have had one cesarean section to give birth vaginally?*

Definitely know the position of both your provider and the hospital about vaginal birth after cesarean. If you have already had a cesarean, this will be the most important determining factor in considering who will be your provider.

*Do you have specific recommendations concerning weight gain, diet, and exercise?*

Doctors are less likely today to insist on a restricted weight gain and more likely to recommend a healthy diet and exercise plan. Keeping active throughout pregnancy will enhance your ability to labor and give birth and decrease your chances of gestational diabetes.

*Do you require or suggest that I take a childbirth class?*

All first-time couples benefit greatly from taking an informative and practical birth preparation class, and doctors are recognizing the value of preparation. If you encounter a doctor who doesn't think childbirth classes are important, keep looking.

*How often will I see you?*

Visits are usually scheduled once a month until the seventh month, every two weeks until thirty-six weeks, and once a week after that. Extra appointments can be scheduled at any time between regular visits. Depending on how busy the practice is, you might only be seeing your doctor for as little as five minutes at each appointment. If you want longer prenatal visits or find that you have more questions than can be answered in one visit, look for a new provider, especially a midwife.

*Do you return calls personally or ask your nurses to call?*

If the nurses on staff in the doctor's office can handle normal questions, it can be pleasant to develop a relationship with them. But it is good to know how calls and questions are handled before they arise.

*If there is more than one doctor in the practice, what is your rotation policy? How often are you on call? Will I be seen by each doctor in the practice? Who will actually be at my birth? Do I have a choice? Will the other doctors respect the agreements you make with me?*

It is very important to meet either the other partners in your doctor's practice or whoever covers the practice when he or she is out of town or unavailable. If your doctor has a busy practice, it is not reasonable to assume that he or she can attend every birth. Therefore, interview the other doctors and make sure they share your philosophies and goals and that they understand how you want your birth to be. Don't wait until you are in labor to be disappointed.

*Where do you have hospital privileges? Can I choose which hospital if you have privileges at more than one?*

Take a tour of each hospital and choose the one you want to birth in. Your doctor may not want to travel across town or out of his area. Hospitals often grant privileges to other doctors in special circumstances.

# HOSPITAL QUESTIONS

You can ask your provider about routine procedures or save these questions for a tour of the hospital or a meeting with the nurse manager of the labor and birth unit.

*Does the hospital encourage women to follow written birth plans?*

This is a question for the hospital, but it may also be asked of the physician.

*Could you tell me how a routine vaginal birth is handled at that hospital?*

*When do I need to check into the hospital?*

The longer you stay at home in early labor, the less possibility there will be for interventions.

*Can I labor, give birth, and stay with my baby in the same room?*

The concept of labor, delivery, recovery, and postpartum (LDRP) in the same room has been promoted for the last ten years. If your prospective hospital is one that still transfers women into a delivery room, request that they make an exception in your case. Also be aware of the "cosmetic cover-up" discussed in chapter 8. Not all LDRP rooms are alike, and not all allow women to do what they want.

*Do you routinely require an IV?*

*Do you routinely require electronic fetal monitoring during labor?*

*How often does someone do a vaginal exam to assess progress?*

*What mechanism is in place so that I can refuse routine interventions like vaginal exams?*

*How soon after my labor begins will you (or the doctor on call) come to see me?*

*Will you stay with me during labor?*

*Can my partner stay with me the entire time?*

*Can the rest of my family members, including my children or my mother and father, be present during labor and birth?*

*Does the hospital have showers or baths in each room?*

*Can I eat and drink during my labor?*

*Do you encourage women to walk, squat, or be on their hands and knees during labor?*

Understanding the philosophy behind why you need to remain active during labor encourages women to move. Lying still on a bed during labor is probably the hardest thing for women to cope with.

*Can I birth the baby in the position of my choice?*

Hospital beds often break apart at the foot to "allow" a woman to semi-squat. What some women have found easier is to simply put the mattress on the floor or be supported by their partners while they squat on the floor. Assess early on if those alternatives are acceptable to your doctor and the hospital.

*Can I use a warm bath for pain relief during my labor, even if my water has broken?*

There is absolutely no reason to restrict the bath even with ruptured membranes. One woman at Santa Monica Hospital was promised that she would be able to use the brand-new baths that had been installed for labor. What her doctor did not tell her was his list of restrictions: A woman could not take a bath if her water had not broken and the baby's head had not engaged into the pelvis (for fear of a cord prolapse), and she could not enter the water after her water had broken (for fear of infection). She never once used the new baths and ended up with an epidural and her baby experienced the application of low-forceps.

*Can I stay in the water to birth my baby?*

Find out right away what position your doctor takes on waterbirth. It might be your opportunity to educate him or her.

*What kind of pain medication do you routinely use?*

*What kinds of nonpharmacological pain management techniques do you recommend?*

*If I want an epidural, what are your guidelines?*

Some doctors offer a "walking epidural" which is a different kind of epidural. Question your doctor carefully about the kinds of medication used and the guidelines with which they are administered.

*Do you do episiotomies? Why? In what percentage of births?*

Does your doctor think that episiotomies are necessary? Is he or she willing to allow you to try other techniques? If a doctor cuts more than 10 percent of birthing clients, look for a new doctor.

*Do you ever use a vacuum extractor? In what percentage of births?*

Vacuum extractors were developed to take the place of low forceps. A large suction cup (usually made of hard plastic and sometimes silicone) is placed on the baby's scalp. The cup is attached to a tube that is attached to a vacuum. When a suction on the baby's head has been achieved, constant suction will quite literally pull the baby out within ten to twenty minutes. There are some risks with extraction, such as perineal lacerations, hematomas on the baby's scalp, and pain for both the mother and baby. It requires a fully dilated cervix, a baby with at least some part of the scalp visible in the birth canal, and the cooperation of the mother. Vacuum extraction is preferred over the use of forceps.

*Do you ever use forceps? In what percentage of births?*

*What is your policy concerning stripping or rupturing membranes?*

Rupturing membranes is often the first intervention that doctors do to "get a labor going." Ask your doctor if a labor can progress normally and slowly without rupturing the membranes. Will you be informed of his or her desire to break your water? Do you have the right to refuse this intervention? Assess your doctor's guidelines for ruptured membranes. How long will he or she allow you to go without starting labor? What lab tests are required? Some doctors take white blood counts every twenty-four hours and body temperatures every four hours and leave a woman alone. Others want her hospitalized immediately and induce labor with Pitocin. Studies have shown that women who walk and remain active have fewer cesareans and generally give birth before those who receive Pitocin.

*How long will you allow me to labor before starting interventions?*

Does your doctor go by the book in judging length of labor? What are his or her considerations: maternal exhaustion, nutritional needs, movement?

*How long will you wait to cut the cord and deliver the placenta?*

*Can my partner cut the cord?*

Is cord cutting viewed as a medical procedure or simply part of the process of birth that the couple has shared? Are fathers included in this process?

*Is it necessary put antibiotics in the baby's eyes right away or can we delay that for 24 hours?*

State laws mandate that an antibacterial agent be put into the baby's eyes to reduce the incidence of blindness from venereal disease that has been passed from the mother to the baby. The use of silver nitrate has been abandoned by most hospitals. More common antibiotic agents are now used. Find out from your doctor what he or she recommends, and ask if you can choose not to use anything at all, especially if your baby is not at risk.

*Do you routinely give vitamin K shots to newborns?*

Vitamin K is routinely given to prevent hemorrhagic disease in newborns. The incidence of intracranial hemorrhage is extremely low. The administration of vitamin K has also been given to counteract the possibilities of bleeding after circumcision. There has been an unusually high incidence of childhood cancer linked to vitamin K shots. Oral vitamin K has not shown any relationship to cancer in children. Ask your doctor if oral vitamin K may be substituted and if he or she has access to the latest research.

*Can I breast-feed immediately after birth?*

*Can I delay weighing and measuring the baby for at least an hour?*

*Can the baby stay with me in my room (rooming-in)?*

*Do you routinely recommend circumcision?*

If you doctor is still suggesting circumcision and does not stress the normalcy of the intact penis, take the opportunity to educate him or her before you find another doctor.

*How soon after the birth can we leave the hospital?*

Most doctors recommend a short stay in the hospital. Some are even willing to discharge after twenty-four hours. Find out if your doctor is open to discharge after six to twelve hours, especially if you have given birth vaginally and you have adequate help at home.

# Questions to Ask a Midwife

*What is your education and training as a midwife?*

It is good to discern if you are hiring a certified nurse-midwife (CNM), a certified professional midwife, or a direct-entry midwife. Find out what their training or midwifery school was like. The three groups represent vast differences in educational experience but not necessarily in the way they practice.

*What kind of testing or licensing procedure did you go through to become a midwife?*

*How many years have you been practicing?*

Do you want to trust a midwife who is just starting out in independent practice or do you continue your search for a more experienced midwife? Find this out right away.

*What is your general philosophy about pregnancy and birth?*

Midwives in general hold the philosophy that normal birth is not a medical event and needs to be respected for the creative process that it is. I would be surprised if you found a midwife who viewed birth as a potential emergency to be prepared for.

*Are you a mother yourself? How old are your children now?*

If you are choosing a midwife with young children, how will she be able to attend your birth if there are family needs? Are you open to her bringing her young children and perhaps nursing child with her to your birth? Ask her to share her birth stories with you. Many women become midwives after a not-so-wonderful birth experience. Find out about your midwife's births. Some argue that midwives who have never given birth cannot be as good as those who have had children. I don't agree with this assumption; I know some wonderful, talented, caring midwives who have not had the opportunity to give birth.

*Do you work alone or with a partner or assistant? If you work with someone, what is his or her experience?*

It is important to meet all the people who will have any responsibility concerning your prenatal care, labor, or birth. Some midwives take on apprentices or students. Find this out in the beginning.

*How many births have you attended as the primary caregiver?*

How long has your midwife been in independent practice? Has she always worked with an experienced partner? You may ask for references from former clients. Some midwives provide a chance for past clients and future clients to meet each other at informal classes or support groups.

*Do you attend births in a birth center or hospital?*

Perhaps this midwife has hospital privileges or attends births at home and in a birth center.

*How many births do you typically attend each month?*

For a home-birth practice, the most births that one midwife with one assistant can possibly attend is six to eight per month. If she tries to attend more, there could be two women in labor at the same time, leaving one with no coverage. Midwives in birth centers can handle many more births per month because they can attend more than one laboring woman at a time.

*Who takes over for you if you go on vacation or get sick?*

A very important consideration is who will take over the midwife's practice if she is unable to continue or needs to leave for a certain period of time. Make these plans with your midwife early on in your pregnancy. Know that you will be covered if anything happens to your midwife.

*Do you have guidelines or restrictions about who can give birth at home?*

*Are these your policies or those that the state licensing requires?*

A midwife should have the same screening criteria as a doctor screening for risk factors. Depending on licensing status, some midwives must refer to a physician for cases of breech or twins or even VBAC. Other states have less restrictive or no guidelines. This must be discussed.

*Do you require that I see a physician during my pregnancy even if everything is all right?*

A visit to a backup physician is usually in order just so you can meet and he or she can establish a chart on you. If your midwife does not have an active relationship with a backup physician, it may be your responsibility to obtain a doctor and see him or her.

*What are your fees and what do they include?*

Just as with a doctor, most midwives' fees cover all prenatal care, birth, newborn assessment, home care, and follow-up for six weeks. Any lab tests, diagnostic tests, or extra doctors' visits are not included. Also not included are the costs of a hospital transfer, including ambulance, hospital, and doctors' fees.

*Can you submit your charges to my insurance company?*

Many CPM and CNM services are covered by health insurance plans or state-funded Medicaid programs.

*What payment arrangements do you make?*

Most midwives will make an affordable arrangement to take payments throughout pregnancy. Many even have payment forms and billing systems on their computers. Payment of services in full is usually required before the birth. Be considerate about the midwife's bill and make clear and early arrangements for payment.

*How often will I see you?*

Visits are scheduled once a month until the seventh month, every two weeks until thirty-six weeks, and once a week after that. Extra appointments can be scheduled at any time between regular visits.

*What are your guidelines concerning weight gain, nutrition, and exercise?*

Nutritional status will be monitored throughout the pregnancy. Most midwives focus on the importance of a healthy balanced diet and work with women to get the most out of what they eat. Many midwives have special education in the use of herbs, food supplements, and home-opathy for pregnancy.

*Do you require that I take a childbirth education class? Do you teach a childbirth preparation class?*

Midwives will often teach their own preparation classes. Some midwives feel that they give so much individualized attention that couples do not need extra classes to prepare for birth.

*If I am planning a home birth, do you visit my home before I go into labor?*

Midwives generally make at least one home visit before they come to the house for labor. They assure that the home is adequate and clean, and they help plan any necessary details with the couples, such as where the birth pool should go.

*When should I call you after my labor begins?*

Each midwife sets her own protocols about when and the reasons why to call after labor begins. Generally midwives want to know as soon as contractions begin so they can plan their day (or night). Some midwives will have apprentices who come right away, others arrive when they are needed. Most encourage women to enjoy the early stages of labor and to get plenty of rest and eat if they are hungry.

*How do you handle emergencies?*

Ask very carefully just what kind of emergencies she is prepared to deal with and has dealt with in different situations. A very experienced midwife may have different answers from someone just graduating from midwifery school, but their protocols should be very similar.

*In what situations would I need to go to the hospital?*

Find out exactly why you might be transported. Transports can sometimes be an emergency, but more than likely they are for women who have been laboring for more than a day and become exhausted. Find out what your midwife's transport rate is and evaluate it. Most home-birth midwives and birth centers have a rate of less than fifteen percent.

*Would you stay with me in the hospital?*

Most midwives can accompany their clients into the hospital and stay with them, but in some states where midwifery is still illegal, the midwife cannot come into the hospital and admit that she has been attending a home birth. Find out if your midwife has a good working relation-ship with a local hospital.

*What is your experience with water for labor and birth?*

Midwives traditionally have used water for pain relief during labor. Many are now advocating its use by all of their clients. It is difficult to find a midwife today who doesn't use water in labor or for birth.

*Can I give birth in water?*

Ask if your midwife has access to a birth pool for her clients or if she knows where you can rent or purchase one. Find out if she truly supports the option of waterbirth. I have talked with many women who have said that their midwives talked about waterbirth prenatally and even encour-aged water labor, but then asked the mother to get out of the birth pool at the last minute.

### How 'hands off' are you during a birth?

Is your midwife willing to "allow" the family to conduct the birth under her supervision? Ask if she is willing to give you complete control. Will she encourage or instruct you and your partner when and how to catch the baby? Will she leave you alone in another room if that is what you want? How involved can your children be in the labor and birth?

### What is your experience with breech births? How many have you attended?

Breech may be beyond the scope of practice for some licensed midwives. Others handle it just like any other birth and specialize in breeches, especially in water.

### What is your experience with twins? How many have you attended?

Twins may also be beyond the scope of practice. Find this out before you make further plans.

### Do you cut episiotomies and suture perineal tears?

Home-birth and birth-center midwives usually have an episiotomy rate of close to zero, but tears do sometimes happen during a birth. Unless your midwife sutures well, you may need to travel to a hospital if you need stitches. This might influence your choice of practitioners.

### What is your experience with a vaginal birth after a cesarean [VBAC]?

### Will you attend a VBAC at home? in the hospital?

Many midwives cannot legally attend a first-time VBAC at home because of licensing restrictions. Some are willing to look the other way in order to give the woman a chance. This is a very serious consideration that requires much discussion with your midwife.

### Have you ever had to resuscitate a baby?

Assess the resuscitation skills of the midwife. Midwifery organizations and nursing schools teach courses in neonatal resuscitations, and your midwife should have a current certificate. Ask to see it. Ask if her resuscitation course focused on the latest information about the consciousness of newborns.

### What kind of equipment do you bring to a birth?

Find out what kind of drugs, oxygen, resuscitation equipment, intravenous (IV) equipment, and other emergency equipment your midwife keeps in her bags.

### Do you examine the baby after birth?

Midwives perform a normal newborn exam on the baby usually an hour or two after the baby has been born and breast-fed. Assess from the midwife what her routines are for newborn exams and what she uses for eye drops and vitamin K. She may use alternatives such as oral vitamin K.

### Will you help me with breast-feeding?

Midwives should be on call twenty-four hours a day, seven days a week, for all problems after birth, especially breast-feeding. Many even have special classes or private sessions to evaluate breast-feeding readiness and answer any questions. Some have great relationships with lactation counselors or consultants for more difficult problems. Babies born without medications usually have an easier time breast-feeding, but that doesn't mean every mother automatically has an easy time.

### How often do you come to see me after I give birth?

Home-birth midwives generally come back for follow-up visits after twenty-four hours, two days, five days, and ten days.

*Do you provide or know of anyone who will help new mothers after birth?*

Some home-birth services provide a postpartum doula or can recommend one for help after the baby's birth. There is generally an extra charge that is well worth every penny.

*Do you have a pediatrician you work with or recommend?*

Some naturopathic doctors who attend home births automatically become the pediatrician. Midwives often have collaborative relationships with pediatricians who support home birth and possibly delayed immunizations or not immunizing at all. Interview pediatricians the same way you would your provider.

*How do you feel about circumcision?*

I don't know of very many midwives who will present both viewpoints about circumcision unless their clients are Jewish or Muslim. If there is a religious consideration, the thoughtful midwife will support her clients' decision.

# Sample Birth Plan

## STEPS TO PREPARING YOUR BIRTH PLAN

1. Inform yourself about all your options.
2. Write a list of some of your wishes for your birth.
3. Arrange them in order of importance.
4. Learn about and understand the policies where you'll be giving birth.
5. Organize your list for each phase of your birth: Labor, Birth, Postpartum, Baby Care.
6. Discuss the plan in depth with your partner.
7. Share the plan with your provider and your doula.
8. Have everyone who will attend the birth, including the pediatrician who will take care of the baby afterward, sign the birth plan.
9. Give copies of the birth plan to the hospital/birth center, and everyone involved.
10. Keep the original with you in your labor bag.
11. Make sure to keep it simple and short!
12. Keep the language positive.
13. Instruct those who will be with you on the best ways to support you.
14. Always be flexible. Choose your battles and don't let the little things bother you.

A simple birth plan appears on the opposite page. Your birth plan should express your preferences, not necessarily those represented here.

I _____ (fill in your name) am preparing to give birth at _____ (fill in the name of the hospital). My care provider is _____, who is fully supportive of my choices.

My support team includes my husband/partner _____ (fill in the name) and my doula _____ (fill in the name). We plan on staying home until labor has been very active for at least two hours.

Upon admission I will consent to a short period of evaluation, which may include electronic fetal monitoring. After that I prefer to have my baby checked with either a fetoscope or fetal Doppler, using the standard ACOG guideline for intermittent monitoring.

My desire is for a drug-free birth experience. I plan on using alternatives to medication, such as walking, shower, bath, and making sounds. I want complete freedom of movement during labor, which will enhance the labor process.

I will be bringing in my own food and drinks for my use and my family's use. I will consent to an IV (intravenous line) only if it becomes medically necessary. I will be wearing my own clothes or no clothes at all. I wish to have my privacy protected by limiting unnecessary intrusions from strangers.

I will control my pushing efforts. I will assume any position that is comfortable for giving birth, including but not limited to, a full squat on the floor; hands and knees on the bed; in the shower; in the bath; sitting on the toilet or any position that feels comfortable. I want to guide my baby out of my own body.

It is very important to me that the umbilical cord be left intact with no cutting or clamping at least until it stops pulsing. I would prefer that the cord not be cut at all until after the placenta is delivered.

I want my baby on my chest at all times with skin to skin contact. I will consent to a newborn exam and weighing only after the first hour. If I am unable to be with my baby during the first hour, I would prefer my partner/husband hold the baby for this critical time.

Only I or my partner/husband will bathe the baby, if we determine that it is necessary. We will be rooming-in with our baby throughout our stay. I am planning to breast-feed. Please honor that intention by providing me with uninterrupted contact with the baby from birth on. I plan on refusing eye ointment and any routine vaccinations at birth.

Thank you in advance for your efforts at our birth.

SIGNATURES:_____

_____

_____

_____

# Sample Letter to Hospital

Contact the hospital early in your pregnancy and plan on at least three months to gain approvals. Hospitals have moved more quickly than that, but the typical request takes several months and deliberation by numerous committees before policies are changed or decisions are made.

It is best to address your letter to the nurse manager of the labor and delivery unit of the hospital. You can find out who that is by calling the hospital operator and asking to be transferred to labor and delivery (some hospitals call their labor floors Birth Centers or Mother-Baby units). When you are connected to the labor unit of the hospital, ask for the nurse manager and before they transfer you to her office, request her name. Don't leave a message if you get an answering machine. Nurse managers have enough to deal with. Make sure you obtain her name, direct phone number, e-mail address if possible, and full position and title.

After getting all of this information, you may want to do the same thing to find the CEO or administrator of the hospital.

Some of this information may be contained in the hospital Web site. Almost every hospital in the country has a Web site. Many of them advertise their maternity units and state what kind of experience you can expect at that hospital.

Be sure to save a copy of the letter for your files and give one to your provider to include in your chart. Wait to hear back from the nurse manager before you send a copy of the letter to the hospital administrator or CEO. You can also develop a press release to give to your local newspaper.

Mary Q. Public
Any Street
Anywhere, Any State 11101
Community Hospital

Any Street
Anywhere, Any State 11101
Attn: (name nurse manager)

Dear _____ (insert name of nurse manager)

   I have decided to use the pain-relieving qualities of warm water immersion during my labor. I have discussed my desires for a drug-free labor with my provider (insert name). He/she is supportive of my choice to labor and possibly give birth in a deep relaxation pool. I understand that _____ (insert name of hospital) does not have a policy for the use of water immersion, nor has anyone brought a portable pool into the hospital prior to this. I have compiled information on the use of warm water during labor and have been consulting with a nonprofit organization that provides evidence-based information as well as the hospital-approved portable pool equipment that I would like to use.

   I have enclosed the flyers for the pool rental, a sample protocol, some journal articles, and the Web site address where you can download more information. My due date is approximately _____ (fill in the number) weeks away. I would like to have everything in place no later than the beginning of my thirty-sixth week of pregnancy.

   I sincerely hope that we can work together to help me achieve a gentle, empowering labor and birth experience and that you honor my request to use a deep relaxation pool in labor. I look forward to your response. Please feel free to call or e-mail me.

Sincerely,

Mary Q. Public

# APPENDIX E

# *Resources*

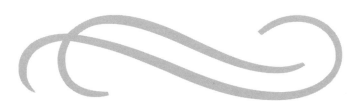

Please visit my Web site for the most up-to-date information about the organizations listed here and more.

**Waterbirth International (Project of Global Maternal/Child Health Association)**
P.O. Box 1400
Wilsonville, OR 97070
(503) 673-0026
Web site: www.gentlebirthchoices.org

Founded by Barbara Harper in 1988 to provide research, information, support, and referrals to places and providers of water immersion. The most extensive Web site on waterbirth information. WBI also provides birth pool equipment for home birth, hospitals, and birth centers as well as consulting on room design and implementation of waterbirth programs.

## U.S. RESOURCES

**The Alliance for Transforming the Lives of Children (ATLC)**
901 Preston Ave, Suite 400
Charlottesville, VA 22903
Web site: http://www.atlc.org

The Alliance is a coalition of organizations and individuals whose desire is to have fun with, learn from, and responsively lovingly interact with children. They support practices and guide people in consciously conceiving, birthing, and nurturing children.

**American Academy of Husband-Coached Childbirth (The Bradley Method)**
P.O. Box 5224
Sherman Oaks, CA 91413
(800) 422-4784
Web site: www.bradleybirth.com

This organization, which began the Bradley method of childbirth preparation, sponsors workshops, publishes a newsletter and pamphlets, and certifies childbirth educators in this method.

**American College of Nurse-Midwives (ACNM)**
8403 Colesville Road, Suite 1550
Silver Spring, MD 20910
(240) 485-1800
Web site: www.acnm.org

ACNM was founded in 1955 to establish and maintain standards for the practice of nurse-

258

midwifery. Information about nurse-midwifery and referrals to nurse-midwives can be received from the national headquarters. For referrals in your area, call or visit the ACNM Web site.

## Association of Labor Assistants and Childbirth Educators (ALACE)

P.O. Box 390436
Cambridge, MA 02139
(888) 222-5223
Web site: www.alace.org

ALACE provides education, training, and certification courses to become a childbirth educator or labor assistant/birth doula.

## Association of Pre- and Perinatal Psychology and Health (APPPAH)

P.O. Box 1398
Forestville, CA 95436
707) 887-2838
Web site: www.birthpsychology.com

Founded in 1983 by Toronto psychiatrist and psychologist Thomas R. Verny, M.D., APP-PAH is a forum for individuals from diverse backgrounds and disciplines interested in psychological dimensions of prenatal and perinatal experiences.

## Attachment Parenting International (API)

2609 Berry Hill Drive
Nashville, TN 37204
615-298-4334
Web site: www.attachmentparenting.org

API is a membership organization which networks with parents and professionals to promote Attachment Parenting concepts.

## Building and Enhancing Bonding & Attachment (BEBA)

Dr. Ray Castellino, Director
1105 N. Ontare Road
Santa Barbara, CA 93105
(805) 687-2897
Web site: www.beba.org

BEBA supports families to resolve prenatal, birth and other early trauma, both physical and emotional, while facilitating the development of compassionate relationships, the healthy growth of children, and effective parenting.

## Birthing the Future

PO Box 1040
Bayfield, CO 81122
970-884-4090
Web site: www.birthingthefuture.com

Internationally acclaimed author, photojournalist, visionary and activist, Suzanne Arms has been a leader in the international birth movement for over 25 years. Birthing the Future is Suzanne's non-profit organization dedicated to promoting the significance of birth in our lives.

## Birthworks

P.O. Box 2045
Medford, NJ 08055
(888) 862-4784
Web site: www.birthworks.org

Provides training and certification for childbirth education and birth and postpartum doulas. Birthworks' Web site houses the Primal Research Database, which is one of the most important tools to promote and protect normal birth.

## Childbirth and Postpartum Professional Association (CAPPA)

(888)-MY-CAPPA
www.cappa.net

CAPPA is a nonprofit international organization that was founded in 1998 to offer the highest level of professional membership and training to childbirth educators, lactation educators, labor doulas, antepartum doulas, and postpartum doulas.

## Circumcision Resource Center (CRC)

P.O. Box 232
Boston, MA 02133
(617) 523-0088
Web site: www.circumcision.org
Wesbiste: www.jewishcircumcision.org

CRC informs the public and professionals about the practice of circumcision in an effort to raise awareness and facilitate healing.

## Citizens for Midwifery (CfM)

P.O. Box 82227
Athens, GA 30608
Phone: (888) 236-4880
Web site: www.cfmidwifery.org

Citizens for Midwifery is the only national consumer-based group promoting the Midwives Model of Care. CfM works to provide information and resources that promote the local midwife, as well as midwives and midwifery care across the country.

## The Coalition for Improving Maternity Services (CIMS)

P.O. Box 2346
Ponte Vedra Beach, FL 32004
888-282-2467
Web site: www.motherfriendly.org

Established in 1996, the Coalition for Improving Maternity Services (CIMS) is a collaborative effort of numerous individuals and more than 50 organizations representing over 90,000 members. Our mission is to promote a wellness model of maternity care that will improve birth outcomes and substantially reduce costs.

## Doctors Opposing Circumcision (D.O.C.)

2442 NW Market Street, Suite 42
Seattle, Washington 98107
http://faculty.washington.edu/gcd/DOC/

Physicians and others who are opposed to routine neonatal circumcision. D.O.C. has members in fifty states, twelve Canadian provinces, and in nations on six continents. They believe that doctors should have no role in this painful, unnecessary procedure inflicted on the newborn.

## DONA International (Formerly Doulas of North America)

811 Newton Street
Jasper, IN 47546
(888) 788-3662
Web site: www.dona.org

DONA International, founded in 1992 by Marshall Klaus M.D., Phyllis Klaus, John Kennell M.D., Penny Simkin and Annie Kennedy, is an international association of doulas who are trained to provide the highest quality emotional, physical, and educational support to women and their families during childbirth and postpartum.

## The Farm

156 Drakes Lane
Summertown, TN 38483
Web site: www.thefarm.org

The Farm, founded by Ina May Gaskin, offers midwifery workshops, childbirth education classes, and an onsite birth center.

## InterNational Association of Parents and Professionals for Safe Alternatives in Childbirth (NAPSAC)

Rt. 4 Box 646
Marble Hill, MO 63764
(573) 238-2010
Web site: www.napsac.org

NAPSAC publishes books and pamphlets supporting the alternative birth movement and offers an international directory of alternative birth services.

## International Center for Traditional Childbearing (ICTC)

2823 N. Portland Blvd.
Portland, OR 97217
(503) 460-9324
Web site: www.blackmidwives.org

ICTC is a nonprofit African-centered organization created to promote the health of women and their families and to train Black women aspiring to become midwives.

## International Cesarean Awareness Network (ICAN)
1304 Kingsdale Avenue
Redondo Beach, CA 90278
(800) 686-4226
Web site: www.ican-online.org

ICAN is striving to improve maternal-child health by preventing unnecessary cesareans through education, providing support for cesarean recovery, and promoting Vaginal Birth After Cesarean (VBAC).

## International Childbirth Education Association (ICEA)
P.O. Box 20048
Minneapolis, MN 55420
(952) 854-8660
Web site: www.icea.org

ICEA certifies childbirth educators and publishes a journal and a catalog of books, pamphlets, and videos on childbirth and family-centered maternity care.

## International Lactation Consultant Association (ILCA)
1500 Sunday Drive, Suite 102
Raleigh, North Carolina, 27607
(919) 861-5577
Web site: www.ilca.org

ILCA provides support and up-to-date material about breast-feeding.

## La Leche League International (LLLI)
1400 N. Meacham Road
P.O. Box 4079
Schaumburg, IL 60168
(847) 519-7730
Web site: www.lalecheleague.org

Offers breast-feeding help and referrals to local LLLI support group. LLLI also publishes many informative books on breast-feeding.

## Lamaze International
2025 M Street, Suite 800
Washington, DC 20036
(800) 368-4404
Web site: www.lamaze.org

Lamaze International is home to The Institute for Normal Birth and works to promote, support and protect normal birth through education and advocacy.

## Maternity Center Association
281 Park Avenue South, 5th Floor
New York, NY 10010
(212) 777-5000
Web site: www.maternitywise.org

Established in 1918, MCA is the oldest organization in the United States continuously supporting safe, effective, and satisfying maternity care for all women and their families through research, education, and advocacy. Their Web site is one of the most complete, well-researched, user-friendly sites for understanding all the implications of mother-friendly and baby-friendly maternity care practices.

## Midwives Alliance of North America (MANA)
375 Rockbridge Road, Suite 172-313
Lilburn, Georgia 30047
(888) 923-6262
Web site: www.mana.org

MANA members primarily provide out-of-hospital midwifery services. They support the midwives model of care with education, regulation and licensing.

**Midwifery Today Magazine**
P.O. Box 2672
Eugene, OR 97402
(800) 743-0974
Web site: www.midwiferytoday.com

This magazine is geared toward birth professionals but has excellent articles about home birth, natural childbirth, and midwifery that parents will also find useful.

**Mothering Magazine**
P.O. Box 1690
Santa Fe, NM 87504
505-984-8116
Web site: www.mothering.com

This quarterly magazine offers a variety of advice for parents about pregnancy, childbirth, infancy, parenting, and education. Excellent interactive Web site and parenting community online.

**Mothers and More**
PO Box 31
Elmhurst, IL 60126
630-941-3553;
Web site:
www.mothersoughttohaveequalrights.com

MOTHERS promotes the economic, social, and political worth and importance of family, child, and dependent care.

**National Association of Childbearing Centers (NACC)**
3123 Gottschall Road
Perkiomenville, PA 18074
(215) 234-8068
Web site: www.birthcenters.org

NACC provides information and support for the utilization, support, and development of free-standing birth centers and midwifery.

**National Association of Mothers' Centers (NAMC)**
64 Division Avenue
Levittown, NY 11756
(800) 645-3828
Web site: www.motherscenter.org

NAMC offers programs and support for families. Assists in establishing local resource centers and provides a list online of 33 current Mothers' Centers.

**National Organization of Circumcision Information Resource Centers (NOCIRC)**
PO Box 2512
San Anselmo, CA 94979
(415) 488-9883
Web site: www.nocirc.org

NOCIRC provides information about the devastating effects of circumcision through newsletter, Web site, conferences, books, and telephone consultations.

**National Women's Health Network**
514 10th Street NW, Suite 400
Washington, DC 20004
(202) 628.7814
Web site: www.womenshealthnetwork.org

The network monitors federal policies that affect women's health, especially in the area of reproductive rights and environmental and occupational health. A newsletter and other publications are available.

**National Organization to Halt the Abuse and Routine Mutilation of Males (NOHARMM)**
PO Box 460795
San Francisco, CA 94146-0795
415-826-9351
Web site: http://www.noharmm.org/home.htm

A nonprofit, educational, and direct-action men's network organized against circumcision of healthy male infants and children.

**Santa Barbara Graduate Institute**
525 E. Micheltorena St. Suite 205
Santa Barbara, CA 93103
(805) 963-6896
Web site: www.sbgi.edu

Offers M.A. and Ph.D. degrees in Clinical Psychology, Prenatal and Perinatal Psychology, and Somatic Psychology.

**The Star Institute**
1426 Toomey Rd.
Austin, Texas 78704
(512) 479-9977
Web site: www.thestarinstitute.com

The Star Institute offers continuing education, infant massage classes, onsite massage and birth services, and doula trainings.

## INTERNATIONAL RESOURCES

**Active Birth Centre**
25 Bickerton Road
London N19 5JT
England
011-44-020-7281-6760
Web site: www.activebirthcentre.com

Active Birth Centre, founded by author Janet Balaskas, offers various prenatal classes, birth pool rentals, and consultations for women seeking alternatives to obstetric birth.

**Association for Improvements in the Maternity Services (AIMS)**
Beverly Lawrence Beech, Chair
5 Ann's Court, Grove Road,
Surbiton, Surrey, KT6 4BE
England
011-44-0870-765-1453
Web site: www.aims.org.uk

Founded in 1960 in direct response to women's demands for change in the maternity care system, AIMS has provided information and support for parents and professionals for almost half a century. They collect data and publish a quarterly journal and a wide range of booklets which enable parents to make informed decisions concerning every aspect of their maternity care.

**Birth International**
87 Percival Rd
Stanmore, NSW 2048
Australia
011-61-2-9564-2388
Web site: www.birthinternational.com

Childbirth education organization that sponsors workshops and publishes books and childbirth materials. Extensive Web site with excellent articles by founder Andrea Robertson.

**Birthlight**
PO Box 148
Cambridge CB4 2GB
England
011-44-01223 362288
Web site: www.birthlight.com

Founded by Francoise Freedman, Birthlight provides training for professionals as well as classes for parents in prenatal yoga, aquatic yoga for mothers and babies, and postpartum classes. The training courses are the most unique and complete system of aquatic preparation.

**Canadian Association of Midwives (CAM)**
For a complete listing of all the midwife associations, education programs and professional organizations within all the provinces of Canada, go to their Web site.
Web site: http://members.rogers.com/
canadianmidwives/home.html

CAM is the national organization representing midwives and the profession of midwifery in Canada.

**Childbirth Education Associations of Australia**
P.O. Box 240
Sutherland, NSW, 2232
011-02-8539-7188
Web site: www.cea-nsw.com.au/

Doula services, childbirth education classes, and early parenting classes.

**The Cochrane Collaboration Library**
**The Cochrane Collaboration Secretariat**
PO Box 726
Oxford OX2 7UX
England
 +44 1865 310138
Web site: www.cochrane.org/index0.htm

The Cochrane Collaboration produces and disseminates systematic reviews of health care interventions and promotes the search for evidence in the form of clinical trials and other studies of interventions. The Cochrane Collaboration was founded in 1993 and named for the British epidemiologist, Archie Cochrane.

**International College of Spiritual Midwifery**
144 Barkers Rd
Hawthorn NSW 3122
Australia
011-61-03 9818-1177
www.womenofspirit.asn.au

A dedicated group of midwives who provide training courses for midwives and prenatal work for parents, and run a birth center. Publications include information about Lotus Birth.

**International Confederation of Midwives (ICM)**
Eisenhowerlaan 138
2517 KN The Hague
The Netherlands
(011) 31-70-3060520
Web site: www.internationalmidwives.org

ICM hosts international conferences every three years and publishes a quarterly newsletter as well as promoting the training and education of midwives throughout the world.

**Midwives Information and Resource Service (MIDIRS)**
9 Elmdale Road
Clifton, Bristol BS8 1SL
England
(011) 44 (0) 117 925 1791
Web site: www.midirs.org

MIDIRS publishes the most comprehensive digest of reprinted articles and abstracts about childbirth, midwifery, and related issues.

**Primal Health Research Centre**
72, Savernake Road
London NW3 2JR
England
Web site: www.birthworks.org/primalhealth/

The groundbreaking research and documentation of the effects of the prenatal and perinatal period on the growth and development of all humans.

**Royal College of Midwives (RCM)**
15 Mansfield Street
London W1G 9NH
England
(011) 44-(0)20-7312-3535
Web site: www.rcm.org.uk

The RCM is the only trade union and professional organization run by midwives for midwives. It is the voice of midwifery, providing excellence in professional leadership, education, influence and representation for and on behalf of midwives

# Notes

## Chapter One: Gentle Beginnings

1. *CIA World Fact Book*
2. Declercq et al., "Listening to mothers."
3. The Public Citizen Health Research Group, *Health Letter* 5:3 (1994): 2.
4. World Health Organization, *Report on Maternal-Child Health Statistics,* May 1990.
5. Healthy People 2010, 16–30.
6. Shearer, "Crisis in Obstetrics."
7. Harper, "Practitioner Survey on Waterbirth Practices."
8. Brace, "Physiology of amniotic fluid volume regulation," 280; and Ross, "Fetal swallowing," 352.
9. Ivell, "Endocrinology: This hormone has been relaxin' too long!" 637.
10. Odent, *Birth and Breastfeeding*, 117–121.
11. Odent, *Birth Reborn*, 15.
12. Simkin and Ancheta, *The Labor Progress Handbook.*
13. Enkin et al., *A Guide to Effective Care in Pregnancy and Childbirth.*
14. Declercq et al.,"Listening to mothers."
15. Caldeyro-Barci et al., "Effect of Position Changes," 284–90.
16. Goldsmith, *Childbirth Wisdom,* 32.
17. Bloom, et al., "Lack of effect of walking." 117–18.
18. Berezin, *Gentle Birth Book.*
19. Dr. Bruce Sutherland, interview with author, July 1990.
20. Brown et al., "Effects of adrenaline," 137–52; and Johnson, "Birth under water," 202–8.
21. Karmer et al., "The contribution of mild and moderate preterm birth to infant mortality," 843–49.
22. Declercq et al.,"Listening to mothers."

23. Pearce, *Evolution's End*.
24. Ibid.
25. Richard and Alade, "Sucking technique and its effect on breastfeeding."
26. International Confederation of Midwives/World Health Organization, Project on Safe Motherhood, April 2002.
27. Haire, *The Cultural Warping of Childbirth*, 14.
28. Odent, *Birth and Breastfeeding*, 117–21.
29. Kroeger and Smith, *Impact of Birthing Practices on Breastfeeding*.
30. Bradley, *Husband-Coached Childbirth*.
31. Kitzinger, *The Complete Book of Pregnancy and Childbirth*, 278.

## Chapter Two: The Medicalization of Childbirth

1. Leavitt, *Brought to Bed*, 23.
2. Ibid., 269.
3. Eastman, *Expectant Motherhood*, 125.
4. *CIA World Fact Book*.
5. Haggard, *Devils, Drugs, and Doctors*, 48.
6. Katz-Rothman, *Giving Birth*, 24.
7. Starr, *The Social Transformation of American Medicine,* 49–50.
8. Ehrenreich and English, *Witches, Midwives, and Nurses,* 20.
9. O'Neill, *Mourning Becomes Electra*. In the play, O'Neill makes references to his mother's drug habits.
10. Eastman, *Expectant Motherhood*, 149–53.
11. Leavitt, *Brought to Bed*, 117.
12. Sullivan and Weitz, *Labor Pain*, 23.
13. Edwards and Waldorf, *Reclaiming Birth*, 153.
14. Ibid., 155.
15. Litoff, *The American Midwife Debate*, 11.
16. Leavitt, *Brought to Bed*, 289.
17. Rooks, *Midwifery and Childbirth in America*.
18. *Webster's Third New International Dictionary*.
19. DeLee, "The Prophylactic Forceps Operation," 34–44.
20. Leavitt, *Brought to Bed*, 12.
21. Eastman, *Expectant Motherhood*.
22. Leavitt, *Brought to Bed*, 174.
23. Armstrong and Feldman, *A Wise Birth*, 95.
24. Leavitt, *Brought to Bed*, 134.
25. Enkin et al., *A Guide to Effective Care in Pregnancy and Childbirth,* 58.
26. Bricker et al., *UK Health Technology Assessment*.
27. Blatt, "An Overview of Genetic Screening and Diagnostic Tests."
28. Ibid.
29. Blatt, *Prenatal Tests*.
30. D'alton and DeCherney, "Prenatal Diagnosis," 114–20.
31. Enkin et al., *A Guide to Effective Care in Pregnancy and Childbirth*, 104.

32. Ibid.

33. Falcao, "Group B Strep."

34. Lukacs, Schoendorf, and Schuchat, "Trends in sepsis-related neonatal mortality," 599–603.

35. Christensen, Dykes, and Christensen, "Reduced colonization of newborns," 239–43.

36. Paltro, "Do Pregnant Women Have Rights?"

37. Ibid.

38. Blume et al., "Focus on Wrongful Birth Cases."

39. Wertz and Wertz, *Lying-In*, 165.

40. Johanson, Newburn, and Macfarlane, "Has the Medicalization of Childbirth Gone Too Far?" 892–95.

## Chapter Three: Dispelling the Medical Myths

1. Chalmers, Enkin, and Keirse, eds., *Effective Care in Pregnancy and Childbirth*.

2. Enkin et al., *A Guide to Effective Care in Pregnancy and Childbirth*.

3. Cochrane Library can be accessed at www.cochrane.org.

4. National Center for Health Statistics, "Birth: Preliminary Data for 2003."

5. *CIA World Fact Book*.

6. National Center for Health Statistics, "Trends in the Attendant, Place and Timing of Births."

7. Odent, *Planned Home Birth in Industrialized Countries*, 2.

8. Healthy People 2010, "Implementation."

9. Sagov et al., *Home Birth: A Practitioners Guide to Birth Outside the Hospital*, 30–32.

10. NHS Department of Health, *Changing Childbirth*.

11. Mehl et al., "Outcomes of Elective Home Births," 281–90.

12. Mehl-Madrona and Madrona, "Physician and midwife attended home births," 91–98.

13. Durand, "The Safety of Home Birth," 450–52.

14. Rooks et al., "Outcomes of Care in Birth Centers," 1804–11.

15. Wiegers et al., "Outcome of planned home and planned hospital births in low risk pregnancies," 1309–13.

16. Phone interview with National Association of Childbearing Centers Executive Director Kate E. Bauer.

17. ACNM Membership Department Statistics 2004 at www.midwives.org and MANA membership statistics at www.mana.org.

18. ACNM Fact sheet. (See note 17 for Web address.)

19. National Vital Statistics Report, 51, No. 2 (December, 2002).

20. Tyson, "The Re-emergence of Canadian Midwifery."

21. Ibid.

22. World Health Organization, "Strengthening Midwifery Within Safe Motherhood."

23. Edwards and Waldorf, *Reclaiming Birth*, 178.

24. Thacker and Stroup, "Continuous electronic fetal heart rate monitoring."

25. Wagner, *Pursuing the Birth Machine*.

26. U. S. Preventive Services Task Force, *Guide To Clinical Preventive Services*, 433–42.

27. Paul and Hon, "Clinical fetal monitoring versus effect on perinatal outcome," 529–33.

28. Zain et al., "Interpreting the fetal heart rate tracing," 367–70.

29. Nelson and Ellenberg, "Antecedents of Cerebral Palsy," 39.

30. Leveno et al., "A prospective comparison of selective and universal electronic fetal monitoring," 10.

31. Freeman, "Intrapartum metal monitoring," 624–25.

32. ACOG, "Fetal heart rate patterns."

33. Morrison et al., "Intrapartum fetal heart rate assessment," 63–66.

34. Maternity Care Health Index, *Mothering* 28 (1992).

35. Mittendorf et al., "The length of uncomplicated human gestation," 929–32.

36. Goer, *The Thinking Woman's Guide to a Better Birth.*

37. Muster, Schmidt, and Helm, "Length and variation in the menstrual cycle," 422–29.

38. Nathanielsz, *A Time to Be Born.*

39. Ibid.

40. ACOG, "Induction of Labor."

41. Goer, *Obstetrical Myths v. Research Realities.*

42. Luthy et al.; Elective induction doubles cesarean risk," 1511–15.

43. Declercq et al., "Listening to mothers: Executive Summary and Recommendations."

44. Curtin and Park, "Trends in the attendant, place, and timing of births," 4.

45. United States Food and Drug Administration, "Cytotec Drug Bulletin."

46. Wagner, "Cytotec induction and off-label use."

47. Buchanan, *Peace of Mind During Pregnancy,* 29.

48. Goer, *The Thinking Woman's Guide to a Better Birth.*

49. Enkin et al., *A Guide to Effective Care in Pregnancy and Childbirth.*

50. Klein, "The Epidural Controversy."

51. Rosenblatt et al., "The influence of maternal analgesia on neonatal behaviours," 407–13.

52. Ramin et al., "Randomized trial of epidural versus intravenous analgesia," 783–89.

53. Jacobson et al., "Opiate addiction in adult offspring," 1067–70.

54. Haire, *Cultural Warping of Childhood,* 6.

55. ABCnews.com, "Oh, the pain, the pain."

56. National Center for Health Statistics, *National Vital Statistics Reports,* 2003.

57. Nygaard and Cruikshank, "Should all women be offered elective cesarean delivery?" 217–19.

58. Cole, "Elective Primary Cesarean Delivery."

59. Belizán; "Rates and implications of caesarean sections in Latin America."

60. Coalition for Improving Maternity Services, "The Risks of Cesarean Delivery to Mother and Baby."

61. National Center for Health Statistics. "Births: Preliminary Data for 2003."

62. Young, "The Push against Vaginal Birth," 149–52.

63. Rosen and Thomas, *The Cesarean Myth,* 23.

64. Rubin, *What If I Have a C-Section?*

65. ACOG, "Maternal and fetal medicine, guidelines for vaginal delivery after cesarean birth."

66. Flamm, *Birth after Cesarean,* 65.

67. Rageth, Juzi, and Grossenbacher, "Delivery after previous cesarean: a risk evaluation." 332–37.

68. Dr. Michael Rosenthal, personal interviews, 1991 and 1995.

69. Rubin, "What If I Have a C-Section?" 162.
70. ACOG, "Vaginal birth after previous cesarean delivery."
71. National Center for Health Statistics,"Births: Preliminary Data for 2003."
72. Helen Bellanka, personal interview with author, November, 2004.
73. Tanja Johnson, telephone interview, October, 2004.
74. Flamm, "Vaginal birth after cesarean." 595–99.
75. Towner et al., "Effect of mode of delivery," 1709–14; Hemminki, "Impact of caesarean section, 366–79; and Rageth, et al., "Delivery after previous cesarean," 332–7.
76. Tulman and Fawcett, "Return of functional ability after childbirth."
77. Klaus, Kennell, and Klaus, *Bonding.*
78. Shah, "Soaring cesarean section rates," 283–84.
79. Jamois, "Women have right to refuse caesarean."
80. National Center for Health Statistics, "National hospital discharge survey." Annual summary with detailed diagnosis and procedure data. www.cdc.gov/nchs/about/major/hdasd/nhds.htm
81. Goer, *Thinking Woman's Guide to a Better Birth,* 153.
82. Mother-Friendly Childbirth Initiative, "Having a Baby? Ten Questions to Ask."
83. Mansfield, "Maternal Age: What Is Really High Risk?" 64–69.
84. Rowe-Finkbeiner, "Juggling Career and Home."
85. Mansfield, "Maternal Age: What Is Really High Risk?"
86. Chalmers, Enkin, et al., *A Guide to Effective Care in Pregnancy,* 355.
87. Sleutel, "Fasting in labor," 507–12.
88. Newton, "Experimental Inhibition of Labor through Environmental Disturbance," 371–77.
89. Klaus, Kennel, and Klaus, "Effect of social support during parturition on maternal and infant morbidity," 585–87.
90. ACOG News Release, "Recommendations on Cesarean Delivery Rates."
91. Wagner, "Hospital Birth Deemed Too Risky."
92. Varney, *Varney's Midwifery.*
93. Fleiss, "The Case Against Circumcision."
94. American Academy of Pediatrics, "Policy Statement on Circumcision."
95. Larson, "The Politics of Newborn Pain," 45.
96. Anand and Hickey, "Pain and Its Effects in the Human Neonate and Fetus," 1321–29.
97. Emde et al., "Stress and Neonatal Sleep," 491–97.
98. Marshall et al., "Circumcision: II. Effects upon mother-infant interaction," 367–74.
99. Anand and Hickey, "Pain and Its Effects in the Human Neonate and Fetus."
100. Grof and Halifax, *The Human Encounter with Death,* 116.
101. Laibow, "Circumcision and Its Relationship to Attachment Impairment," 14.
102. Ritter, *Say No To Circumcision,* 18–19.
103. Fleiss, "The Case Against Circumcision."
104. Ibid.
105. O'Hara, *Sex as Nature Intended It.*
106. Ibid.
107. Reiss, "Circumcision: My Position."
108. John Travis, personal communication with the author December, 2003.
109. Salk, "Keynote Speech."

## Chapter Four: A Gentle Revolution

1. U. S. Department of Labor. "Women at Work: A Visual Essay."
2. Edwards and Waldorf, *Reclaiming Birth*, 32.
3. Gutmann, *The Legacy of Dr. Lamaze*.
4. Karmel, *Thank You, Dr. Lamaze*, 35.
5. Bing, *Six Practical Lessons for an Easier Childbirth*, 139.
6. Leboyer, *Birth without Violence*, 15.
7. Illich, *Medical Nemesis*, 32.
8. Odent, *Birth Reborn*, 36.
9. Odent, *Primal Health*, 265–95.
10. Personal communications with the author, May, 1997.
11. Personal communications with the author, June, 2002.
12. Baker and Baker, *Conscious Conception*.
13. Odent, *The Scientification of Love*.
14. Ibid.
15. Poindron and Neindre, "Endocrine and sensory regulation of maternal behavior in the ewe."
16. Newton and Newton, "Mothers' Reactions to Their Newborn Babies." 206–10.
17. Madrid and Pennington, "Maternal-infant bonding and asthma," 279–89.
18. Madrid et al., "Does Maternal-Infant Bonding Therapy Improve Breathing in Asthmatic Children?" 90–117.
19. Klaus and Kennell, *Maternal-Infant Bonding*.
20. Joseph Chilton Pearce, interview in "The Psychology of Birth: Invitation to Intimacy." DVD (London: Owl Productions, 2005)
21. Edwards and Waldorf, *Reclaiming Birth*, 62–63.
22. Gaskin, *Spiritual Midwifery*.
23. Web site of Baby-Friendly USA, www.babyfriendlyusa.org/
24. Davis-Floyd, *Birth as an American Rite of Passage*.
25. Odent, *The Farmer and the Obstetrician*.

## Chapter Five: Midwifery in America

1. National Center for Health Statistics, "Births: Final Data for 2002."
2. Ibid.
3. American College of Nurse Midwives, press release: "Midwifery patients experience greater continuity of care."
4. Wagner, *Pursuing the Birth Machine*.
5. Davis-Floyd, *Childbirth and Authoritative Knowledge*.
6. Tritten, *Sharing Midwifery Knowledge*.
7. Odent, "Primal Health Research."
8. Ibid.
9. Jarrett, "Gestational diabetes," 37–38.
10. Gaskin, *Spiritual Midwifery*.
11. Personal communication with Ina May Gaskin via Carol Nelson, MANA and NARM Board representative, January, 2005.
12. Canadian Association of Midwives Annual Report.

13. Mitford, *The American Way of Birth*, 225.
14. Varney, *Varney's Midwifery*, 156.
15. Edwards and Waldorf, *Reclaiming Birth*.
16. Arms, *Immaculate Deception*.
17. Becker et al., *Midwifery and the Law*, 14.
18. Personal communication with Stephen Keller, 1995.
19. Korte, "Midwives on Trial," 52–59.
20. Pratt, "The Role of a Midwife."
21. Wilker, "Mennonite Midwife Behind Bars."
22. Elizabeth Davis, *Heart and Hands*, 2.

## Chapter Six: Waterbirth

1. Watson and Derbyshire, *The Water Planet*, 111.
2. Brownridge, "The nature and consequence of childbirth pain," 9–15.
3. Otigbah et al., "A retrospective comparison," 15–20.
4. Odent, "Birth under Water," 67.
5. Harper, "Survey of Waterbirth Practice," 86.
6. Garland, "Collaborative Waterbirth audit," 508–11.
7. I found this book at Samuel Weiser's Bookstore in the rare book collection, where it was priced at $800. I left it on the bookshelf but only after poring over it for several hours.
8. Grandfather Semu, personal communication, November. 1987.
9. Embry, "Observations sur un accouchement termine," 185–91.
10. Sidenbladh, *Water Babies*.
11. Leboyer, *Birth without Violence*.
12. Odent, "Lessons from the first hospital birthing pool."
13. Michel Odent, M. D., interviews with author, July 1987, Aug. 1989, May 1990.
14. Odent, *Birth Reborn*, 36.
15. Odent, "The fetus ejection reflex."
16. Odent, "Birth under Water," 24, 31.
17. Ray, *Ideal Birth*.
18. Rosenthal, "Warm-water immersion in labor and birth," 16, 35–37, 40–41, 44, 46.
19. Michael Rosenthal, interviews with author, April, 1995; September, 1999.
20. Church, "Water birth: One birthing center's observations," 165–70.
21. Lisa Stolper, Carmen Carignan, and Sarah Ellsworth. "The Cheshire Experience: Changing Minds and Hearts." Recorded presentation to International Waterbirth Congress, Chicago, April, 2004.
22. Ken Johnson, MANA Stats Epidemiology Analyst; personal communication with author, October, 2004.
23. Declercq et al., "Listening to mothers."
24. Lichy and Herzberg, *The Waterbirth Handbook*.
25. Balaskas and Meeus, *The Water Birth Book*.
26. Garland, "Supporting practice with audit," 508–11.
27. Garland, *Water Birth: An Attitude to Care*.

28. NHS Department of Health, *Changing Childbirth*.

29. Beech, *Water Birth Unplugged*.

30. Royal College of Midwives "Position Paper 1a: The use of water in labour and birth," *Midwives Journal*, vol. 3, no. 12 (2000).

31. Royal College of Obstetricians and Gynaecologists. "Birth in water."

32. Garland, *Water Birth: An Attitude to Care*.

33. The United Kingdom Parliament Select Committee on Health: Written Evidence, "Memorandum by the National Childbirth Trust," (MS 47). www.parliament.the-stationery-office.co.uk/pa/cm200203/cmselect/cmhealth/464/4

34. Dr. Bruce Sutherland, interview with author, May 1990.

35. Rachana, *Lotus Birth*.

36. Sei, "A Study of Waterbirths after Informed Consent of Client."

37. Jin, Dong, Liu, et al., "Delivery in Water: The Field Report of 51 Cases."

38. Josie Muscat, "Waterbirth in Malta," recorded presentation, 1st International Waterbirth Congress, London (April, 1995).

39. Zina Bakhareva, "Waterbirth in the Far East of Russia," recorded presentation, International Waterbirth Congress, Chicago, (April, 2004).

40. Appelt and Huber-Lange, *Geburten*.

41. Geissbuehler and Eberhard, "Waterbirths: A comparative study," 291–300.

42. Johnson, "Birth under water," 202–8.

43. Harding, Johnson, and McClelland, "Liquid sensitive laryngeal receptors in the developing sheep, cat, and monkey," 409–22.

44. Karlberg, et al., "Alteration of the infant's thorax during vaginal delivery," 202–8.

45. Personal interviews by author, 1990.

46. Rosenthal, "Warm-water immersion in labor and birth," 44–51.

47. Eriksson, Mattsson, and Ladfors, "Warm tub bath during labour," 642–44.

48. Siegel, "Does bath water enter the vagina?"

49. Katz et al., "A comparison of bed rest and immersion for treating the edema of pregnancy," 147–51.

50. Gutkowska, Antunes-Rodrigues, and McCann, "Atrial natriuretic peptide in brain and pituitary gland," 465–515.

51. Cluett et al., "Randomised controlled trial of labouring."

52. Odent, "Can immersion stop labor?" 414–16.

53. Krista Lewis, personal communication with author, November, 2004.

54. Nikodem, "Immersion in water in pregnancy, labour and birth."

55. H. Ponette, "Water births: My experience of 1600 waterbirths, including breeches and twins;" abstract published for the World Waterbirth Conference, London, (1995), appearing in *Waterbirth Unplugged*, Beverly Beech, ed.

56. Napierala, *Waterbirth: A Midwife's Perspective*.

## Chapter Seven: The Mind-Body Connection

1. Dick-Read, *Childbirth without Fear*, 16.

2. Brewer, *What Every Pregnant Woman Should Know*.

3. Lawson, "Eating Smart for Two."

4. Steingraber, *Having Faith*.
5. Steingraber, *How Mercury-Tainted Tuna Damage Fetal Brains*.
6. Renesch and DeFoore, *The New Bottom Line*.
7. Chopra, *Quantum Healing*.
8. Lee and Gay, "Sleep in late pregnancy," 2041–46.
9. Cohen and Estner, *Silent Knife*, 6.
10. Lipton, *Nature, Nurture and the Power of Love*.
11. Vines, "There is more to heredity than DNA," 16.
12. Deepak Chopra, telephone interview with author, December, 1991.
13. Cheek, "Are telepathy, clairvoyance and hearing possible in utero?" 125–37.
14. McCarty, "Welcoming Consciousness."
15. Chamberlain, "The significance of birth memories."
16. English, "Different Doorway," 22.
17. Chamberlain, *The Mind of Your Newborn Baby*, 211.
18. Ibid., 153.
19. Wirth, *Prenatal Parenting*.
20. Campbell, *The Mozart Effect*.
21. Odent, *Midwives, Lullabies and Mother Earth*.
22. Winsor, *The Pilates Pregnancy*.
23. Peterson, *An Easier Childbirth*, 17.
24. Ibid.
25. Mongan, *HypnoBirthing*.
26. Martin, Schauble, Rai, and Curry. "The Effects of Hypnosis," 441–43.
27. Fekety, *The Pocket Midwife*.
28. Maser, *Blessingways*.
29. G. Shah, "How Indian Women Prepare for Birth." Oral presentation, International Waterbirth Congress, Chicago, April 2004
30. Simkin and Klaus, *When Survivors Give Birth*.
31. Ibid.
32. Siegel and Hartzell, *Parenting From the Inside Out*.
33. Mehl and Peterson, *Pregnancy as Healing*, 58.
34. Gayle Peterson, personal communication, May 1992.
35. Bardsley and Capacchoione, *Creating a Joyful Birth*.
36. England and Horowitz, *Birthing From Within*.
37. Dr. Robert Doughton, interview with author, June, 1989.

## *Chapter Eight: Creating Gentle Birth Choices*

1. Anderson, R., and D. Anderson, "The cost effectiveness of home birth," 30–35. (Note: Figures from article were extrapolated to allow for a 3.3 percent inflation rate.)
2. NHS Department of Health, *Changing Childbirth*.
3. Crompton, "Hard labour wards."
4. Goorchenko and Goorchenko, *Psalm and Zoya: The Unassisted Homebirth of Our Twins*.
5. Kate Bauer, personal communication, June, 2004.
6. Sosa et al., "The effect of a supportive companion," 597–600.

7. Dr. William Tuxton, keynote speech at annual convention of American College of Nurse-Midwives, Atlanta, May 1990.

8. *CIA World Fact Book.*

9. Singh et al., *Prenatal Care in the United States.*

10. U. S. Census Bureau data, 2003. http://factfinder.census.gov/servlet/ACSSAFFFacts?

11. Declercq et al., "Listening to mothers: Executive Summary and Recommendations."

12. Barton, "Survey shows."

13. Ibid.

14. *California Association of Midwives Newsletter,* Summer 1991.

15. Hawken and Lovins, *Natural Capitalism.*

# Bibliography

ABC News. "Oh, the pain, the pain." February, 2001. www.ABCnews.com.

American Academy of Pediatrics. "Policy Statement on Circumcision." *Pediatrics* 103, no. 3 (March 1999): 686–93.

American College of Nurse-Midwives (ACNM). "Midwifery patients experience greater continuity of care and fewer interventions." www.midwife.org press release (November 20, 2003).

———. "Births attended by certified nurse-midwives on the rise." ACNM Fact sheet. www.midwife.org/press/cnmattendedfacts.pdf.

——— and S. Jacobs. *Having Your Baby with a Nurse-Midwife.* New York: Hyperion, 1993.

American College of Obstetricians and Gynecologists (ACOG). "OB-GYNS issue recommendations on cesarean delivery rates," news release, August 9, 2000.

———. Committee on Obstetrics. "Maternal and fetal medicine, guidelines for vaginal delivery after cesarean birth, committee opinion," no. 64 (October 1988).

———. "Fetal heart rate patterns: monitoring, interpretation, and management." *ACOG Technical Bulletin,* no. 207 (July 1995).

———. "Induction of labor," *ACOG Technical Bulletin,* no. 217 (December 1995).

———. "Vaginal birth after previous cesarean delivery." *ACOG Practice Bulletin,* no. 5 (July 1999).

Anand, K. J. S., and P. R. Hickey. "Pain and its effects in the human neonate and fetus." *New England Journal of Medicine,* no. 317 (1987): 1321–29.

Anderson, G. C., E. Moore, J. Hepworth, and N. Bergman. "Early skin-to-skin contact for mothers and their healthy newborn infants." *The Cochrane Database of Systematic Reviews* 2003, issue 2.

Anderson, R., and D. Anderson. "The cost effectiveness of home birth." *Journal of Nurse-Midwifery* 44, no. 1 (January 1999): 30–35.

Appelt, Michael, and Wolfgang Huber-Lang. *Geburten.* Berlin: Schwarzkopf and Schwarzkopf, 2003.

Arid, A., M. Luckas, and W. Buchett. "Effects of intrapartum hydrotherapy on labour related parameters." *Australian and New Zealand Journal of Obstetrics and Gynaecology* 37, no. 2 (May 1997): 137–42.

Arms, Suzanne. *Immaculate Deception.* Boston: Houghton-Mifflin, 1975.

Armstrong, Penny, and Sheryl Feldman. *A Wise Birth.* New York: William Morrow, 1990.

Baby-Friendly USA. "Baby Friendly Hospital Initiative." www.babyfriendlyusa.org.

Baker, Jeannine Parvati, and Frederick Baker. *Conscious Conception.* Joseph, Utah: Freestone Press, 1986.

Balaskas, Janet. *New Natural Pregnancy: Practical Wellbeing from Conception to Birth.* Sussex, U.K.: Gaia Books, 2004.

———. *Active Birth: The New Approach to Giving Birth Naturally,* rev. Boston: Harvard Common Press, 1991.

Balaskas, Janet, and Cathy Meeus. *The Water Birth Book.* London: Thorsons, 2004.

Barbira-Freedman, Francoise. *Yoga for Pregnancy: Birth and Beyond.* London: DK Publishing, 2004.

———. *Water Babies: Teach Your Baby the Joys of Water—From Newborn Floating to Toddler Swimming.* London: Lorenz Books, 2001.

Bardsley, Sandra, and Lucia Capacchoione. *Creating a Joyful Birth Experience.* New York: Fireside, 1994.

Barlett, Donald L., and James B. Steele. *Critical Condition: How Health Care in America Became Big Business and Bad Medicine.* New York: Doubleday, 2004.

Barton, Laura. "Survey shows that mothers' dreams of holistic experience end in hospital shock." January 13, 2005. www.guardian.co.uk/uk_news/story/0,3604,1389192,00.html.

Baumann, E., K. Brock, S. Cochran et al. *From Calling to Courtroom: A Survival Guide for Midwives.* Mount Prospect, Ill.: From Calling to Courtroom, Inc., 1994. www.fromcallingtocourtroom.net.

Becker, Ellie, et al. *Midwifery and the Law.* Santa Fe: Mothering, 1990.

Beech, Beverly. *Water Birth Unplugged.* London: Books for Midwives Press, 1996.

Belizán, J. M., et al. "Rates and Implications of Caesarean Sections in Latin America: Ecological Study." *British Medical Journal* (November 1999): 1397–1402.

Berezin, Nancy. *Gentle Birth Book.* New York: Simon and Schuster, 1980.

Bing, Elizabeth. *Six Practical Lessons for an Easier Childbirth.* New York: Bantam Books, 1977.

Blatt, Robin J. R. *Prenatal Tests.* New York: Vintage Books, 1988.

———. "An Overview of Genetic Screening and Diagnostic Tests in Health Care." www.geneletter.org/0996/screening.htm (accessed December 18, 2003).

Bloom, S. L., D. D. McIntire, M. A. Kelly et al. "Lack of effect of walking." *The New England Journal of Medicine* 2, no. 339 (1998): 117–18.

Blume, J., et al. "Focus on Wrongful Birth Cases, Firm Develops New Area of Expertise." (2001). www.njatty.com/whatsnew/wrongbirth.html (accessed November 13, 2004)

Brace, R. A. "Physiology of amniotic fluid volume regulation." *Clinical Obstetrics and Gynecology* 40, no. 2 (June 1997): 280–89.

Bradley, Robert. *Husband-Coached Childbirth: The Bradley Method of Natural Childbirth,* 4th ed. New York: Bantam, 1996.

Brewer, Gail. *What Every Pregnant Woman Should Know: The Truth About Diet and Drugs in Pregnancy,* rev. ed. East Rutherford, N. J.: Penguin, 1985.

Bricker, L., et al. "Ultrasound screening in pregnancy: A systematic review of the clinical effectiveness, cost-effectiveness and women's views." *Health Technology Assessment 2000* 4, no. 16 (2003).

Brown, M. J., R. E. Olver, C. A. Ramsden, L. B. Strang, and D. V. Walters. "Effects of adrenaline and of spontaneous labour on the secretion and absorption of lung liquid in the fetal lamb." *Journal of Physiology* 344 (1993): 137–52.

Brownridge, P. "The nature and consequence of childbirth pain." *European Journal of Obstetrics Gynecology and Reproductive Biology* 32 (1995): 9–15.

Buchanan, Kelley. *Peace of Mind During Pregnancy.* New York: Dell, 1989.

*CIA World Fact Book.* Updated November 30, 2004. www.cia.gov/cia/publications/factbook/index.html.

Caldeyro-Barcia, R., et al. "Effect of Position Changes on the Intensity and Frequency of Uterine Contractions during Labor." *American Journal of Obstetrics and Gynecology* 10, no. 80 (1960): 284–90.

*California Association of Midwives Newsletter,* Summer 1991.

Campbell, Don. *The Mozart Effect.* New York: Avon Books, 1997.

Canadian Association of Midwives. "Annual Report 2003." http://ca.geocities.com/canadianmidwives@rogers.com/papers.html

Caton, D., M. A. Frolich, and T. Euliana. "Anesthesia for childbirth: Controversy and change." *American Journal of Obstetrics and Gynecology,* no. 186 (May 2002): 25–30.

Chalmers, Iain, Murray Enkin and Mark J. N. C. Keirse, eds. *Effective Care in Pregnancy and Childbirth.* Oxford: Oxford University Press, 1989.

Chamberlain, David. "The significance of birth memories." *Journal of Prenatal and Perinatal Psychology and Health* 14, no. 1–2 (1999): 65–84.

———. *The Mind of Your Newborn Baby.* Berkeley: North Atlantic Books, 1998.

Cheek, David. "Are telepathy, clairvoyance and hearing possible in utero? Suggestive evidence as revealed during hypnotic age-regression studies of prenatal memory." *The International Journal of Pre- and Perinatal Psychology and Medicine* 7, no. 2 (Winter 1992): 125–37.

Chopra, Deepak. *Quantum Healing: Exploring the Frontiers of Mind/Body Medicine.* New York: Bantam, 1989.

Christensen, K. K., A. K. Dykes, and P. Christensen. "Reduced colonization of newborns with Group B Streptococci following washing of the birth canal with chlorhexidine." *Journal of Perinatal Medicine* 13 (1985): 239–43.

Christensson, K., T. Cabrera, E. Christensson, K. Uvnas-Mobert, and J. Winberg. "Separation distress call in the human neonate in the absence of maternal body contact." *Acta Paediatricia* 84, no. 5 (1995): 468–73.

Church, Linda. "Water birth: One birthing center's observations." *Journal of Nurse-Midwifery* 34, no. 4 (1989): 165–70.

Cluett, E., R. Pickering, K. Getliffe, and N. Saunders. "Randomised controlled trial of labouring in water compared with standard of augmentation for management of dystocia in first stage of labour." *British Medical Journal* 328 (February 2004): 315.

Cluett, E. R., V. C. Nikodem, R. E. McCandish, and E. E. Burns. "Immersion in water in pregnancy, labour and birth." *The Cochrane Database of Systematic Reviews* 2004, Issue 1. Art. No. CD000111.

Coalition for Improving Maternity Services (CIMS) Fact Sheet. "The Risks of Cesarean Delivery to Mother and Baby." September 2003. www.motherfriendly.org/Downloads/csec-fact-sheet.pdf.

Cohen, Nancy Wainer, and Lois Estner. *Silent Knife: Cesarean Prevention and Vaginal Birth after Cesarean.* South Hadley, Mass.: Bergin and Garvey, 1983.

Cole, D. S., M.D. "Elective Primary Cesarean Delivery: What's the Big Deal?" *Highlights in Obstetrics from the 50th Annual Meeting of the American College of Obstetricians and Gynecologists.* Los Angeles: May 4–8, 2002. www.medscape.com/viewarticle/434586.

Conkling, Winifred. *Hypnosis for a Joyful Pregnancy and Pain-Free Labor and Delivery.* New York: St. Martin's Press, 2002.

Crompton, Simon. "Hard labour wards." *Times Online.* January 15, 2005. www.timesonline.co.uk/article/0,,589-1439263,00.html.

Curtin, L., and M. Park. "Trends in the Attendant, Place, and Timing of Births, and in the Use of Obstetric Interventions: United States, 1989–97." *National Vital Statistics Reports.* U. S. Department of Health and Human Services, CDCP (December 2, 1999): 4.

D'Alton, M. E., and A. H. DeCherney. "Prenatal Diagnosis." *New England Journal of Medicine* 328 (January 14, 1993): 114–20.

Davis, Elizabeth. *Heart and Hands: A Midwife's Guide to Pregnancy and Birth,* 2nd ed. Berkeley: Celestial Arts, 1987.

Davis-Floyd, Robbie. *Birth as an American Rite of Passage.* Berkeley: University of California Press, 1992.

Davis-Floyd, Robbie, and Carolyn F. Sargent. *Childbirth and Authoritative Knowledge: Cross-Cultural Perspectives.* Berkeley: University of California Press, 1997.

Davis-Floyd, Robbie, Ivy Lynn Bourgeault, and Cecilia Benoit. *Reconceiving Midwifery.* Toronto: McGill-Queen's University Press, 2004.

Davis-Floyd, Robbie, and Gloria St. John. *From Doctor to Healer: The Transformative Journey.* New Brunswick: Rutgers University Press, 1998.

Davis-Floyd, Robbie, and Sven P. Arvidson. *Intuition: The Inside Story: Interdisciplinary Perspectives.* New York: Routledge, 1997.

Declercq, E., C. Sakala, M. P. Coirry, S. Applebaum, and P. Risher. *Listening to Mothers: Report on the First National U.S. Survey of Women's Childbearing Experiences.* New York: Maternity Center Association, October 2002. www.maternitywise.org/pdfs/LtMreport.pdf.

DeLee, J. B. "The Prophylactic Forceps Operation." *American Journal of Obstetrics and Gynecology* 1, no. 1 (1920): 34–44.

Department of Health (U.K.). *Changing Childbirth: The Report of the Expert Maternity Group.* London: HMSO, 1993.

DeVries, Raymond. *Birth By Design: Pregnancy, Maternity Care, and Midwifery in North America and Europe.* London: Routledge, 2001.

Dick-Read, Grantly. *Childbirth without Fear: The Principles and Practices of Natural Childbirth.* New York: Harper and Row, 1944.

Durand, M. "The Safety of Home Birth: The Farm Study." *Journal of the American Public Health Association* 82 (March 1992): 450–52.

Eastman, Nicholson J., M.D. *Expectant Motherhood,* 2nd ed. Boston: Little, Brown and Company, 1947.

Edwards, Margot, and Mary Waldorf. *Reclaiming Birth: History and Heroines of American Childbirth Reform.* Freedom, Calif.: Crossing Press, 1984.

Ehrenreich, Barbara, and Dierdre English. *Witches, Midwives, and Nurses.* New York: Feminist Press, 1973.

Embry, M. "Observations sur un accouchement termine dans le bain." *Annales de la Societe de Medicine Pratique de Montpelier* 1805, no. 53: 185–91.

Emde, R. N., et al. "Stress and Neonatal Sleep," *Psychosomatic Medicine,* no. 33 (1971): 491–97.

Emoto, Masaru. *The Hidden Messages in Water.* Hillsboro, Ore.: Beyond Words Publishing, 2004.

England, Pam, and Rob Horowitz. *Birthing From Within: An Extra-Ordinary Guide to Childbirth Preparation.* Santa Fe: Partera Press, 1998.

English, Jane. *Different Doorway: Adventures of a Cesarean Born.* Point Reyes Station, Calif.: Earth Heart, 1985.

Enkin, M., M. J. Keirse, J. Neilson et al. *A Guide to Effective Care in Pregnancy and Childbirth,* 3rd ed. New York: Oxford University Press, 2000.

Enning, Cornelia. *Waterbirth Midwifery: A training book.* Stuttgart, Germany: Hippokrates, 2003.

Falcao, R. "Group B Strep." www.gentlebirth.org/archives/gbs.html#Alternatives/GroupBStrep (accessed December 23, 2004).

Fekety, Susan. *The Pocket Midwife.* Falmouth, Me.: Fekety, 2003.

Flamm, B. "Vaginal birth after cesarean: What's new in the new millennium?" *Current Opinions in Obstetrics and Gynecology,* no. 14 (2002): 595–99.

———. "Once a cesarean, always a controversy." *Obstetrics and Gynecology* 90 (August 1997): 312–15.

———. *Birth after Cesarean.* New York: Prentice Hall, 1990.

Fleiss, P. "The Case Against Circumcision." *Mothering.* no. 85 (Winter 1997). www.mothering.com/articles/new_baby/circumcision/against-circumcision.html.

Freeman, R. "Intrapartum Fetal Monitoring: A Disappointing Story." *New England Journal of Medicine* 322, no. 9 (March 1, 1990): 624–25.

Garland, D. *Waterbirth: An Attitude to Care,* 2nd ed. London: Books for Midwives Press, 2000.

——— "Collaborative Waterbirth audit—Supporting practice with audit." *MIDIRS Midwifery Digest* 12, no. 4 (December 2002): 508–511. (MIDIRS is an acronym for Midwives Information and Resource Service, a United Kingdom publication.)

Garland, D., and S. Crook. "Is the use of water in labour an option for women following a previous LSCS?" *MIDIRS Midwifery Digest* 14, no. 1 (March 2004): 63–67.

Gaskin, Ina May. *Spiritual Midwifery.* 4th ed. Summertown, Tenn.: The Book Publishing Co., 2002.

Geissbuehler, V., and J. Eberhard. "Waterbirths: A comparative study: a prospective study on more than 2000 waterbirths." *Fetal Diagnosis and Therapy* 15, no. 5 (September-October 2000): 291–300.

Ghetti, C., B. K. S. Chan, and J. Guise. "Physicians' Responses to Patient-Requested Cesarean Delivery." *Birth: Issues in Perinatal Care* 31, no. 4 (2004): 280.

Gilbert, R. E., and P. A. Tookey. "Perinatal mortality and morbidity among babies delivered in water: surveillance study and postal survey." *British Medical Journal* 319 (August 21, 1999): 483–487.

Goer, H. *Obstetrical Myths versus Research Realities.* Westport, Conn.: Bergin and Garvey, 1995.

———. *The Thinking Woman's Guide to a Better Birth.* Berkeley: Berkeley Publishing Group, 1999.

———. "Humanizing Birth: A Global Grassroots Movement." *Birth: Issues in Perinatal Care* 31, no. 4 (December 2004): 308.

Goldsmith, Judith. *Childbirth Wisdom*. Brookline, Mass.: East-West Health Books, 1990.

Goorchenko, Mindy, and Alex Goorchenko. *Psalm & Zoya: The Unassisted Homebirth of Our Twins*. Hermosa Beach, Calif.: Earth Birth Productions, 2004.

Gordon, Yehudi. *Birth and Beyond: The Definitive Guide to Your Pregnancy, Your Birth, Your Family—From Minus 9 to Plus 9 Months*. London: Vermillion, 2002.

Graham, I., J. Logan, B. Davies, and C. Nimrod. "Changing the use of electronic fetal monitoring and labor support: A case study of barriers and facilitators." *Birth: Issues in Perinatal Care*, 31, no. 4 (December 2004): 293.

Grof, Stanislav, and Joan Halifax. *The Human Encounter with Death*. New York: E. P. Dutton, 1977.

Gurevich, Rachel. *The Doula Advantage: Your Complete Guide to Having an Empowered and Positive Birth with the Help of a Professional Childbirth Assistant*. Roseville, Calif.: Prima Publishing, 2003.

Gutkowska, J., J. Antunes-Rodrigues, and S. M. McCann. "Atrial natriuretic peptide in brain and pituitary gland." *Physiological Reviews* 77, no. 2 (April 1997): 465–515.

Gutmann, Caroline. *The Legacy of Dr. Lamaze: The Story of the Man Who Changed Childbirth*. New York: St. Martin's Press, 2001.

Haggard, Howard. *Devils, Drugs, and Doctors*. New York: Blue Ribbon Books, 1929.

Haire, Doris. *The Cultural Warping of Childbirth*. Minneapolis: International Childbirth Education Association Publications, 1973.

Hamilton, B., J. Martin, and P. D. Sutton. "Birth: Preliminary Data for 2003." *National Vital Statistics Reports* 53, no. 9 (2003). www.cdc.gov/nchs/data/nvsr/nvsr53/nvsr53_09.pdf.

Harding, R., P. Johnson, and M. McClelland. "Liquid sensitive laryngeal receptors in the developing sheep, cat, and monkey." *Journal of Physiology* 277 (1978): 409–22.

Harper, Barbara. "Taking the plunge: reevaluating water temperature." *MIDIRS Midwifery Digest* 12, no. 4 (December 2002): 506–8.

———. "Waterbirth Basics: from newborn breathing to hospital protocols." *Midwifery Today* 54 (Summer 2000): 9–15, 68.

———. "Practitioner survey on waterbirth practices." Wilsonville, Ore.: Global Maternal/Child Health Association, 1992.

———. "Survey of Waterbirth Practice." *Journal of Nurse-Midwifery* 34, no. 4 (1989): 86.

Hawken, Paul, and Amory Lovins. *Natural Capitalism: Creating the Next Industrial Revolution*. Cambridge: Back Bay Books, 2000.

Healthy People 2010. "Implementation." Washington, D.C.: Office of Disease Prevention and Health Promotion, U.S. Department of Health and Human Services. www.healthypeople.gov/Implementation/

Hemminki, E. "Impact of caesarean section on future pregnancy—a review of cohort studies." *Paediatric Perinatal Epidemiology* 10, no. 4 (October 1996): 366–79.

Hodnett, E. "Pain and women's satisfaction with the experience of childbirth: a systematic review." *American Journal of Obstetrics and Gynecology* 186, no. 5 (2002): 160–72.

Hodnett, E., S. Gates, G. J. Hofmeyr, and C. Sakala. "Continuous support for women during childbirth." *The Cochrane Database of Systematic Reviews* 2003, issue 3. Art. No. CD003766.

Illich, Ivan. *Medical Nemesis: The Expropriation of Health*. New York: Random House, 1976.

Ivell, R. "Endocrinology. This hormone has been relaxin' too long!" *Science*, no. 295 (2002): 637.

Jacobson, B., K. Nyberg et al. "Opiate Addiction in Adult Offspring through Possible Imprinting after Obstetric Treatment." *British Journal of Medicine*, no. 3011 (November 1990): 1067–70.

Jamois, Tanya. "Women have right to refuse Caesarean." *North County Times*, April 13, 2004. www.nctimes.com/articles/2004/04/14/opinion/commentary/21_27_324_13_04.txt.

Jarrett, R. J. "Gestational diabetes: a non-entity?" *British Medical Journal*, no. 306 (1993): 37–38.

Jin, W., S. Dong, P. Liu et al. "Delivery in Water: The Field Report of 51 Cases." Department of Gynaecology and Obstetrics, Shanghai Changning Maternity and Infant Hospital. Paper presented at International Waterbirth Congress, Chicago (April 2004).

Johanson, R., M. Newburn, and A. Macfarlne. "Has the Medicalization of Childbirth Gone Too Far?" *British Medical Journal* 324, no. 13 (April 2004): 892–95.

Johnson, P. "Birth under water: to breathe or not to breathe." *British Journal of Obstetrics and Gynaecology* 103 (1996): 202–8.

Karlberg, P., et al. "Alteration of the infant's thorax during vaginal delivery." *Acta Obstetrica Gynecologica Scandinavia* 41 (1987): 223.

Karmel, Marjorie. *Thank You, Dr. Lamaze.* Garden City, N.Y.: Doubleday, 1965.

Karmer, M. D., K. Demissie, R. W Platt, R. Suave, and R. Liston. "The contribution of mild and moderate preterm birth to infant mortality." *Journal of the American Medical Association* 7, no. 284 (2000): 843–49.

Katz, V., R. Ryder, R. Cefalo, S. Carmichael, and R. Goolsby. "A comparison of bed rest and immersion for treating the edema of pregnancy." *Obstetrics and Gynecology* 75, no. 2 (February 1990): 147–51.

Katz-Rothman, Barbara. *Giving Birth: Alternatives in Childbirth.* Harmondsworth, U.K.: Penguin, 1982.

Kitzinger, Sheila. *The Complete Book of Pregnancy and Childbirth,* 11th ed. New York: Alfred A. Knopf, 1986.

———. *Rediscovering Birth.* New York: Pocket Books, 2000.

———. *Birth Your Way: Choosing Birth at Home or in a Birth Center.,* rev. ed. London: DK Books, 2001.

Klaus, Marshall H., and John H. Kennell. *Maternal-Infant Bonding.* St. Louis: Mosby, 1976.

Klaus, Marshall H., John H. Kennell, and Phyllis H. Klaus. *The Doula Book: How a Trained Labor Companion Can Help You Have a Shorter, Easier and Healthier Birth.* Cambridge, Mass.: Perseus Publishing, 2002.

———. *Bonding: Building the Foundations of Secure Attachment and Independence.* Boston: Addison Wesley, 1996.

———. "Effects of social support during parturition on maternal and infant morbidity." *British Medical Journal* 293 (1986): 585–87.

Klein, M. "The Epidural Controversy: Do epidurals increase the c-section rate?" *British Columbia Women's and Childrens' Hospital Newsletter* 5, no. 2 (1995).

Korte, D. "Midwives on Trial." *Mothering* (Fall 1995).

Kozak, L. J., and J. D. Weeks. "U.S. Trends in Obstetric Procedures, 1990–2000." *Birth: Issues in Perinatal Care* 29, no. 3 (2002): 157–161.

Kroeger, Mary and Linda Smith. *Impact of Birthing Practices on Breastfeeding: Protecting the Mother and Baby Continuum.* Sudbury, Mass.: Jones and Bartlett, 2004.

Laibow, R. "Circumcision and Its Relationship to Attachment Impairment." Paper presented at the Second International Symposium on Circumcision, San Francisco, April 30, 1991.

Larson, J. "The Politics of Newborn Pain." *Mothering* (Fall 1990): 45.

Lawson, W. "Eating Smart for Two: Boosting a Baby's Brain." *Psychology Today* (April 1, 2003). http://cms.psychologytoday.com/articles/pto-20030401–000008.html.

Leavitt, Judith. *Brought to Bed: Childbearing in America 1750–1950.* New York: Oxford University Press, 1986.

Leboyer, Frederick. *Birth without Violence.* Rochester, Vt.: Healing Arts Press, 2002.

Lee, K. and Gay, C. L. "Sleep in late pregnancy predicts length of labor and type of delivery." *American Journal of Obstetrics and Gynecology* 191 (2004): 2041–46.

Leveno, K., et al. "A Prospective Comparison of Selective and Universal Electronic Fetal Monitoring in 34,995 Pregnancies." *New England Journal of Medicine,* no. 315 (1986): 10.

Lichy, Roger, and Eileen Herzberg. *The Waterbirth Handbook.* London: Gateway Books, 1993.

Lipton, B. "Nature, Nurture and the Power of Love." *Journal of Prenatal and Perinatal Psychology and Health,* no. 13 (1998): 3–10.

Litoff, Judith, ed. *The American Midwife Debate.* Westport, Conn.: Greenwood Press, 1986.

Lothian, J. "Childbearing Women's Fears: at the Heart of Choice." *The Journal of Perinatal Education* 12, no. 4 (2003): 36–39.

———. "Lamaze International Position Paper: Promoting, Protecting and Supporting Normal Birth." *The Journal of Perinatal Education* 13, no. 2 (Spring 2004): 1–5.

Lukacs, S. L., K. C. Schoendorf, and A. Schuchat. "Trends in sepsis-related neonatal mortality in the United States, 1985–1998." *Pediatric Infectious Disease Journal* 23, no. 7 (July 2004): 599–603.

Luthy, D., et al. "Elective Induction Doubles Cesarean Risk." *American Journal of Obstetrics and Gynecology,* no. 191 (2004): 1511–15.

Madrid, A., and D. Pennington. "Maternal-infant bonding and asthma." *Journal of Prenatal and Perinatal Psychology and Health* 14, no. 3–4 (Spring/Summer 2000): 279–89.

Madrid, A., R. Ames, S. Skolek, and G. Brown. "Does Maternal-Infant Bonding Therapy Improve Breathing in Asthmatic Children?" *Journal of Prenatal and Perinatal Psychology and Health* 15, no. 2 (Winter 2000): 90–117.

Mansfield, P. "Maternal Age: What Is Really High Risk?" *Mothering,* no. 41 (Fall 1986): 64–69.

Marshall, R. E., F. L. Porter, A. G. Rogers et al. "Circumcision: II. Effects upon mother-infant interaction." *Early Human Development* 7, no. 4 (December 1982): 367–74.

Martin, A., P. Schauble, S. Rai, and R. W. Curry. "The Effects of Hypnosis on the Labor Processes and Birth Outcomes of Pregnant Adolescents." *Journal of Family Practice,* no. 50 (2001): 441–43.

Maser, Sheri. *Blessingways: A Guide to Mother-Centered Baby Showers.* Greenbrae, Calif.: Moondance Press, 2004.

McCarty, Wendy Anne. *Welcoming Consciousness: Supporting Babies' Wholeness from the Beginning of Life.* Santa Barbara, Calif.: Wondrous Beginnings, 2004.

Mehl, Lewis, and Gayle Peterson. *Pregnancy as Healing.* Berkeley, Calif.: Mind Body Press, 1984.

Mehl, L., G. H. Peterson, M. Whitt, and W. E. Hawes. "Outcomes of Elective Home Births: A Series of 1,146 Cases." *The Journal of Reproductive Medicine* 19, no. 5 (November 1977): 281–90.

Mehl-Madrona, L. and M. M. Madrona. "Physician and midwife attended home births: Effects of breech, twin, and post-dates outcome data on mortality rates." *Journal of Nurse Midwifery,* no. 2 (1997): 91–98.

Midwives Alliance of North America *Annual Report* 2004.

Mitford, Jessica. *The American Way of Birth.* New York: Penguin Books, 1992.

Mittendorf, R., M. A. Williams, C. S. Berkey, and P. F. Cotter. "The Length of Uncomplicated Human Gestation." *Obstetrics and Gynecology* 6, no. 75 (1990): 929–32.

Mongan, Marie. *HypnoBirthing: A Celebration of Life,* 3rd ed. Deerfield Beach, Fla.: Health Communications, 2005.

Morrison, J.C., B. F. Chez, I. D. Davis et al. "Intrapartum Fetal Heart Rate Assessment: Monitoring by Auscultation or Electronic Means." *American Journal of Obstetrics and Gynecology,* no. 168 (1993): 63–66.

Motha, Gowri, and Karen Swan Macleod. *The Gentle Birth Method: The Month-by-month Jeyarani Way Programme.* London: HarperCollins, 2004.

Mother-Friendly Childbirth Initiative. "Having a Baby? Ten Questions to Ask." Coalition for Improving Maternity Services, 2003. www.motherfriendly.org/resources/10Q/

Muster, K., L. Schmidt, and P. Helm. "Length and Variation in the Menstrual Cycle: A Cross-Sectional Study from a Danish County." *British Journal of Obstetrics and Gynecology,* no. 99 (1992): 422–29.

Napierala, Susanna. *Waterbirth: A Midwife's Perspective.* New York: Bergin and Garvey, 1994.

Nathanielsz, Peter W. *A Time to Be Born: The Life of the Unborn Child.* Oxford: Oxford University Press, 1995.

National Center for Health Statistics. "National Hospital Discharge Survey: Annual Summary with Detailed Diagnosis and Procedure Data." (2003). www.cdc.gov/nchs/about/major/hdasd/nhds.htm.

———. "Trends in the Attendant, Place and Timing of Births and in the Use of Obstetric Interventions, United States, 1989–1997." *National Vital Statistics Reports* 47, no. 27.

———. "Births: Preliminary Data for 2003." *National Vital Statistics Reports* 53, no 9.

———. "Births: Final Data for 2001." *National Vital Statistics Report* 51, no 2.

Nelson, K., and J. Ellenberg. "Antecedents of Cerebral Palsy." *American Journal of Diseases of Children,* no. 1 (1985): 39.

Newton, Niles. "Experimental Inhibition of Labor through Environmental Disturbance," *Obstetrics and Gynecology* 27, no. 3 (March 1966): 371–77.

Newton, Niles, and M. Newton. "Mothers' Reactions to Their Newborn Babies." *Journal of the American Medical Association* 181 (July 21, 1962): 206–10.

Nissen, E., G. Lilja, A. M. Widstrom, and K. Uvnas-Moberg. "Elevation of oxytocin levels early post partum in women." *Acta Obstetrica Gynecologico Scandinavia* 74 (1995): 530–533.

Nygaard, I., and D. P. Cruikshank. "Should all women be offered elective cesarean delivery?" *Obstetrics and Gynecology,* no. 102 (2003): 217–219

Odent, Michel. *Birth and Breastfeeding: Rediscovering the Needs of Women During Pregnancy and Childbirth.* East Sussex, U.K.: Clairview Books, 2004.

———. *Birth Reborn.* New York: Pantheon, 1984.

———. "Birth under Water." *Lancet* 2, no. 147 (1983): 67.

———. "Can immersion stop labor?" *Journal of Nurse Midwifery* 42, no. 5 (1997): 414–16.

———. *The Caesarean.* London: Free Association Books, 2004.

———. *The Farmer and the Obstetrician.* London: Free Association Books, 2002.

———. "The fetus ejection reflex." *Birth: Issues in Perinatal Care* 14, no. 2 (1987).

———. "Lessons from the first hospital birthing pool." *Midwifery Today* 54 (2000).

———. "Midwives, Lullabies and Mother Earth." BBC video production, 1994.

———. *Planned Home Birth in Industrialized Countries.* Copenhagen: World Health Organization, 1991.

————. "Primal Health Research: Four Essays." *Journal of Prenatal and Perinatal Psychology and Health* 16, no. 3 (Spring 2002): 265–95.

————. *Primal Health: Understanding the Critical Period between Conception and the First Birthday.* East Sussex, U.K.: Clairview Books, 2002.

————. *The Scientification of Love.* London: Free Association Books, 1999.

————. "Use of water during labour: updated recommendations." *MIDIRS Midwifery Digest* 8, no. 1 (March 1998): 68–69.

Odent, Michel, and Jessica Johnson. *We Are All Water Babies.* Berkeley: Celestial Arts, 1995.

O'Hara, Kristen. *Sex as Nature Intended It: The Most Important Thing You Need to Know about Making Love, But No One Could Tell You Until Now,* 2nd ed. Hudson, Mass.: Turning Point Publications, 2002.

O'Mara, Peggy. *Having A Baby Naturally: The Mothering Magazine Guide to Pregnancy and Childbirth.* New York: Atria Books, 2003.

O'Neill, Eugene. "Mourning Becomes Electra." In *Eugene O'Neill: Complete Plays 1920–1931.* New York: Library of America, 1988.

Otigbah, C. M., M. K. Dhanjal, G. Harmsworth, and T. Chard. "A retrospective comparison of water births and conventional vaginal deliveries." *European Journal of Obstetrics, Gynecology & Reproductive Biology* 91, no. 1 (July 2000): 15–20.

Paltro, L. "Do Pregnant Women Have Rights?" *AlterNet,* December 8, 2004. www.alternet.org/story/18493.

Paul, R. H., and E. H. Hon. "Clinical fetal monitoring versus effect on perinatal outcome." *American Journal of Obstetrics and Gynecology* 118, no. 4 (February 15, 1974): 529–33.

Pearce, Joseph Chilton. *Evolution's End: Claiming the Potential of Our Intelligence.* New York: HarperCollins, 1995.

Perkins, Barbara Bridgman. *The Medical Delivery Business: Health Reform, Childbirth, and the Economic Order.* New Brunswick, N.J.: Rutgers University Press, 2004.

Peterson, Gayle. *An Easier Childbirth.* Los Angeles: Jeremy Tarcher, 1991.

Poindron, P., and P. Neindre. "Endocrine and sensory regulation of maternal behavior in the ewe." In *Advances In The Study Of Behavior.* J. S. Rosenblatt et al., eds. New York: Academic Press, Inc., 1980.

Popovic, J. R. "National Hospital Discharge Survey: Annual summary with detailed diagnosis and procedure data." *Vital Health Statistics 2000* 151, no. 13: 7.

Pratt, C. L. "The Role of a Midwife." *The Daily Record.* Wooster, Ohio. March 17, 2002. www.the-daily-record.com/past_issues/03_mar/020317dr1.html.

Public Citizen Health Research Group. *Health Letter* 3, no. 5 (1994): 2.

Rachana, Shivam. *Lotus Birth.* Sydney: Greenwood Press, 2000.

Rageth, J. C., C. Juzi, and H. Grossenbacher. "Delivery after previous cesarean: a risk evaluation." *Obstetrics and Gynecology* 3, no. 93 (1999): 332–37.

Ramin, S. M., et al. "Randomized trial of epidural versus intravenous analgesia during labor." *Obstetrics and Gynecology* 5, no. 86 (November 1995): 783–89.

Ransjo-Arvidson, A., et al. "Maternal analgesia during labor disturbs newborn behavior: Effects on breastfeeding, temperature, and crying." *Birth* 28, no. 1 (March 2001): 5–12.

Ray, Sondra. *Ideal Birth.* Berkeley: Celestial Arts, 1985.

Reiss, M. "Circumcision: My Position," rev. 2003. *Doctors Opposing Circumcision.* http://faculty.washington.edu/gcd/DOC/mposition.html.

Renesch, John, and Bill DeFoore, eds. *The New Bottom Line: Bringing Heart and Soul to Business.* Lanham, Md.: National Book Network, 1998.

Richard, L., and M. O. Alade. "Sucking technique and its effect on breastfeeding." *Birth* 19, no. 185 (December 1992): 189.

Ritter, Thomas J. *Say No to Circumcision.* Aptos, Calif.: Hourglass, 1992.

Robbins, John. *Reclaiming Our Health: Exploding the Medical Myth and Embracing the Sources of True Healing.* Tiburon, Calif.: H.J. Kramer, 1998.

Rooks, J. P., et al. "Outcomes of Care in Birth Centers." *New England Journal of Medicine* 321 (1989): 1804–11.

Rooks, Judith, Ph.D. *Midwifery and Childbirth in America.* Philadelphia: Temple University Press, 1999.

Rosen, M., and L. Thomas. *The Cesarean Myth: Choosing the Best Way to Have Your Baby.* Harmondswork, U.K: Penguin Books, 1989.

Rosenblatt, D., et al. "The influence of maternal analgesia on neonatal behaviour: II. Epidural bupivacaine." *British Journal of Obstetrics and Gynaecology* 88 (April 1981): 407–13.

Rosenthal, Michael. "Warm-water immersion in labor and birth." *The Female Patient* (1991): 16, 35–37, 40–41, 44, 46.

Ross, M. G., and M. J. Nijland. "Fetal Swallowing: Relation to Amniotic Fluid Regulation." *Clinical Obstetrics and Gynecology,* no. 40 (1997): 352.

Rowe-Finkbeiner, K. "Juggling Career and Home: Albright, O'Connor, and You." *Mothering,* no. 117 (March/April 2003).

Royal College of Obstetricians and Gynaecologists. "Birth in water." London: RCOG, 2001. www.rcog.org.uk.

Rubin, Rita. *What If I Have a C-Section?* Emmaus, Penn.: Rodale Press, 2004.

Sagov, S., et al; *Home Birth: A Practitioner's Guide to Birth Outside the Hospital.* Rockville, Md.: Aspen Systems, 1984.

Salk, Lee. Keynote speech to Prenatal and Perinatal Psychology Association of North America Conference, Amherst, Mass., 1989.

Scheepers, H., M. Thans, P. de Jong et al. "Eating and Drinking in Labor: The Influence of Caregiver Advice on Women's Behavior." *Birth: Issues in Perinatal Care* 28, no. 2 (June 2001): 119.

Schultz, G. D. "Cruelty in the maternity wards." *Ladies' Home Journal* (May 1958): 44–45, 152–55.

Scrutton, M. J., G. A. Metcalfe, C. Lowry et al. "Eating in labor: A randomized controlled trial assessing the risks and benefits." *Anesthesia* 54, no. 4 (1999): 329–34.

Sei, Fuseiko. "A Study of Waterbirths after Informed Consent of Client." Paper presented at the International Confederation of Midwives conference, Kobe, Japan, October, 1990.

Shah, M. "Soaring Cesarean Section Rates: A Cause for Alarm." *Journal of Obstetric, Gynecological, and Neonatal Nursing* 32, no. 3 (May/June 2003): 283–84.

Shearer, B. "Crisis in Obstetrics," *C/SEC Newsletter* 3, no. 13 (1988).

Sidenbladh, Erik. *Water Babies.* New York: St. Martin's Press, 1983.

Siegel, Daniel J. *The Developing Mind: How Relationships and the Brain Interact to Shape Who We Are.* New York: The Guilford Press, 1999.

Siegel, Daniel, and Mary Hartzell. *Parenting From the Inside Out.* Los Angeles: Jeremy Tarcher, 2003.

Siegel, P. "Does bath water enter the vagina?" *Obstetrics and Gynecology* 15 (May 1960): 660–61.

Simkin, Penny. *Pregnancy, Childbirth, and the Newborn: The Complete Guide,* rev. and updated. Minnetonka, Minn.: Meadowbrook, 2001.

Simkin, Penny, and Ruth Ancheta. *The Labor Progress Handbook.* Malden, Mass.: Blackwell Science, 2005.

Simkin, Penny, and Phyllis Klaus. *When Survivors Give Birth: Understanding and Healing the Effects of Early Sexual Abuse on Childbearing Women.* Las Vegas: Classic Day Publishers, 2004.

Simkin, P., and M. O'Hara. "Nonpharmacologic relief of pain during labor: Systematic reviews of five methods." *American Journal of Obstetrics and Gynecology* 186, no. 5 (2002): 131–59.

Singh, Susheela, Jacqueline Darroch Forrest, and Aida Torres. *Prenatal Care in the United States: A State and County Inventory.* New York; Washington, D. C.: Alan Guttmacher Institute, 1989.

Sleutel, M., and S. S. Golden. "Fasting in labor: Relic or requirement?" *Journal of Obstetric, Gynecologic and Neonatal Nursing* 77, no. 28 (1999): 507–12.

Solter, Aletha J. *The Aware Baby,* rev. ed. Goleta, Calif.: Shining Star Press, 2001.

Sosa, R., J. Kennel, S. Robertson, and J. Urrutia. "The Effect of a Supportive Companion on Perinatal Problems, Length of Labor, and Mother-Infant Interaction." *The New England Journal of Medicine* 11, no. 303 (1980): 597–600.

Starr, Paul. *The Social Transformation of American Medicine.* New York: Basic Books, 1982.

Steingraber, Sandra. *Having Faith: An Ecologist's Journey to Motherhood.* Berkeley: Berkeley Publishing Group, 2001.

———. "How Mercury-Tainted Tuna Damages Fetal Brains." *In These Times.* December 27, 2004.

Strong, Thomas H. *Expecting Trouble: The Myth of Prenatal Care in America.* New York: New York University Press, 2002.

Sullivan, Deborah, and Rose Weitz. *Labor Pains: Modern Midwives and Home Birth.* New Haven, Conn.: Yale University Press, 1988.

Thacker, S. B., and D. F. Stroup. "Continuous Electronic Fetal Heart Rate Monitoring Versus Intermittent Auscultation for Assessment During Labor." *The Cochrane Database of Systematic Reviews* 2001, issue 2.

Towner, D., M. A. Castro, E. Eby-Wilkens, and W. M. Gilbert. "Effect of mode of delivery in nulliparous women on neonatal intracranial injury." *New England Journal of Medicine* 341, no. 23 (Dec 2, 1999): 1709–14.

Tritten, Jan, ed. *Sharing Midwifery Knowledge: Tricks of the Trade,* vol. 4. Eugene, Oreg.: Midwifery Today, 2004.

Tulman, L. and J. Fawcett. "Return of Functional Ability after Childbirth." *Nursing Research* 37, no. 2 (1988).

Tyson, H. "The Re-emergence of Canadian Midwifery: A New Profession Dedicated to Normal Birth." *Birth International.* www.acegraphics.com.au/articles/holliday01.html.

United Kingdom Parliament Select Committee on Health: Written Evidence. "Memorandum by the National Childbirth Trust," (MS 47). www.parliament.the-stationery-office.co.uk/pa/cm200203/cmselect/cmhealth/464/4.

U.S. Census Bureau. "2003 American Community Survey Data Profile Highlights." http://factfinder.census.gov/servlet/ACSSAFFFacts?

U. S. Department of Labor. "Women at Work: A Visual Essay." *Monthly Labor Review.* Bureau of Labor Statistics, October 2003. www.bls.gov/opub/mlr/2003/10/ressum3.pdf.

U.S. Food and Drug Administration (FDA). "Cytotec Drug Bulletin." Center for Drug Evaluation and Research. www.fda.gov/cder/foi/label/2002/19268slr037.pdf.

U. S. Preventive Services Task Force. *Guide To Clinical Preventive Services,* 2nd ed. Baltimore: Williams and Wilkins, 1996.

Varney, Helen, Jan M. Kriebs, and Carolyn L. Gegor. *Varney's Midwifery,* 4th ed. Sudbury Mass.: Jones and Bartlett, 2004.

Vines, G. "There is more to heredity than DNA." *New Scientist,* no. 16 (1997).

*Vital Statistics Reports* 52, no. 10. Hyattsville, Md.: National Center for Health Statistics (December 17, 2003).

Wagner, M. "Hospital Birth Deemed Too Risky." *Chicago Sun Times.* April 2, 1989. As reported in *Mothering* 55 (Fall 1989): 75.

Wagner, Marsden. *Pursuing the Birth Machine: The Search for Appropriate Birth Technology.* Camperdown, NSW, Australia: Ace Graphics, 1994.

———. "Cytotec induction and off-label use." *Midwifery Today,* no. 57 (Fall 2003).

Walker, M. "Do labor medications affect breastfeeding?" *Journal of Human Lactation* 13 (1997): 131–37.

Watson, Lyall, and Jerry Derbyshire. *The Water Planet: A Celebration of the Wonder of Water.* New York: Crown, 1988.

Wertz, Dorothy, and Richard Wertz. *Lying-In: A History of Childbirth in America.* New Haven, Conn.: Yale University Press, 1989.

"What Every Pregnant Woman Needs to Know About Cesarean Section." Maternity Center Association (April 2004). www.maternitywise.org/cesareanbooklet/.

Wiegers, T. A., M. J. Kierse, J. van der Zee, and G. A. H. Berghs. "Outcome of Planned Home and Planned Hospital Births in Low Risk Pregnancies: Prospective Study in Midwifery Practices in the Netherlands." *British Medical Journal,* no. 313 (1996): 1309–13.

Wilker, B. "Mennonite Midwife Behind Bars: A Case of Overreach." *National Review Online.* December 3, 2002. www.nationalreview.com/comment/comment-wiker120302.asp.

Winsor, Mari. *The Pilates Pregnancy.* Cambridge: Perseus, 2001.

Wirth, Fred. *Prenatal Parenting.* New York: HarperCollins/ReganBooks, 2001.

Wolfe, S., and M. Gabay. "Unnecessary Cesarean Sections: Curing a National Epidemic." Washington, D.C: Public Citizens Health Research Group, 1994.

World Health Organization. "Project on Safe Motherhood." International Confederation of Midwives, April 2002.

———. "Strengthening Midwifery within Safe Motherhood: Report of a Collaborative ICM/WHO/UNICEF Pre-Congress Workshop." May 1996. www.safemotherhood.org.

———. "Report on Maternal-Child Health Statistics." May 1990.

Young, D. "The Push against Vaginal Birth." *Birth: Issues in Perinatal Care* 30, no. 3 (September, 2003): 149–52.

Zain, H. A., J. W. Wright, G. E. Parrish, and S. J. Diehl. "Interpreting the Fetal Heart Rate Tracing: Effect of Knowledge of Neonatal Outcome." *Journal of Reproductive Medicine* 43 (1998): 367–70.

# About the Photographs and the Photographers

**Suzanne Arms** is an internationally acclaimed author, photojournalist, visionary, and activist who has been a leader in the natural birthing movement and a midwifery advocate in the United States for over 25 years. Her second book, *Immaculate Deception: A New Look at Women and Childbirth,* stirred a national social change movement and became a *New York Times* "Best Book of the Year" in 1975. Her Web site is www.birthingthefuture.com  Her photographs appear on pages 40, 63, 79, 91, 126, 138, 209, and 239.

**Christy Scherrer** is a Bay Area childbirth activist who has attended births in the capacity of doula, midwife assistant, and photographer. She is the mother of three, two born at home. Her dynamic and insightful images of motherhood, in all its forms, evoke an awareness about the sacredness of birth. Her work can be viewed at www.bellymotherbaby.com  Her photographs appear on pages vi, 5, 13, 19, 37, 49, 57, 83, 95, 108, 119, 196, 220, and 243.

**Anna Verwaal** is a maternal-child health nurse, certified lactation educator, and doula. Educated in nursing in her native Holland, she has worked for a number of years in a Los Angeles hospital. She is now a birth consultant and photographer. Her beautiful and sensitive glimpses of babies at birth communicate the consciousness of newborns. Her photos appear on pages x, 23, 25, 29, 101, 131, 136, 150, 154, 203, 227, and 233.

**Patti Ramos** lives in the Tacoma, Washington area, but her photographs of birth, families, end of life, and everyday miracles have been published in books, journals, greeting cards, and catalogs worldwide.  A skilled childbirth educator and doula, she has helped over 10,000 couples prepare for birth. Her work can be viewed at www.pattiramos.com  Her photographs appear on the title page and on pages 98 and 216.

Photograph on page 167 used with the permission of Michael Appelt.

Photograph on title page used with the permission of Ankur Aras.

Photographs on pages 8, 114, 171, 180, and 215 courtesy of Waterbirth International.

Photographs on pages 114 and 180 courtesy of Jennifer Gallardo, Andaluz Waterbirth Center.

Photographs on pages 141 and 147 courtesy of the American College of Nurse-Midwives

Photographs on pages ii, xiv, xvii, and 163 are from the author's personal collection.

# *Index*

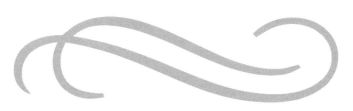

# BOOKS OF RELATED INTEREST

**Birth without Violence**
by Frederick Leboyer, M.D.

**Labor Pain**
*A Natural Approach to Easing Delivery*
by Nicky Wesson

**Parenting Begins Before Conception**
*A Guide to Preparing Body, Mind, and Spirit For You and Your Future Child*
by Carista Luminare-Rosen, Ph.D.

**When a Child Is Born**
*The Natural Child Care Classic*
by Wilhelm zur Linden, M.D.

**Reclaiming the Spirituality of Birth**
*Healing for Mothers and Babies*
by Benig Mauger

**Natural Mothering**
*A Guide to Holistic Therapies for Pregnancy, Birth, and Early Childhood*
by Nicky Wesson

**Vaccinations: A Thoughtful Parent's Guide**
*How to Make Safe, Sensible Decisions about the Risks, Benefits, and Alternatives*
by Aviva Jill Romm

**Natural Health after Birth**
*The Complete Guide to Postpartum Wellness*
by Aviva Jill Romm

Inner Traditions • Bear & Company
P.O. Box 388
Rochester, VT 05767
1-800-246-8648
www.InnerTraditions.com

Or contact your local bookseller